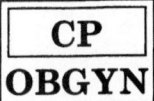 Clinical Perspectives in Obstetrics and Gynecology

Series Editor:

The late Herbert J. Buchsbaum, M.D.

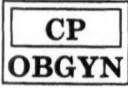
perspective *noun:* . . . the capacity to view subjects
in their true relations or relative importance.

Each volume in Clinical Perspectives in Obstetrics and
Gynecology will cover in depth a major clinical area in
the health care of women. The objective is to present to
the reader the pathophysiologic and biochemical basis
of the condition under discussion and to provide a
scientific basis for clinical management. These volumes
are not intended as "how to" books, but as a ready
reference by authorities in the field.

Though the obstetrician and gynecologist may be the
primary provider of health care for the female, this
role is shared with family practitioners, pediatricians,
medical and surgical specialists, and geriatricians. It is
to all these physicians that the series is addressed.

Series Editor: The late Herbert J. Buchsbaum, M.D.

Published Volumes:

Buchsbaum (ed.): *The Menopause*
Aiman (ed.): *Infertility*
Futterweit: *Polycystic Ovarian Disease*
Lavery and Sanfilippo (eds.): *Pediatric and Adolescent
                              Obstetrics and Gynecology*
Galask and Larsen (eds.): *Infectious Diseases in the Female
                          Patient*
Buchsbaum and Walton (eds.): *Strategies in Gynecologic
                            Surgery*
Szulman and Buchsbaum (eds.): *Gestational Trophoblastic
                             Disease*
Sanfillipo and Levine (eds.): *Operative Gynecologic
                             Endoscopy*
Cibils (ed.): *Surgical Diseases in Pregnancy*
Collins (ed.): *Ovulation Induction*

Forthcoming:

Altchek and Deligdisch (eds.): *The Uterus*

Ovulation Induction

Robert L. Collins
Editor

With 63 Illustrations

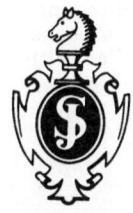

Springer-Verlag
New York Berlin Heidelberg London
Paris Tokyo Hong Kong Barcelona

Editor:
Robert L. Collins, M.D., Director of Education, Section of Reproductive Endocrinology and Infertility/A81, The Cleveland Clinic Foundation, Cleveland, Ohio, USA

Series Editor:
The late Herbert J. Buchsbaum, M.D.

Library of Congress Cataloging-in-Publication Data
Ovulation induction / Robert L. Collins
   editor
       p.   cm.—(Clinical perspectives in obstetrics and
  gynecology)
   Includes bibliographical references.
   Includes index.
   1. Ovulation—Induction.   2. Human reproduction—Endocrine
  aspects.   I. Collins, Robert L.   II. Series.
   [DNLM: 1. Fertilization In Vitro.   2. Ovulation Induction.   WP
  540 0954]
  RG133.7.O98   1990
  DNLM/DLC
  for Library of Congress   90-9933

Printed on acid-free paper

© 1991 Springer-Verlag New York, Inc.
Softcover reprint of the hardcover 1st edition 1991

Typeset by Asco Trade Typesetting Ltd., Quarry Bay, Hong Kong.

9 8 7 6 5 4 3 2 1

ISBN-13: 978-1-4612-7766-8   e-ISBN-13: 978-1-4612-3026-7
DOI: 10.1007/978-1-4612-3026-7

To the memory of
my father and my sister,
who both departed this life prematurely
but left a legacy for those to follow.
And to my family.
Vickie, Nicole, and Robbie,
whose love and support made this book
possible.

Preface

There have been several major milestones in the field of reproductive endocrinology. The first milestone for ovulation induction was the discovery in the early 1920s that the human gonads were gonadotropin-dependent. This led to the development of commercial gonadotropins derived from human pituitaries and, ultimately, to the commercial preparation of exogenous gonadotropins derived from urinary extracts. Ever since the marketing of human menopausal gonadotropins, ovulation has been achieved successfully in suitable candidates. There has been an explosion of information since ovulation has first induced in the human using exogenous gonadotropins.

The next major milestone for ovulation was the isolation and subsequent characterization of gonadotropin-releasing hormone (GnRH) in the early 1970s. No milestone has achieved greater clinical significance. The significance of that discovery led to two separate investigators being awarded the Nobel Prize in medicine. The initial enthusiasm for GnRH as a replacement for ovulation-inducing exogenous gonadrotropins was dampened by the lack of knowledge of the physiology of the decapeptide, which led to poor clinical responses. There was considerable delay in the realization of GnRH's therapeutic potential. In primate experiments, Knobil and other investigators in his laboratory demonstrated the endogenous pulsatility of GnRH and the requisite delivery in a pulsatile manner during replacement. Ovulation could be achieved consistently in suitable candidates when technical advances led to the production of small, programmable pump delivery systems.

The development of agonistic analogs of GnRH was the next major milestone. Modifications of the GnRH decapeptide led to various analogs with longer half-lives in the serum and greater potencies. Paradoxically, the longer-acting analog led to pituitary down-regulation after a brief period of activation. Several investigators have taken advantage of this medically induced hypophysectomy to treat a variety of ovulatory disorders, in addition to treating estrogen-dependent conditions, such as pelvic endometriosis. Combinations of the GnRH analogs and exogenous gonadotropins have proved to be suitable in certain clinical conditions such as polycystic ovarian disease (PCO). Patients with PCO often demonstrate extreme ovarian hypersensitivity with exogenous gonadotropins alone. The combination of a GnRH analog and exogenous gonadotropins has also been used successfully during ovulation induction or assisted ovulation during in vitro fertilization therapies in patients with poor follicular responses and premature LH surges.

This book was written with the intent of presenting the state of the art of ovulation induction and luteal function after induced ovulation. The book is for those interested in an understanding of the basic neuroendocrinology, ovarian physiology, folliculogenesis, ovulation, and luteal function. It is written for those interested in understanding complex anovulatory states. It is also intended to provide sufficient core information on various therapies for specific conditions that can be incorporated into clinical practice. As a comprehensive text, it should serve as a clinical reference for medical students, residents in obstetrics and gynecology, and clincians. Considerable attention is given to the newest agents and techniques for clinical monitoring.

This book represents the collaborative effort of outstanding contributors who have distinguished themselves as investigators in the field of reproductive endocrinology. Much of the data presented represents original research by each of the individual authors. I am deeply indebted to each of the contributing authors for his or her presentation of original data and critical analysis of the literature. The authors' scientific approach coupled with their practical clinical experience and ability to disseminate factual information on the problems of patient management is combined in what may be considered a reference book.

The book presents normal physiology, a discussion of abnormal ovulatory conditions, and subsequent therapeutics. The first chapter reviews our current understanding of the neuroendocrine physiological events that lead to successful ovulation. The second chapter, presents original data generated from Dr. Hodgen's laboratory, and deals with the interrelationships between neuroendocrinology and ovarian physiology that result in ovulatory menstrual cycles. Only with this basic understanding of hypothalamic–pituitary–ovarian interrelationships can we then approach various anovulatory states and rationally consider treatment options.

The third chapter deals with various anovulatory states, and presents a contemporary approach to categorization, differential diagnosis, and the management of chronic anovulatory disorders.

The next chapter, written by Dr. Austin, considers various techniques for the clinical monitoring of the follicular response during ovulation induction. Dr Austin focuses on the use of serial ultrasounds but she also discusses other modalities and the appropriateness, the advantages, and the disadvantages of each technique.

The next three chapters deal with various treatment modalities for anovulatory disorders. An up-to-date and comprehensive review of clomiphene citrate, including indications, dosages, and complications, follows. Then we proceed to a chapter on exogenous gonadotropin therapy. Adjunctive therapies such as pure FSH and the use of GnRH analogs are also discussed, especially as they relate to PCO. The next chapter gives a contemporary review of pulsatile GnRH therapy and how it may be used in the hypothalamic amenorrheic patient.

An extensive chapter is devoted entirely to the luteal phase after induced ovulation. The chapter includes information on luteal-phase function following various treatment modalities. The following chapter discusses bromocriptine and related compounds and how they may be used for hyperprolactinemic states.

A chapter dealing with the surgical approach to anovulatory states such as PCO is next. Wedge resection has become something of historical interest since the appearance of pharmaceutical agents that successfully produce ovulation in suitable patients, yet there is an argument that laparoscopic management of anovulatory disorders still may be appropriate in certain patients. The last chapter is an update regarding ovulation induction in normal women undergoing assisted reproductive technologies. It discusses the goals of assisted folliculogenesis and the management of the poorly responding patient.

This book could not have been completed without considerable help from certain individuals. I gratefully acknowledge Helen Thams for her diligence and scientific editorial assistance. Very special thanks are due to Sara Pingeon for her patience and her secretarial and administrative aid. Thanks are also due to JoAnn Patterson and Roberta Woodman for their expert technical assistance.

I wish to thank my colleague, Dr. Josef Blankstein, for his expert advice. I also wish to express my gratitude to the editorial staff at Springer-Verlag for their helpful suggestions, patience, and advice. Finally, I am most appreciative of our patients, nurses, family, and friends. Without their forbearance and support this book would not have been written.

Robert L. Collins

Contents

Contents

Contributors

CYNTHIA MILES AUSTIN, M.D.
Assistant Professor, Case Western University, and Co-Director, In Vitro Fertilization Department, MacDonald Hospital, Cleveland, Ohio 44106, USA

JOSEF BLANKSTEIN, M.D.
Director, Department of Obstetrics/Gynecology, The Mount Sinai Medical Center, Cleveland, Ohio 44106, USA

ROBERT L. COLLINS, M.D.
Director of Education, Section of Reproductive Endocrinology and Infertility, Department of Gynecology, The Cleveland Clinic Foundation, Cleveland, Ohio 44195-5037, USA

BRYAN COWAN, M.D.
Associate Professor and Director, Division of Reproductive Endocrinology, Department of Obstetrics and Gynecology, University of Mississippi Medical Center, Jackson, Mississippi 39216-4505, USA

JAMES F. DANIELL, M.D.
Clinical Associate Professor, Department of Obstetrics and Gynecology, Vanderbilt Medical School, Nashville, Tennessee 37232, USA

MARC A. FRITZ, M.D.
Associate Professor, Department of Obstetrics and Gynecology, Uniformed Services, University of the Health Sciences, F. Edward Wébert School of Medicine, Bethesda, Maryland 20814, USA

GARY D. HODGEN, PH.D.
Professor and Scientific Director, The Jones Institute for Reproductive Medicine, Department of Obstetrics and Gynecology, Eastern Virginia Medical School, Norfolk, Virginia 23510, USA

DANIEL KENIGSBERG, M.D.
Long Island IVF, Mather Hospital, Port Jefferson, New York 11777, USA

VIVIAN LEWIS, M.D.
Department of Gynecology, Kaiser Permanente Medical Center, San Francisco, California 94115, USA

CYNTHIA H. MEYERS-SEIFER, M.D.
Chief, Division of Pediatric Endocrinology, Department of Pediatrics, Yale University School of Medicine, New Haven, Connecticut 06510, USA

ANNA K. PARSONS, M.D.
Assistant Professor, Department of Obstetrics and Gynecology, University of South Florida College of Medicine, Tampa, Florida 33606, USA

MARTIN M. QUIGLEY, M.D.
Chief, Section of Reproductive Endocrinology and Infertility, Department of Obsterics/Gynecology, The Mount Sinai Medical Center, Cleveland, Ohio 44106, USA

DAVID B. SEIFER, M.D.
Division of Reproductive Endocrinology, Department of Obstetrics and Gynecology, Yale University School of Medicine, New Haven, Connecticut 06510, USA

1
The Neuroendocrine Regulation of the Menstrual Cycle

CYNTHIA H. MEYERS-SEIFER and DAVID B. SEIFER

Neuroendocrinology is the study of the relationship between the nervous and endocrine systems, which together regulate the organism. The neuron typically transmits information along an axon, communicating with a target cell across a synapse. An endocrine cell secretes its chemical message, or hormone, into the circulation to affect a specific target organ. Both the neuron neurotransmitter and the endocrine hormone activate target cells through specific cell receptors. Furthermore, several kinds of peptides and neurotransmitters, synthesized by neurons, are also secreted by endocrine glands.

Neurosecretion refers to release of a hormone into circulation from a nerve terminal. For example, oxytocin and vasopressin are formed in hypothalamic neurons, transported to the posterior pituitary by axoplasmic flow, and secreted into the systemic circulation. In addition, hypothalamic hypophysiotropic hormones are released from nerve terminals into the pituitary portal system to regulate the anterior pituitary. These neurosecretions, which enter circulating blood, are termed neurohormones. With the discovery of the endogenous opioids and extensive extrahypothalamic peptidergic neurons in the central nervous system (CNS), neurosecretion now includes the release of any secretory product from a nerve terminal.

Peptidergic neurons are those that synthesize and release peptides, either into circulation (neurohormones) or between neurons (neurotransmitters or neuromodulators). The peptidergic neurons that secrete hormones are believed to "transduce" neural into endocrine information.[1] These neuroglandular neurons are modulated by other neurons, all of which respond to changes in the CNS neural, hormonal, and metabolic milieu.

This chapter focuses on the hypothalamic and pituitary mechanisms responsible for the menstrual cycle and the influence of ovarian steroid hormones, CNS neuromodulators, and neurotransmitters. Also included is a brief summary of the neuroendocrine events leading to the onset and progression of puberty.

Functional Anatomy of the Hypothalamus and Pituitary

The hypothalamic neurons form during the second and third months of gestation and migrate to the adult location of the base of the brain, becoming the floor and part of the lateral walls of the third ventricle. The posterior lobe of the pituitary and the pituitary stalk develop from the ventral diencephalon of the brain, retaining their neural connections into adulthood. The anterior pituitary grows upward from a tubular diverticulum of the primitive oral cavity called Rathke's pouch. The intermediate lobe is rudimentary in humans. As the anterior and posterior lobes fuse, the anterior portion develops buds that grow to envelop the base of the hypothalamus and pituitary stalk with a layer of cells called the pars tuberalis. A funnel-shaped structure called the infundibulum connects the hypothalamus with the pituitary stalk and the neural pituitary lobe.

The tuberoinfundibular (pituitary) stalk descends from the central portion of the basal hypothalamus called the median eminence. The median eminence is a neural, vascular, and epithelial complex comprised of the central portion of the infundibulum, a capillary plexus that drains into the hypophyseal portal circulation and the pars tuberalis of the anterior pituitary gland.

The hypothalamus contains many cellular nuclei that synthesize and secrete hormones (Fig. 1-1). Vasopressin and oxytocin are synthesized in the supraoptic and paraventricular nuclei, transported along pituitary stalk axons to the posterior lobe, and secreted into the systemic circulation. Other hypothalamic nuclei synthesize hypophysiotropic hormones that act on the anterior pituitary. Five hypophysiotropic hormones have been characterized: gonadotropin-releasing hormone (GnRH), thyrotropin-releasing hormone (TRH), growth hormone-inhibiting hormone (somatostatin), growth hormone-releasing hormone (GHRH), and corticotropin-releasing hormone (CRF). These hormones are transported by axoplasmic flow to the median eminence and secreted into the long portal vessels of the hypophyseal portal venous system to regulate anterior pituitary activity. Evidence suggests that pituitary-to-hypothalamus secretion may occur as well, via short portal vessels.[2]

Hypothalamic activity may also be influenced via the cerebrospinal fluid (CSF). Special ependymal cells called tanycytes line the third ventricle over the median eminence, terminating at the hypophyseal portal vessels, thus providing a communication between CSF and the pituitary–hypothalamic axis.

The hypothalamus has extensive internuclear connections as well as functional and anatomical extrahypothalamic connections with the limbic system, amygdala, hippocampus, thalamus, and pons. Altered activity in these areas may influence hypothalamic neurosecretion[3] (Fig. 1-1).

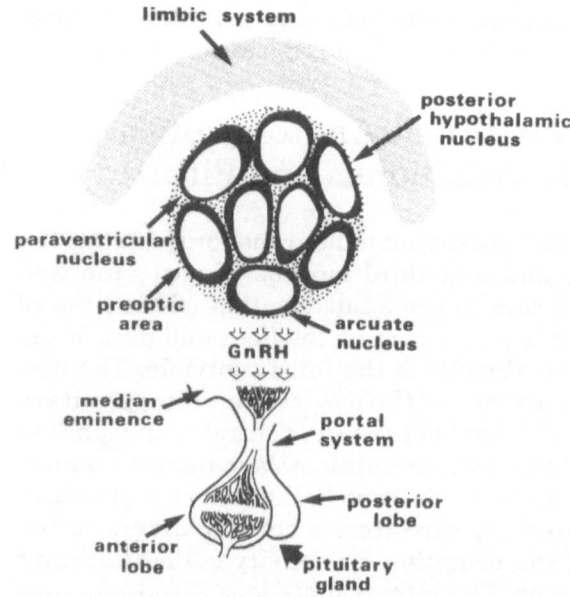

FIGURE 1-1. Schematic representation of the anatomic relationships of the limbic system, the nuclear organization of the hypothalamus, the portal system, and the pituitary. From ref. 85, with permission.

Characterization of GnRH

Our current understanding of the neuroendocrine control of the female reproductive system began following the isolation, characterization, and synthesis of gonadotropin-releasing hormone (GnRH), also known as luteinizing hormone-releasing hormone (LHRH). It is a decapeptide responsible for the synthesis and secretion of both pituitary gonadotropins, luteinizing hormone (LH) and follicle-stimulating hormone (FSH). Gonadotropin-releasing hormone has a brief half-life of 2 to 4 minutes (Fig. 1-2). A single injection of synthetic or native GnRH in human females results in a rise in both LH and FSH within 5 minutes, with peaking of LH in 25 minutes and peaking of FSH in 45 minutes.[4,5] Infusion of a submaximal dose of GnRH results in an initial LH peak at 25 minutes, followed by another sustained release at 90 minutes. This biphasic response is thought to

pyroGLU——HIS——TRP——SER——TYR——GLY——LEU——ARG——PRO——GLY—NH₂

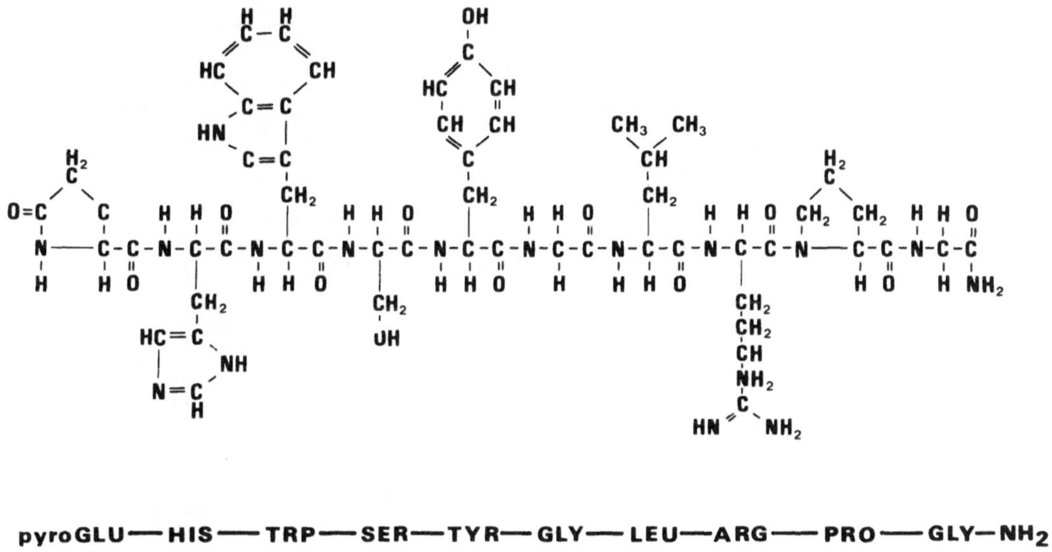

FIGURE 1-2. The amino acid sequence of the decapeptide gonadotropin-releasing hormone (GnRH). From ref. 85, with permission.

represent a readily releasable pool and a second reserve pool of gonadotropins.[6,7] The relative activity of these two pools that determines pituitary sensitivity and reserve is regulated by GnRH and ovarian steroids.

At the pituitary gonadotrope, GnRH binds to membrane receptors to stimulate synthesis and release of gonadotropins. Both LH and FSH are synthesized on the rough endoplasmic reticulum and packaged into secretory granules by the Golgi apparatus. Gonadotropin release involves activation of adenylate cyclase and increased intracellular cAMP, ultimately resulting in alteration of cell membrane permeability. The alteration in membrane permeability allows exocytosis of LH and FSH secretory granules[8] (Fig. 1-3).

Responses of FSH are less obvious and tend to parallel the LH responses to GnRH stimulation.[6] No specific FSH-releasing hormone has been identified, although there are instances of separate LH and FSH secretion. For example, stimulation of the preoptic area in the rat results in selective FSH secretion.[9] The dissociated release of FSH and LH is generally explained by alterations in hormonal environment and GnRH administration, selecting one gonadotropin over the

other. For example, a brief high pulse of GnRH, given to pentobarbital-blocked proestrus rats, releases LH, whereas low prolonged GnRH releases FSH.[5,9] Rabbit antiserum to GnRH suppresses LH and FSH secretion in ovariectomized rhesus monkeys, reinforcing the role of GnRH in gonadotropin release and confirming that a single hypophysiotropic hormone controls both FSH and LH.[10] Presently, it is believed that the majority of LH and FSH activity is the result of GnRH.

Gonadotropin-releasing hormone is produced in neurons. Antiserum to GnRH and immunohistochemical techniques have shown primate GnRH neurons predominantly localized to the arcuate nucleus of the medial basal hypothalamus (MBH). These neuron cell bodies project axons to GnRH neuron terminals in the median eminence (Fig. 1-1). The presence of an axonal pathway projecting to the median eminence suggests that the origin of this pathway, the MBH, is involved in the control of GnRH release.[11] Immunoreactive axons to GnRH are found in the anterior and posterior hypothalamus in rhesus monkeys but do not appear to effect gonadotropin release. The function of GnRH-

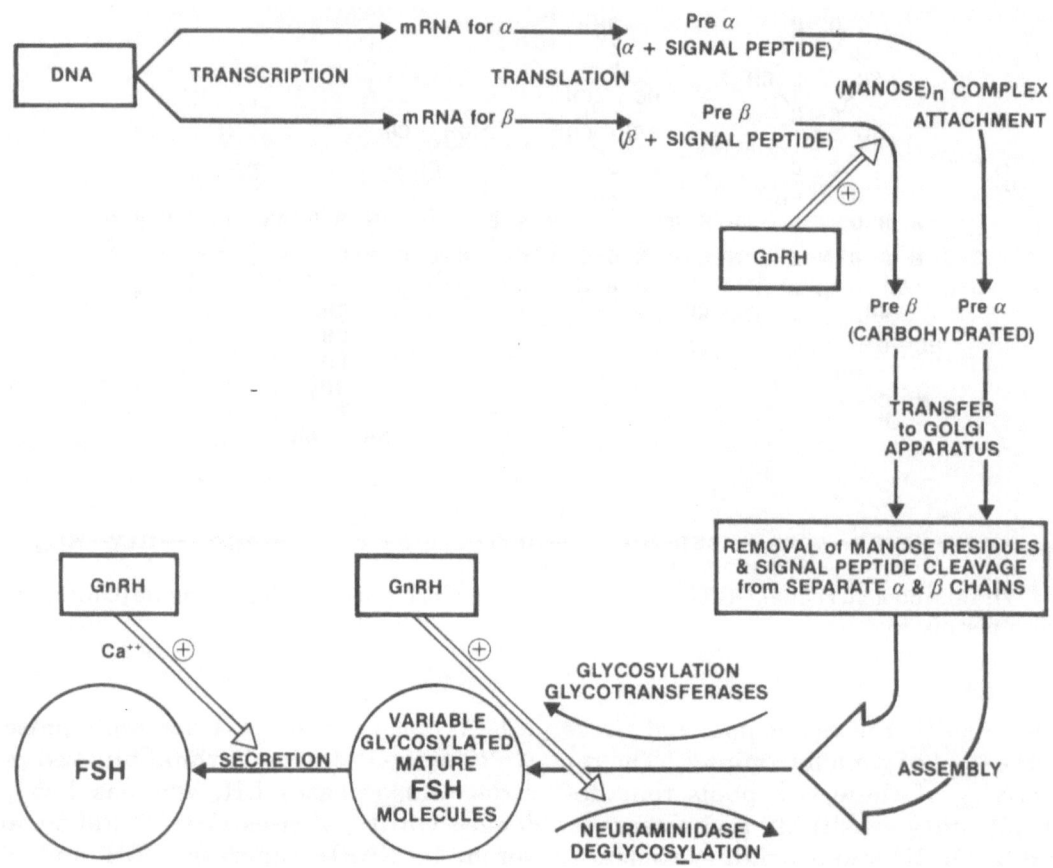

FIGURE 1-3. The actions of GnRH within gonadotrophic cells. The GnRH action involves a second messenger, adenylate cyclase, and mobilization of calcium cations. From ref. 85, with permission.

containing structures outside of the MBH remains to be clarified.[5]

The arcuate nucleus continuously generates GnRH, integrating hypothalamic and extrahypothalamic neural and hormonal input. The placement of radiofrequency lesions in the arcuate nucleus results in a rapid decrease in gonadotropin secretion, further localizing the hypothalamic control of gonadotropins to the arcuate nucleus within the MBH.[12] The menstrual cycle depends on the pulsatile secretion of GnRH as well as the modulating effects of gonadotropins and gonadal steroids via feedback mechanisms. The long feedback loop includes the stimulatory and inhibitory effects of target gland hormones on the hypothalamus and pituitary. Short feedback refers to negative feedback of gonadotropins on GnRH to affect pituitary secretion, and an ultrashort feedback loop regulates inhibition of GnRH by GnRH itself.[13] Hormonal feedback, along with CNS alternations, may influence the secretion of GnRH through various neurotransmitters.

Pulsatile Secretion of Gonadotropins and GnRH

Frequent sampling in ovariectomized rhesus monkeys demonstrates circhoral pulses of LH that contribute to elevated circulating LH levels.[14,15] Luteinizing hormone also demonstrates circhoral release during the follicular phase in intact monkeys with some variation in frequency over the remainder of the menstrual cycle.[16] In addition, pulsatile secretion of gonadotropins is found in human females with and without ovarian function.[17-21] Women with gonadal dysgenesis or who are postmenopausal demonstrate elevated LH and FSH maintained by gonadotropin pulses every 1 to 2 hours.[17,18] Rhythmic gonadotropin secretion is well characterized in normal women. A pulsatile secretion of gonadotropins is superimposed on a low level of continuous release.[18,19] Luteinizing hormone pulsation occurs every 1 to 2 hours in the follicular phase, but amplitude and frequency vary during the menstrual cycle, modulated by ovarian steroids.[19-21]

Radiofrequency ablation of the arcuate nucleus results in rapid decline of circhoral LH secretion in ovariectomized rhesus monkeys.[12] Pulsatile hourly replacement with synthetic GnRH (1 μg/min for 6 minutes) restores FSH and LH to levels prior to the arcuate lesions, whereas a constant infusion fails to sustain LH and FSH levels after a brief elevation[21,22] (Fig. 1-4). It is believed that continuous GnRH infusion may result in a phenomenon called "down-regulation," that is, a reduction in the number of available unoccupied GnRH receptors. This renders the gonadotrope refractory to GnRH stimulation[22,23] and produces a reversible hypogonadotropic state.

Pituitary portal blood sampling shows that GnRH is released in a pulsatile fashion into the pituitary portal vessels of intact and ovariectomized monkeys. Pulse frequency is similar to that of LH in peripheral blood.[24] Recently, measurements of peripheral plasma GnRH have shown a circhoral pulsatile pattern in women.[25] These studies suggest that pulsatile gonadotropin secretion is not intrinsic to the pituitary but originates with pulsatile GnRH activity in the hypothalamus. Recording electrodes implanted in the

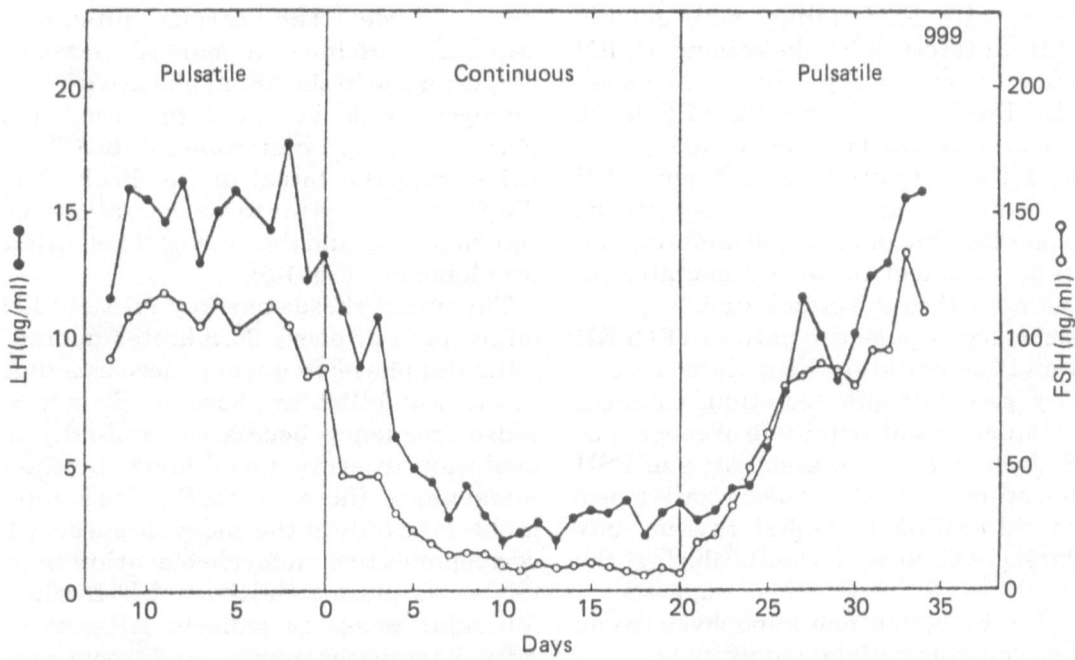

FIGURE 1-4. Suppression of plasma LH and FSH concentrations after initiation, on day 0, of a continuous GnRH infusion (1 μg/min) in an ovariectomized rhesus monkey with a radiofrequency lesion in the hypothalamus; gonadotropin secretion had been reestablished by the intermittent (pulsatile) administration of the decapeptide (1 μg/min for 6 minutes once per hour). The inhibition of gonadotropin secretion was reversed after reinstitution of the intermittent mode of GnRH stimulation on day 20. From Belchetz et al.,[22] reproduced with permission of the publisher. Copyright 1978 by the AAAS.

medial basal hypothalamus reveal sharply increased electrical activity concomitant with each peripheral LH pulse.[26] A hypothalamic neural oscillator or pulse generator rhythmically releases GnRH, which stimulates circhoral secretion of LH and FSH.

During the menstrual cycle, pulsatile function of FSH is less well defined than that of LH, presumably because of the smaller amounts of FSH released as well as the longer half-life of FSH, which tends to obscure measurement of pulses. Pulsatile activity of both LH and FSH are well defined in women without ovarian function, suggesting that FSH is more sensitive than LH to ovarian steroid negative feedback.[17,18,20]

Alteration in GnRH pulse frequency or amplitude changes the gonadotropin response in the rhesus monkey. In castrate rhesus monkeys with arcuate nucleus lesions, raising GnRH frequency to between two and five pulses per hour decreases LH and FSH. The rate of decline is proportional to GnRH pulse frequency, with FSH falling more quickly than LH. Interestingly, decreasing GnRH frequency to once every 3 hours decreases mean LH level while increasing FSH level. The 3-hour interval between GnRH pulses increases the magnitude of LH and FSH pulses twofold and fourfold respectively. The longer half-life of FSH (220 minutes) versus LH (65 minutes) allows accumulation of FSH but not LH in the circulation.[27]

In summary, a pulsatile pattern of GnRH secretion is essential to the maintenance of pituitary gonadotropin secretion. Changes in the frequency and amplitude of exogenous GnRH alters absolute plasma LH and FSH concentrations as well as their relative proportion. Alteration in GnRH rhythm may modulate physiological events during the menstrual cycle, and this suggests a mechanism by which one hypophysiotropic hormone controls both gonadotropins.

Regulation of GnRH Secretion During the Menstrual Cycle

The hypothalamus rhythmically generates GnRH, stimulating the synthesis and release of gonadotropins that orchestrate ovarian follicle development and steroid production. In the early follicular phase, estrogen is low, and plasma FSH is higher than LH, allowing for recruitment and maturation of ovarian follicles. The combined effects of FSH and LH stimulate E_2 secretion, which is produced by the dominant ovarian follicle during the midfollicular phase.[28] During the follicular phase, estrogen increases, peaking just prior to the preovulatory gonadotropin surge in midcycle. Rising E_2 inhibits FSH secretion and to a lesser degree LH secretion during the follicular phase. Inhibin, a protein produced in the ovarian follicle, may potentiate the selective E_2 inhibition of FSH.[28]

At midcycle, an E_2 level of 200 to 500 pg/mL sustained for 36 to 48 hours stimulates the LH and FSH surge, resulting in ovulation. The preovulatory follicle produces a slight rise in progesterone prior to ovulation, which augments the preovulatory gonadotropin surge. The corpus luteum subsequently produces a marked increase in progesterone in the luteal phase with a small estrogen peak in the late luteal phase. Estrogen and progesterone inhibit FSH and LH during the luteal phase. Both steroids drop 2 to 3 days prior to menses, allowing the return of FSH and the next cycle of follicular development (Fig. 1-5).

The intact rhesus monkey releases LH on an average of every 60 minutes during the follicular phase; frequency increases slightly in the late follicular phase, as E_2 increases. Pulse frequency decreases gradually after ovulation to every 4 to 6 hours by the late luteal phase. Increase in LH pulse amplitude is observed only at the midcycle surge, which corresponds to a midcycle elevation in pituitary stalk plasma GnRH.[16,29,30] During the follicular phase in women, LH pulse frequency increases from every 60 to 90 minutes in the early follicular phase to every 50 to 70 minutes in the late follicular phase, as E_2 rises.[20,21] Several reports show that LH pulse frequency decreases from every 90 to 100 minutes to every 3 to 4 hours during the luteal phase,[17,21,29,30] with increasing expo-

FIGURE 1-5. The temporal relationship of gonadotropin and ovarian steroid secretion in the normal menstrual cycle. From Fritz and Speroff,[47] reproduced with permission of the publisher, the American Fertility Society.

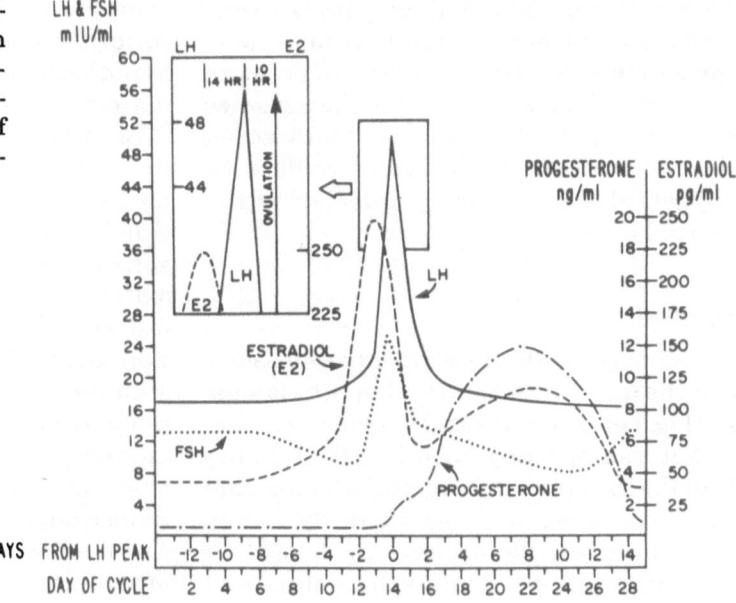

sure to progesterone. One recent study suggests that LH pulse frequency may not vary during the luteal phase but remains constant at every 90 minutes.[20] The faster frequency relates to the observation of small LH pulses occurring between previously noted larger pulses and may reflect a variation in GnRH amplitude or hypothalamic pituitary response to E_2 and progesterone.[20,30] Pulse amplitude remains constant during the follicular phase,[17,20] although one study suggests a decreased amplitude in the mid follicular phase, possibly related to negative estrogen feedback.[21] The LH pulse amplitude is markedly increased at midcycle in women. Mean LH amplitude is greater in the luteal phase than in the follicular phase but decreases from early to late luteal phase.[20,21] Secretion of FSH correlates with LH secretion, although pulsatile release is often obscured by low amplitude and long FSH half-life.[20,21] In summary, pulsatility of LH during the menstrual cycle is characterized as high frequency, low amplitude during the follicular phase and low frequency, high amplitude during the luteal phase.

Interestingly, measurement of human peripheral blood GnRH shows hourly pulses without variation during the menstrual cycle. A

TABLE 1-1. LHRH levels (pg/mL)[a]

	Mean ± SEM	Range
Normal male	1.6 ± 0.4	<0.3 to 4.9
Normal cycling women		
Follicular phase	1.4 ± 0.1	<0.3 to 4.7
Luteal phase	2.0 ± 0.2	<0.3 to 10.7
Periovulatory phase	10.0 ± 3.5	0.64 to 34.7

[a] Modified from Elkind-Hirsch et al.,[25] © 1982, by The Endocrine Society.

significant increase in peripheral GnRH amplitude is noted only during the periovulatory period, as depicted in Table 1-1. Given factors of dilution and rapid metabolism, the relationship of peripheral GnRH pulses to pituitary portal activity remains to be clarified in humans.[25]

The pulsatile pattern of gonadotropin release in women without ovarian function underscores the role of ovarian steroids. Postmenopausal women demonstrate secretory LH and FSH patterns with follicular-phase pulse frequency and midcycle pulse amplitude. Accounting for this rise in gonadotropins is the absence of estrogen.[17] In patients with gonadal dysgenesis, ethinyl estradiol infusion obscures the pulsatile release of LH and FSH and rapidly reduces previously elevated circulating gonadotropin levels. During the period of suppression, intramuscular progesterone and estradiol benzoate promote a surge of LH and FSH.[18] Further studies attempt to clarify the anatomic and biochemical interactions of ovarian steroids with the hypothalamic–pituitary axis during the menstrual cycle.

Estrogen

Estradiol may modulate gonadotropin secretion at the anterior pituitary, hypothalamus, and other central nervous system sites (Fig. 1-6). Autoradiography localizes E_2-binding cells to the preoptic area, hypothalamus, and limbic structures, with particularly heavy staining noted in the arcuate nucleus.[31] In the anterior pituitary many basophils and acidophils also bind estrogen. Thus, cells concentrating E_2 in both the medial basal hypothalamus and the pituitary may modulate gonadotropin secretion.[32–34]

Because estrogen activity is present in both the CNS and anterior pituitary, studies attempt to define the site and mechanism by which estrogen either enhances or diminishes gonadotropin secretion. In both rats and primates, sustained midcycle elevation of E_2 initiates the gonadotropin surge and ovulation. In ovariectomized rhesus monkeys with arcuate nucleus ablation on pulsatile GnRH replacement, administration of E_2 results in an abrupt decline in LH and FSH followed by a rise in gonadotropins. This biphasic response suggests that both negative and positive feedback effects of E_2 occur at the level of the pituitary gland.[32] Finally, the admin-

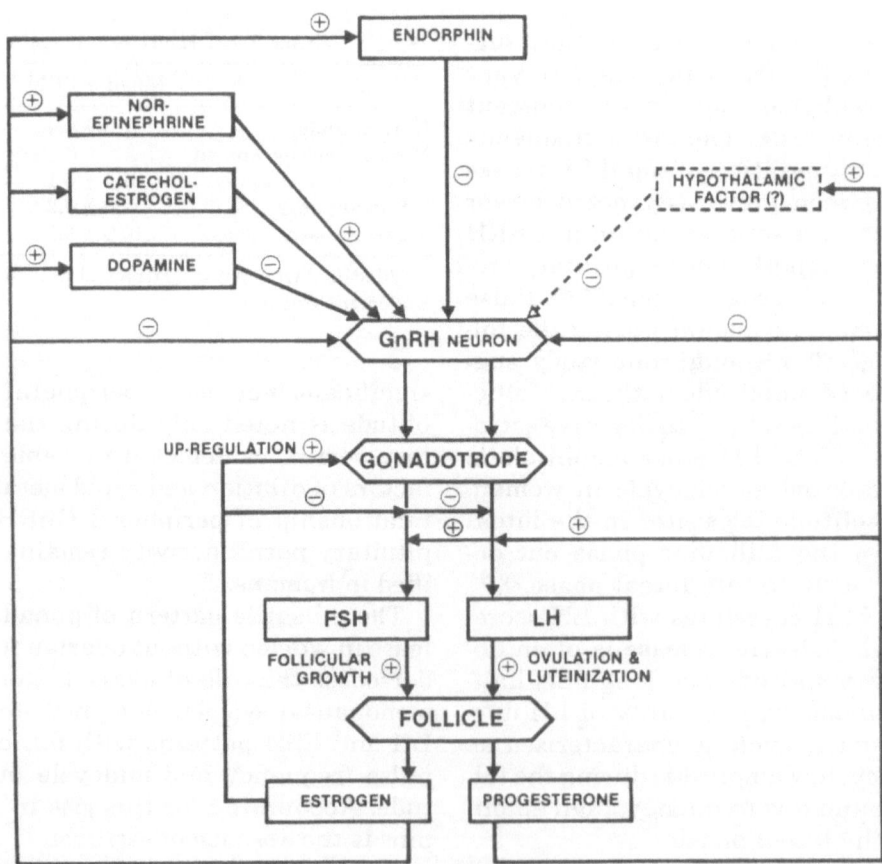

FIGURE 1-6. Diagrammatic representation of the hormonal interrelationships in the regulation of the hypothalamic–pituitary–ovarian axis. From ref. 85, with permission.

istration of GnRH every 2 hours to a patient with Kallmann's syndrome results in ovulatory menstrual cycles.[35] These experiments demonstrate that gonadotropin responses may change without alteration in GnRH pulsatility, suggesting that estrogen acts directly at the pituitary to control gonadotropin secretion, particularly at midcycle. The GnRH pulses provide a permissive but necessary basis for LH and FSH surges.[33] Although there is general agreement that pulsatile GnRH is requisite for basal gonadotropin secretion, the role of a GnRH surge and the sites of estrogen positive feedback remain controversial.

Ovarian estrogen stimulates the secretion of pituitary gonadotropin surges. Evidence suggests that estrogen may act at the hypothalamus to increase periovulatory GnRH secretion. Pituitary portal GnRH shows a significant preovulatory elevation compared with the follicular phase in the rhesus monkey. In addition, portal blood GnRH levels correlate with peripheral LH levels, indicating that estrogen may stimulate the hypothalamus to increase GnRH secretion and produce the LH surge.[29] A recent study in ovariectomized rhesus monkeys confirms the increase in GnRH secretion, measured at the median eminence in estrogen-induced gonadotropin surges.[36] As noted previously, mean peripheral GnRH and GnRH pulse magnitude are increased during the periovulatory period.[25] Thus, numerous studies have explored the steroid influence on midcycle central and pituitary alterations. As noted earlier, estrogen has a well-established negative feedback effect on gonadotropin secretion during the follicular and luteal phases of the menstrual cycle. The particular sites of E_2 inhibition on LH and FSH have also been investigated.

Peripheral E_2 administered to ovariectomized monkeys decreases peripheral LH concentration. Estradiol injected directly into the suprachiasmatic, arcuate, ventral medial, and mamillary nuclei of the MBH also decreases LH secretion by negative feedback. Injection into other hypothalamic sites does not reduce LH secretion.[37] Infusion of E_2 into the third ventricle (which concentrates in the rostral hypothalamus and MBH) of ovariectomized rhesus monkeys decreases serum gonadotropin levels and inhibits pulsatile LH release. Infusion of E_2 into the anterior pituitary also decreases FSH and LH levels but preserves pulsatile gonadotropin rhythm. An intravenous bolus of GnRH given after the CNS estrogen infusion results in a significant increase in FSH and LH levels, but in anterior-pituitary-treated monkeys, no increase in gonadotropins results from a terminal GnRH challenge.[38] These experiments suggest that E_2 inhibits the pulsatile neurosecretory mechanism for GnRH release and decreases responsiveness to GnRH at the pituitary level.

Many studies support the role of E_2 at the level of the gonadotrope in modifying gonadotropin response to GnRH. Both concentration and duration of E_2 exposure determine whether pituitary response to GnRH will be augmented or blunted. A single brief infusion of E_2 designed to approximate either late follicular or midcycle level blunts gonadotropin response to exogenous GnRH in normal women.[39] Sustained exposure of the pituitary to late follicular levels of E_2 over several days results in an augmented gonadotropin response to GnRH.[40] Varying the level of sustained E_2 exposure demonstrates a critical concentration at which exogenous GnRH produces a gonadotropin surge. This level is lower for LH than FSH, although very low sustained E_2 levels have no effect on the pituitary response to GnRH.[41] In summary, these studies suggest that estrogen modulates pituitary sensitivity to GnRH and that this mechanism contributes to the pattern of gonadotropin release during the menstrual cycle.

Estradiol may modify the gonadotrope response to GnRH through quantitative change in pituitary GnRH receptors. In ovariectomized monkeys with E_2 replaced to midcycle level, GnRH receptors steadily increase, peaking at 36 hours and declining after that. In contrast, pituitary LH response is depressed at 12 and 24 hours of estrogen exposure, increasing significantly at 36 hours. Thus, although GnRH receptor content apparently contributes to the LH surge, the preceding negative-feedback component of estrogen does not appear to involve the hormone–receptor complex.[42]

Estradiol pretreatment potentiates GnRH-stimulated release of LH from cultured rat pituitary cells, which is at least in part related to an increase in pituitary cell GnRH receptors.[43] Hypophyseal GnRH receptors are noted to be increased during the preovulatory LH surge in sheep, and this may be related to GnRH-induced increase in GnRH binding capacity.[44] The ability of repetitive GnRH stimulation to facilitate pituitary response, "self-priming" or up-regulation, may be necessary for the preovulatory surge. Estradiol may be important for GnRH self-priming. Estrogen administered to postmenopausal women amplifies the LH and FSH response to the second of paired GnRH pulses. Maximal self-priming is seen after 5 and 10 days of E_2 replacement with attenuation at 30 days.[45] Injection of GnRH into proestrus rats magnifies the LH surge in association with a dramatic loss of pituitary GnRH receptors. Thus, besides follicular-phase self-priming ability, GnRH may produce a decrease or "down-regulation" of its own pituitary receptors[46] after or at the midcycle surge.

In summary, E_2 serves to inhibit gonadotropin secretion in the follicular phase in a manner unrelated to the GnRH receptor, perhaps by decreasing GnRH at the hypothalamus level or by acting directly at the gonadotrope. Receptors for GnRH increase during the follicular phase, coinciding with rising E_2 and somewhat low GnRH and gonadotropins. Rising E_2 potentiates the midcycle gonadotropin surge, at least in part by GnRH self-priming at the pituitary gland. Although ovulatory menstrual cycles can be produced with constant unvarying GnRH pulses, physiological alterations in GnRH frequency and amplitude are present throughout the cycle.[47] In addition, many studies showing ovulation with fixed GnRH pulses use a supraphysiological dose, possibly obviating the need for increasing midcycle GnRH.[28] The role of GnRH alteration (and the role of hypothalamic steroid feedback) in maintaining ovulation and cyclicity remains uncertain.[28]

Progesterone

The role of progesterone (P_4) secretion prior to the midcycle LH surge is still undefined. At midcycle, small amounts of progesterone are released from the dominant preovulatory follicle. While in the luteal phase, the corpus luteum produces high levels of progesterone, which peak in mid- to late luteal phase. Progesterone may stimulate or inhibit gonadotropin secretion with apparent activity at both the pituitary and hypothalamus, and its effect may be dose dependent.

Exogenous E_2 induces a gonadotropin surge when administered to early follicular-phase rhesus monkeys. This estrogen-induced surge is completely blocked by the simultaneous administration of progesterone, although the concentration is somewhat lower than luteal-phase levels. If the exogenous progesterone is given 12 hours after the estrogen, a modified gonadotropin surge occurs, and it is advanced by 24 hours when compared to E_2 alone.[48] In monkeys with arcuate lesions on GnRH replacement, the gonadotropin surge occurs despite simultaneous progesterone and E_2 administration and is again advanced by 24 hours.[49] These studies support progesterone inhibition of gonadotropin release at the hypothalamus and possible stimulation of the preovulatory surge at the pituitary level at lower concentrations. Studies in women who are status post bilateral oophorectomy also indicate that whereas E_2 is required for the gonadotropin surge, progesterone inhibits or stimulates midcycle FSH and LH in a time- and dose-dependent manner.[50]

Midfollicular and hypogonadal women given E_2 followed with progesterone demonstrate that a requisite sustained E_2 peak signals the midcycle gonadotropin surge, and a small (periovulatory level) increment of progesterone establishes the normal surge duration and amplitude.[51] In the early follicular phase, E_2 augments the LH and FSH response to exogenous GnRH. A low level of progesterone added after 4 days of E_2 amplifies the estrogen-augmented response to GnRH. Progesterone amplification of the midcycle surge appears to be mediated at the pituitary, as this study shows no evidence of endogenous GnRH alteration from progesterone.[52] Neutralization of the preovulatory secretion of progesterone by a progesterone antagonist (RU486) administered at midcycle to monkeys blocked the expected midcycle LH surge.[53] The data from that study suggest that P_4 plays a pivotal role in initiating a timely midcycle gonadotropin surge of normal amplitude and duration, although a direct inhibitory effect of the progesterone antagonist on the gonadotrope cannot be excluded completely.

Women treated with luteal-phase levels of progesterone in the follicular phase develop a slowing of LH pulse frequency, augmented pulse amplitude, and decreased mean plasma LH levels when compared with untreated follicular-phase women. Progesterone appears to mediate LH secretion during the luteal phase, presumably modulating the changes in frequency at the hypothalamic level. However, modulation of gonadotropin amplitude at the pituitary cannot be excluded.[54]

The frequency of LH pulses declines progressively over the luteal phase and is significantly correlated with the duration of progesterone exposure, although not with actual progesterone level. The mean amplitude also declines across the luteal phase but is correlated with neither steroid exposure nor absolute level. Frequent sampling techniques document small-amplitude LH pulses occurring between larger pulses. The smaller pulses occur most often in the midluteal phase and are significantly correlated with progesterone level. The heterogeneity of luteal-phase gonadotropin pulses may reflect varying GnRH amplitude or varying pituitary responses to constant GnRH amplitude. The LH pulse frequency and amplitude may be separately modulated, with LH pulse frequency altered by chronic progesterone exposure at the hypothalamus

and pulse amplitude influenced by acute progesterone changes at the pituitary.[30]

Progesterone exhibits varying roles at midcycle and in the luteal phase. Progesterone augments the preovulatory effect of E_2 on gonadotropin release, presumably at the pituitary. Progesterone activity at the hypothalamus and pituitary alter gonadotropin frequency, amplitude, and plasma concentration during the luteal phase, causing a slowing of pulsatility.

Pulsatile secretion of GnRH results in gonadotropin release, ovarian follicle maturation, and steroid production. These components interact in a precisely timed fashion to culminate in the menstrual cycle. Various neurotransmitters, endogenous opioids, and catecholestrogens synthesized in the CNS serve to modulate GnRH secretion. These molecules provide a basis on which pharmacological and psychological input may affect GnRH and the menstrual cycle (Fig. 1-6).

Neurotransmitters

The catecholamines, particularly norepinephrine and dopamine, are considered the predominant neurotransmitters regulating GnRH. They are synthesized in nerve terminals from dihydroxyphenylalanine (DOPA), with dopamine being the immediate precursor of norepinephrine. These catecholamines are believed to alter GnRH pulse frequency and possibly amplitude and duration.[11,49,55]

Most of the neuron cell bodies that secrete norepinephrine are located in the mesencephalon and lower brainstem, ascending to several areas of the brain including the hypothalamus. These cells also synthesize serotonin, whose effect on GnRH is largely unknown.[13]

Norepinephrine has been found to stimulate gonadotropin secretion. Peripheral administration of the α-adrenergic blockers phentolamine and phenoxybenzamine to ovariectomized rhesus monkeys acutely interrupts pulsatile LH release, resulting in a sustained decline in LH concentration. In contrast, β-adrenergic blockade shows no effect on LH.[56] In rhesus monkeys with arcuate lesions on GnRH replacement, α-adrenergic blockade fails to inhibit LH secretion.[57] α-Adrenergic blockers arrest or significantly reduce both arcuate nucleus electrical pulses and pituitary LH pulses in ovariectomized monkeys. These studies indicate that LH inhibition from adrenergic blockade occurs at a suprahypophyseal level.[57,58] Studies regarding catecholamines and gonadotropin response are limited in primates. In the rat, both inhibitors of norepinephrine synthesis and the α-adrenergic blocker phenoxybenzamine significantly reduce the induced portal GnRH and peripheral LH secretion.[59] Thus, norepinephrine synthesis is required for the GnRH (and LH) surge in rats.

The dopaminergic mechanism is more complicated than noradrenergic activity. Dopaminergic cell bodies are found in the arcuate and paraventricular nuclei, while dopamine neuron terminals are located in the arcuate nucleus and the median eminence. Dopamine and GnRH nerve terminals are in close proximity in the medial basal hypothalamus, geographically allowing axoaxonic contact and interneural interaction.[47]

Conventional wisdom has stated that dopamine, in contrast to norepinephrine, inhibits GnRH release. Intravenous dopamine has been found to inhibit the release of FSH, LH, and prolactin in women.[60] However, physiological and pharmacological dopamine infusions have been shown to suppress basal LH levels significantly without altering FSH levels in the follicular phase of women.[61] The gonadotropin sensitivity to exogenous dopamine inhibition varies during the follicular phase of the human menstrual cycle. Between days 2 and 12, there is a relative insensitivity to exogenous dopamine inhibition. On day 14, however, there is increased LH and FSH sensitivity, both of which decline dramatically in response to dopamine. The sensitivity of LH and FSH to dopamine, which peaks at 14 days, suggests that decreased dopamine activity at midcycle facilitates GnRH release and the gonadotropin surge.[60] The midcycle rise in estrogen and the presence of estrogen receptors on arcuate dopaminergic neurons suggest a potential

mechanism for central estrogen modulation of GnRH.[47] One confounding point is that dopamine blunts exogenous GnRH-induced LH release, suggesting that dopamine may inhibit gonadotropins at the pituitary level as well.[60]

Furthermore, the influence of dopamine on gonadotropins may not be completely inhibitory. Administration of metoclopramide, a dopamine antagonist, has been shown to block electrical pulsatile activity in the arcuate nucleus and LH secretion in the rhesus monkey.[58] The dopamine receptor antagonist pimozide increases the height of pregnant mare serum gonadotropin (PMSG)-induced GnRH and LH surges in the rat. However, haloperidol, another dopamine antagonist, reduces the height of induced GnRH and LH surges. Also, dopamine perfusion releases GnRH from the human hypothalamus in vitro through a mechanism that is blocked by haloperidol.[62] These findings suggest the possibility of pharmacological stimulatory and inhibitory dopamine receptors that modulate GnRH neurons.[59,62]

The hypothesis most useful in a clinical setting has been that norepinephrine stimulates GnRH and dopamine inhibits GnRH, with the GnRH secretory pattern reflecting the balance of noradrenergic and dopaminergic effects (Fig. 1-6). However, studies suggest that dopamine activity may vary via inhibitory and stimulatory receptors, which are pharmacologically distinct. Although evidence predominantly supports suprahypophyseal catecholamine activity, direct gonadotrope modulation has not been excluded.

Dopamine is transported to the pituitary portal system via tuberoinfundibular neurons to inhibit prolactin release at the lactotrope. Evidence suggests that dopamine is the hypothalamic inhibitor of prolactin secretion.[13,47] The activity of dopamine suggests a relationship to certain clinical situations. Prolactin is believed to stimulate dopaminergic activity in the median eminence by a short feedback loop mechanism.[47,63] In hyperprolactinemia, increased dopamine may result in abnormal GnRH secretion, altered LH and FSH, and a spectrum of reproductive dysfunctional states ranging from inadequate luteal phase to anovulation and amenorrhea. Other neurotransmitters, including melatonin, γ-aminobutyric acid, and acetylcholine, have been shown to alter the activity of GnRH experimentally.[47,63]

Endorphins

Endogenous opioid peptides represent a group of opiate-like substances that bind to specific brain receptors to effect various physiological functions. Opioid receptors are found throughout the brain, spinal cord, and specifically in the limbic system, brainstem, and sensory neuronal terminals. Certain opioid peptides, the endorphins, appear to be particularly involved in the regulation of the hypothalamic–pituitary axis and the menstrual cycle (Fig. 1-6).

Endorphins are derived from a precursor molecule, proopiomelanocortin (POMC), which gives rise to ACTH and β-lipotropin (Fig. 1-7). β-Lipotropin is broken down to several molecules, including endorphins. Proopiomelanocortin is found in many tissues, including the CNS. The expression of POMC and derivatives is dependent on hormonal input, which varies with the tissue type. The major synthetic products in the brain are opiates, and in the hypothalamus, the major derivative is β-endorphin. Ovarian steroids are thought to be necessary for POMC expression in the hypothalamus.

The highest concentrations of β-endorphin-containing neurons are found in the hypothalamus, specifically in the arcuate nucleus and median eminence, in proximity to the GnRH pulse generator and dopaminergic neurons.[64] β-Endorphin is delivered to the pituitary via the hypophyseal portal circulation, which in monkeys has been shown to contain 10 to 100 times the β-endorphin concentration of simultaneous peripheral blood samples.[65] In addition, portal β-endorphin concentration varies with the menstrual cycle, suggesting ovarian steroid influence.[66]

Administration of β-endorphin to humans results in a decrease in LH concentration.[67] Naloxone, an opiate receptor antagonist, competitively inhibits opiate effects, resulting in increased LH at certain phases of the menstrual cycle. Follicle-stimulating hormone is affected in parallel with LH, but to a lesser degree.[64,68,69]

β-Endorphin's influence on gonadotropin secretion is apparently modulated by the ovarian steroids. Hypophyseal portal β-endorphin concentration varies at different phases of the primate menstrual cycle, showing mild elevation in the mid- and late follicular phase and higher elevation in the luteal phase while becoming undetectable at menstruation. In addition, portal β-endorphin

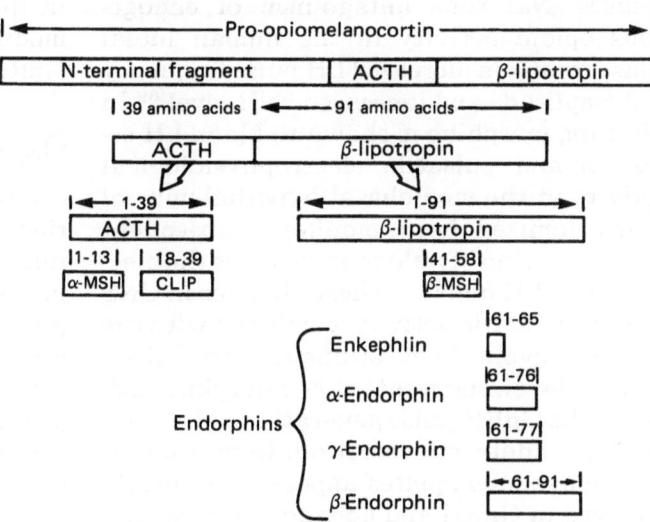

FIGURE 1-7. The molecule proopiomelanocortin (POMC) and its derivatives. From Fritz and Speroff,[47] reproduced with the permission of the publisher, the American Fertility Society.

is undetectable in ovariectomized monkeys. Thus, ovarian steroids are necessary for release of hypothalamic β-endorphin.[67]

The inhibitory effect of opiates on gonadotropin secretion may vary with the changes in ovarian steroids during the menstrual cycle. The effect of naloxone administration on peripheral LH concentration parallels the cyclic changes in portal β-endorphin level. Naloxone causes rapid elevation of LH during the luteal phase (when portal β-endorphin level is highest), moderate elevation of LH in mid- to late follicular phase, and no LH release at menstruation (when β-endorphin is undetectable).[70,71] Naloxone also fails to release LH in oophorectomized women unless estrogen or estrogen and progesterone are replaced.[71] Replacement of E_2 in ovariectomized monkeys results in increased portal β-endorphin, which increases further with the addition of progesterone.[72] These studies and others suggest that ovarian steroids influence the anterior pituitary secretion in part by a mechanism involving β-endorphin secretion.

The cyclic inhibitory effect of opiates on gonadotropin secretion suggests that β-endorphin may be involved in modulating gonadotropin pulse frequency or amplitude. The LH pulse frequency, under the control of GnRH, is circhoral in the follicular phase, decreasing during the luteal phase as progesterone increases and β-endorphin increases. Naloxone antagonism of endogenous opioid activity in the human luteal phase results in increased LH pulse frequency and amplitude and increased FSH level.[69] In addition, morphine is shown to block LH secretion and pulsatile electrophysiological activity in the mediobasal hypothalamus of ovariectomized rhesus monkeys. Subsequent administration of naloxone reverses the electrical and LH block.[73] These changes in CNS and LH pulsatile activity, combined with the observed cyclic fluctuations in portal β-endorphin level, suggest that β-endorphin modulates the GnRH pulse generator to alter pulsatile gonadotropin secretion. In particular, the endogenous opiates appear particularly involved in GnRH and gonadotropin regulation during the high-estrogen and estrogen–progesterone phases of the menstrual cycle, suggesting a mechanism for steroid feedback at the hypothalamus.[69] β-Endorphin may modify hypothalamic activity directly or with involvement of catecholamines. A comprehensive review of β-endorphin physiology and its role in reproductive dysfunction is available.[74]

Catecholestrogens

Hydroxylation of estrogen at the 2 position, which occurs in the hypothalamus, produces molecules with structural similarity to catecholamines, called catecholestrogens. These molecules may alter hypothalamic dopamine and norepinephrine levels by inhibiting tyrosine hydroxylase and thereby decreasing catecholamine synthesis. In competing for catechol-O-methyltransferase (COMT), which degrades catecholamines, the catecholestrogen may function to maintain or increase catecholamine levels. The catecholestrogens may mediate the interactions of ovarian steroids and catecholamines in the regulation of GnRH and gonadotropin secretion (Fig. 1-6).[13,47]

Prostaglandins

Although prostaglandins are not neurotransmitters, they are synthesized and released in the brain. Brain prostaglandins may be modified by estrogen to affect the release of GnRH.[63]

Oxytocin

Oxytocin is produced with its transport peptide, neurophysin I, in the paraventricular nucleus of the hypothalamus and is transported through the median eminence to the posterior pituitary. Oxytocin may also be secreted into the CSF and directly into the pituitary portal system to reach the anterior pituitary and influence gonadotropin secretion.[13] In women, the midcycle peak of estrogen is associated with peak peripheral levels of oxytocin and neurophysin I (also called estrogen-stimulated neurophysin), suggesting a possible role for oxytocin in ovulation.[75] In addition, oxytocin competes with GnRH for degradation enzymes such that, at midcycle, oxytocin may increase available GnRH in pituitary portal blood.[13]

The neuroendocrine control of gonadotropin secretion and the menstrual cycle is initiated by pulsatile GnRH release and modulated by many substances including ovarian steroids, central neurotransmitters, opioid peptides, and others. Figure 1-6 summarizes and illustrates the regulatory mechanisms that have been discussed.

The Initiation of Menarche During Puberty

Gonadotropin-releasing hormone is detectable in the hypothalamus, and LH and FSH in the pituitary, by 11 weeks of gestation, peaking at 20 to 24 weeks. In late gestation, GnRH, LH, and FSH levels decrease as a result of increasing central nervous system inhibition and increasing steroid negative feedback from the fetoplacental unit. The fetal ovary does not produce significant circulating hormones.

With loss of placental estrogen at birth, serum gonadotropins increase in the early neonatal period. Luteinizing hormone remains elevated for several months, and FSH is sustained for most of infancy. In response to elevated gonadotropins, particularly the relatively high FSH, ovarian follicles develop, resulting in E_2 production. In late infancy, gonadotropins fall, which is believed to reflect increasing hypothalamic–pituitary sensitivity to estrogen negative feedback and increasing hypothalamic–pituitary gonadostat inhibition from the maturing central nervous system.[76]

Relatively high FSH persists in early childhood, although both gonadotropins reach their nadir at approximately 6 years of age. The gonadostat is many times more sensitive to steroid negative feedback in childhood than during adulthood. In addition, in early childhood, central inhibition is maximal, as even agonadal children may not show elevated gonadotropins. Girls with gonadal dysgenesis show elevated gonadotropins at age 2 to 3 but show a sharp decline in early childhood as in normal girls. At age 10 to 11, however, gonadotropins are again abnormally elevated in these agonadal girls.[13] Late in the first decade, GnRH and gonadotropins begin to rise, with FSH in relative excess of LH, preceding the onset of puberty.[76] One of the earliest signs of pubertal commencement is the demonstration of nocturnal LH pulsatility.

The precise nature of the signal that initiates puberty is not known. The first steroids to rise in the prepubertal girl are dehydroepiandrosterone (DHEA) and dehydroepiandrosterone sulfate (DHEAS), heralding the onset of adrenarche. Evidence suggests, however, that control of adrenarche (growth of pubic and axillary hair) is separate from that of hypothalamic–pituitary–ovarian maturation or gonadarche.[13]

A major change initiating gonadarche is decreased central inhibition, allowing increased GnRH and gonadotropin secretion. Exogenous GnRH can initiate the cascade of events necessary during puberty. Administration of pulsatile GnRH to immature rhesus monkeys results in anovulatory bleeding initially, followed by monthly ovulatory menstrual cycles.[77] Pubertal maturation of gonadotropin secretion can be induced in response to pulsatile GnRH in prepubertal girls with anorexia nervosa.[78]

The second alteration is decreased gonadotropin sensitivity to E_2 negative feedback. In rhesus monkeys, a developmental increase in serum growth hormone, independent of its growth-promoting action, appears related to the maturational decrease in E_2 negative feedback.[79] Reactivation of gonadotropin synthesis and secretion in puberty requires the reversal of both central suppression and estrogen negative feedback. The specific factor(s) involved in the loss of suppression and activation of gonadotropin secretion are not known. General observations regarding the timing of human puberty have been made, however.

Several factors including genetics, geography, health, nutrition, and psychological state are thought to influence the timing of puberty. Children with a family history of early puberty tend to have early puberty.[13] Studies of twins demonstrate that genetic factors predominate when environment is optimal. Puberty is coordinated with a certain level of skeletal maturation or bone age.[76] Nutrition influences maturation and body mass and is probably responsible for the earlier age of menarche in developed countries. One theory suggests that a critical body weight or critical percentage of body fat must be reached for menarche to occur.[80] Subsequent studies have presented conflicting evidence regarding weight, body fat, and menarche.

Although adequate nutrition precludes normal menstrual cycles, recent studies support the theory that central maturation reduces gonadostat inhibition, which then contributes to growth and changes in body fat. Studies in normal children and children with precocious puberty demonstrate that pubertal growth results from elevated estrogen, growth hormone, and somatomedin-C. The pubertal rise in somatomedin-C is better correlated with pubertal stage than age in normal children. Suppression of gonadal sex steroids in precocious puberty results in decreased somatomedin-C, growth hormone, and height velocity. The pubertal change in somatomedin-C level appears dependent on sex-steroid-induced changes in growth hormone secretion.[81,82] Thus, although normal prepubertal growth may allow for the reversal of gonadostat suppression, normal pubertal growth coincides with steroid hormone changes themselves.

In prepubertal girls, FSH response to GnRH is pronounced, decreasing throughout puberty. In early puberty, LH, and, to a lesser degree, FSH levels rise with sleep and decrease to prepubertal levels during wakefulness.[83] As the child matures, daytime gonadotropins increase, obscuring the diurnal pattern and establishing the mature adult pattern.[76] Follicle-stimulating hormone reaches a plateau at midpuberty, whereas LH and E_2

do not rise until later in puberty. The early pubertal elevation of the FSH to LH ratio may be caused by relatively infrequent GnRH pulses, which have been shown to raise FSH preferentially.[27]

Pituitary response to GnRH increases with puberty. GnRH enhances its own receptors in the pituitary gonadotrope, enhancing synthesis and release of gonadotropins.[7,76] In addition, the bioactivity of plasma LH is augmented over the course of puberty. Bioactive LH increases fivefold over LH measured by radioimmunoassay (immunoreactive LH). The disproportionate rise in bioactive LH is thought to be related to an alteration in the molecular structure.[84]

In response to enhanced GnRH and gonadotropin function, ovarian steroid synthesis is stimulated, producing estrogen peaks and menarche. Initially, the steroid production may not achieve levels sufficient for ovulation. In late puberty, approximately 12 to 18 months after menarche in humans, a high sustained level of estrogen is achieved, resulting in positive hypothalamic–pituitary feedback and ovulatory cycles.

Summary

The neuroendocrine regulation of the menstrual cycle is the integration of a multitude of physiological and psychological influences that modulate a variety of neurohormones and neurotransmitters, resulting in characteristic pulsatility of GnRH. The arcuate nucleus of the medial basal hypothalamus is the major site of GnRH synthesis and release. The GnRH is transported to the median eminence, the portal circulation, and the anterior pituitary, resulting in pulsatile LH and FSH secretion and synthesis. The pulsatile pattern of GnRH is essential to pituitary gonadotropin secretion, and changes in GnRH frequency and amplitude alter absolute and relative LH and FSH concentrations. Gonadotropin-releasing hormone determines cyclic pituitary gonadotropin secretion, which in turn is responsible for the maturation and transformation of ovarian follicles into high-

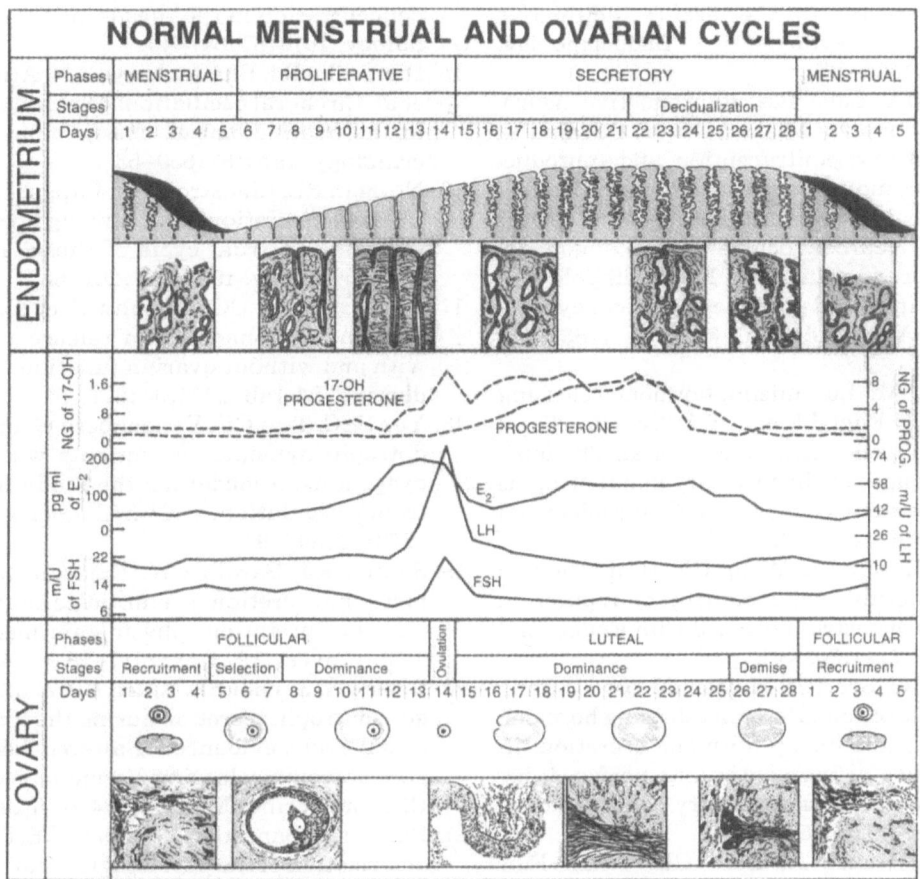

FIGURE 1-8. The functional and temporal relationship of the menstrual and ovarian cycle. From Healy and Hodgen,[86] reproduced with permission of the publisher, © 1983 by Williams & Wilkins, Baltimore.

ly steroidogenic corpora lutea from puberty to menopause.

The pulsatile patterns of GnRH and gonadotropins change with the menstrual cycle under the influence of ovarian steroids. Catecholamines, β-endorphins, and other neurotransmitters and neuromodulators mediate the central and pituitary estrogen and progesterone effects.

The onset of puberty represents the loss of suppression of a system that is active during fetal life and infancy. An unknown signal allows renewed GnRH pulsatile secretion and decreased sensitivity to estrogen negative feedback, resulting ultimately in ovulatory menstrual cycles.

Many reproductive problems may center on an alteration of this exquisitely timed and integrated sequence of events. A basic understanding of the normal physiology described in this chapter allows an appreciation of the pathophysiology and rationale for treatment in various female reproductive dysfunctional states. Figure 1-8 depicts both the ovarian and menstrual cycles. The time-dependent relationships necessary to establish normal hypothalamic–pituitary–ovarian–uterine function are shown.

References

1. Reichlin S. Neuroendocrinology. In: Wilson JD, Foster DW, eds. Williams textbook of endocrinology. Seventh edition. Philadelphia: W. B. Saunders, 1985:492–567.
2. Berglund RM, Page RB. Can the pituitary

secrete directly to the brain? (affirmative anatomical evidence). Endocrinology. 1978;102:1325–38.

3. Kletzky OA, Lobo RA. Reproductive neuro-endocrinology. In: Mishell DR Jr, Davajan V, eds. Infertility, contraception and reproductive endocrinology. Second edition. Oradell, NJ: Medical Economics, 1986:3–30.

4. Kase NG. Neuroendocrine control of gonadotropin secretion. In: Kase NG, Weingold AB, eds. Principles and practice of clinical gynecology. New York: John Wiley & Sons, 1983:125–36.

5. McCann SM. Luteinizing-hormone-releasing hormone. N Engl J Med. 1977;296:797–802.

6. Wang CF, Lasley BL, Lein A, et al. The functional changes of the pituitary gonadotropins during the menstrual cycle. J Clin Endocrinol Metab. 1976;42:718–28.

7. Hoff JD, Lasley BL, Wang CF, et al. The two pools of pituitary gonadotropin: regulation during the menstrual cycle. J Clin Endocrinol Metab. 1977;44:302–12.

8. Borges JLC, Scott D, Kaiser DL, et al. Ca^{++} dependence of gonadotropin releasing hormone stimulated luteinizing hormone secretion: in vitro studies, using continuous perfused dispersed rat antiserum pituitary cells. Endocrinology. 1983;113:557–62.

9. Wise PM, Rance N, Barr GD, et al. Further evidence that luteinizing hormone-releasing hormone also is follicle-stimulating hormone-releasing hormone. Endocrinology. 1979;104:940–47.

10. McCormack JT, Plant TM, Hess L, et al. The effect of luteinizing hormone releasing hormone (LHRH) antiserum administration on gonadotropin secretion in the rhesus monkey. Endocrinology. 1977;100:663–67.

11. Silverman AJ, Antunes JL, Ferin M, et al. The distribution of luteinizing hormone-releasing hormone (LHRH) in the hypothalamus of the rhesus monkey. Light microscopic studies using immunoperoxidase technique. Endocrinology. 1977;101:134–42.

12. Knobil E. The neuroendocrinology of the menstrual cycle. Recent Prog Horm Res. 1980;36:53–88.

13. Speroff L, Glass RH, Kase NG. Clinical gynecologic endocrinology and infertility. Fourth edition. Baltimore: Williams & Wilkins. 1989:51–90.

14. Atkinson LE, Bhattacharya AN, Monroe SE, et al. Effects of gonadectomy on plasma LH concentration in the rhesus monkey. Endocrinology. 1970;87:847–49.

15. Dierschke DJ, Bhattacharya AN, Atkinson LE, et al. Circhoral oscillations of plasma LH levels in the ovariectomized rhesus monkey. Endocrinology. 1970;87:850–53.

16. Norman RL, Lindstrom SA, Bangsberg D, et al. Pulsatile secretion of luteinizing hormone during the menstrual cycle of rhesus macaques. Endocrinology. 1984;115:261–66.

17. Yen SSC, Tsai CC, Naftolin F, et al. Pulsatile patterns of gonadotropin release in subjects with and without ovarian function. J Clin Endocrinol Metab. 1972;34:671–75.

18. Yen SSC, Tsai CC, Vandenberg G, et al. Gonadotropin dynamics in patients with gonadal dysgenesis: a model for the study of gonadotropin regulation. J Clin Endocrinol Metab. 1972;35:897–904.

19. Santen RJ, Bardin CW. Episodic luteinizing hormone secretion in man: pulse analysis, clinical interpretation, physiologic mechanisms. J Clin Invest. 1973;52:2617–28.

20. Reame N, Sauder SE, Kelch RP, et al. Pulsatile gonadotropin secretion during the human menstrual cycle: evidence for altered frequency of gonadotropin-releasing hormone secretion. J Clin Endocrinol Metab. 1984;59:328–37.

21. Filicori M, Santoro N, Merriam GR, et al. Characterization of the physiological pattern of episodic gonadotropin secretion throughout the human menstrual cycle. J Clin Endocrinol Metab. 1986;62:1136–44.

22. Belchetz PE, Plant TM, Nakai Y, et al. Hypophysial responses to continuous and intermittent delivery of hypothalamic gonadotropin releasing hormone. Science. 1978;202:631–32.

23. Ferin M. Neuroendocrine control of ovarian function in the primate. J Reprod Fertil. 1983;69:369–81.

24. Carmel PN, Araki S, Ferin M. Pituitary stalk blood collection in rhesus monkeys: evidence for pulsatile release of gonadotropin releasing hormone (GnRH). Endocrinology. 1976;99:243–48.

25. Elkind-Hirsch K, Ravnikar V, Schiff I, et al. Determinations of endogenous immunoreactive luteinizing hormone-releasing hormone in human plasma. J Clin Endocrinol Metab. 1982;54:602–07.

26. Wilson RC, Kesner JS, Kaufman JM, et al. Central electrophysiologic correlates of pulsatile luteinizing hormone secretion in the rhesus

monkey. Neuroendocrinology. 1984;39:256–60.

27. Wildt L, Hausler A, Marshall G, et al. Frequency and amplitude of gonadotropin-releasing hormone stimulation and gonadotropin secretion in the rhesus monkey. Endocrinology. 1981;109:376–85.

28. Marshall JC, Kelch RP. Gonadotropin-releasing hormone: role of pulsatile secretion in the regulation of reproduction. N Engl J Med. 1986;315:1459–68.

29. Neill JD, Patton JM, Dailey RA, et al. Luteinizing hormone releasing hormone (LHRH) in pituitary stalk blood of rhesus monkeys: Relationship to level of LH release. Endocrinology. 1977;101:430–34.

30. Filicori M, Butler JP, Crowley WF. Neuroendocrine regulation of the corpus luteum in the human evidence for pulsatile progesterone secretion. J Clin Invest. 1984;73:1638–47.

31. Pfaff DN, Gerlach JL, McEwen BS, et al. Autoradiographic localization of hormone-concentrating cells in the brain of the female rhesus monkey. J Comp Neurol. 1976;170:279–94.

32. Nakai Y, Plant TM, Hess DL, et al. On the sites of the negative and positive feedback activity of estradiol in the control of gonadotropin secretion in the rhesus monkey. Endocrinology. 1978;102:1008–14.

33. Knobil E, Plant TM, Wildt L, et al. Control of the rhesus monkey menstrual cycle: Permissive role of hypothalamic gonadotropin-releasing hormone. Science. 1980;207:1371–73.

34. Ferin M, Rosenblatt H, Carmel PW, et al. Estrogen-induced gonadotropin surges in female rhesus monkeys after pituitary stalk section. Endocrinology. 1979;104:50–52.

35. Crowley WF Jr, McArthur JW. Stimulation of the normal menstrual cycle in Kallmann's syndrome by pulsatile administration of luteinizing hormone-releasing hormone (LHRH). J Clin Endocrinol Metab. 1980;51:173–75.

36. Levine JE, Norman RL, Gliessman PM, et al. In vivo gonadotropin-releasing hormone release and serum luteinizing hormone measurements in ovariectomized, estrogen-treated rhesus macaques. Endocrinology. 1985;117:711–21.

37. Ferin M, Carmel PN, Zimmerman EA, et al. Location of intrahypothalamic estrogen-responsive sites influencing LH secretion in the female rhesus monkey. Endocrinology. 1974;95:1059–68.

38. Chappel SC, Resko JA, Norman RL, et al. Stud-

ies in rhesus monkeys on the site where estrogen inhibits gonadotropin: delivery of 17-β-estradiol to the hypothalamus and pituitary gland. J Clin Endocrinol Metab. 1981;52:1–8.

39. Keye WR Jr, Jaffe RB. Modulation of pituitary gonadotropin response to gonadotropin releasing hormone by estradiol. J Clin Endocrinol Metab. 1974;38:805–10.

40. Jaffe RB, Keye WR Jr. Estradiol augmentation of pituitary responsiveness to gonadotropin-releasing hormone in women. J Clin Endocrinol Metab. 1974;39:850–55.

41. Young JR, Jaffe RB. Strength duration characteristics of estrogen effects on gonadotropin response to gonadotropin-releasing hormone in women II. Effects of varying concentrations of estradiol. J Clin Endocrinol Metab. 1976;42:432.

42. Adams TE, Norman RL, Spies HG. Gonadotropin-releasing hormone receptor binding and pituitary responsiveness in estradiol-primed monkeys. Science. 1981;213:1388–90.

43. Menon M, Peegel H, Katta V. Estradiol potentiation of gonadotropin-releasing hormone responsiveness in the anterior pituitary is mediated by an increase in gonadotropin-releasing hormone receptors. Am J Obstet Gynecol. 1985;151:534–40.

44. Crowder ME, Nett TM. Pituitary content of gonadotropins and receptors for gonadotropin-releasing hormone (GnRH) and hypothalamic content of GnRH during the periovulatory period of the ewe. Endocrinology. 1984;114:234–39.

45. Veldhius JD, Evans WS, Rogal AD, et al. Pituitary self-priming action of gonadotropin-releasing hormone kinetics of estradiol's potentiating effects on gonadotropin-releasing hormone-facilitated luteinizing hormone and follicle-stimulating hormone release in healthy postmenopausal women. J Clin Invest. 1986;77:1849–56.

46. Ferland L, Marchetti B, Seguin C, et al. Associated changes of pituitary luteinizing hormone-releasing hormone (LHRH) receptors and responsiveness to the neurohormone induced by 17-β-estradiol and LHRH in vivo in the rat. Endocrinology. 1981;109:87–93.

47. Fritz MA, Speroff L: The endocrinology of the menstrual cycle: the interaction of folliculogenesis and neuroendocrine mechanisms. Fertil Steril. 1982;38:509–29.

48. Dierschke DJ, Yamaji T, Karsch FJ, et al. Blockade by progesterone of estrogen-induced

LH and FSH release in the rhesus monkey. Endocrinology. 1973;92:1496–1501.

49. Wildt L, Hutchinson JS, Marshall G, et al. On the site of action of progesterone in the blockade of the estradiol-induced gonadotropin discharge in the rhesus monkey. Endocrinology. 1981;109:1293–94.

50. March CM, Goebelsmann V, Nakamura RM, et al. Roles of estradiol and progesterone in eliciting the midcycle luteinizing hormone and follicle-stimulating hormone surges. J Clin Endocrinol Metab. 1979;49:507–13.

51. Liu JH, Yen SSC. Induction of midcycle gonadotropin surge by ovarian steroids in women: a critical evaluation. J Clin Endocrinol Metab. 1983;57:797–802.

52. Lasley BL, Wang CF, Yen SSC. The effects of estrogen and progesterone on the functional capacity of the gonadotrophs. J Clin Endocrinol Metab. 1975;41:820–26.

53. Collins RL, Hodgen GD. Blockade of the spontaneous midcycle gonadotropin surge in monkeys by RU 486: a progesterone antagonist or agonist? J Clin Endocrinol Metab. 1986;63:1270–76.

54. Soules MR, Steiner RH, Clifton DK, et al. Progesterone modulation of pulsatile luteinizing hormone secretion in normal women. J Clin Endocrinol Metab. 1984;58:378–83.

55. Schnatz PT. Neuroendocrinology and the ovulation cycle—advances and review. Adv Psychosom Med. 1985;12:4–24.

56. Bhattacharya AN, Dierschke DJ, Yamaji T, et al. The pharmacologic blockade of the circhoral mode of LH secretion in the ovariectomized rhesus monkey. Endocrinology. 1972;90:778–86.

57. Plant TM, Nakai Y, Belchetz P, et al. The sites of action of estradiol and phentolamine in the inhibition of the pulsatile, circhoral discharges of LH in the rhesus monkey (*Macaca mulatta*). Endocrinology. 1978;102:1015–18.

58. Kaufman JM, Kesner JS, Wilson RC, et al. Electrophysiological manifestation of luteinizing hormone-releasing hormone pulse generator activity in the rhesus monkey: influence of alpha-adrenergic and dopaminergic blocking agents. Endocrinology. 1985;116:1327–33.

59. Sarkar DK, Fink G. Gonadotropin-releasing hormone surge: possible modulation through post-synaptic adrenoreceptors and two pharmacologically distinct dopamine receptors. Endocrinology. 1981;108:862–67.

60. Judd HJ, Rakoff JS, Yen SSC. Inhibition of

gonadotropin and prolactin release by dopamine: effect of endogenous estradiol levels. J Clin Endocrinol Metab. 1978;47:494–98.

61. Andersen AN, Hagen C, Lange P, et al. Dopaminergic regulation of gonadotropin levels and pulsatility in normal women. Fertil Steril. 1987;47:391–97.

62. Rasmusen DD, Liu JU, Wolf PL, et al. Gonadotropin-releasing hormone neurosecretion in the human hypothalamus: *in vitro* regulation by dopamine. J Clin Endocrinol Metab. 1986;62:479–83.

63. Futterweit W. Polycystic ovarian disease. New York: Springer-Verlag, 1984:1–21.

64. Gindoff PR, Ferin M. Brain opioid peptides and menstrual cyclicity. Semin Reprod Endocrinol. 1987;5:125–33.

65. Wardlaw SL, Wehrenberg WB, Ferin M, et al. High levels of β-endorphin in hypophysial portal blood. Endocrinol. 1980;106:1323–26.

66. Wehrenberg WB, Wardlaw SL, Frantz AG, et al. β-endorphin in hypophyseal portal blood: variations throughout the menstrual cycle. Endocrinology. 1982;111:879–81.

67. Reid RL, Hoff JD, Yen SSC, et al. Effects of exogenous β-endorphin on pituitary hormone secretion and its disappearance rate in normal human subjects. J Clin Endocrinol Metab. 1981;52:1179–83.

68. Quigley ME, Yen SSC. The role of endogenous opiates on LH secretion during the menstrual cycle. J Clin Endocrinol Metab. 1980;51:179–87.

69. Ropert AF, Quigley ME, Yen SSC. Endogenous opiates modulate pulsatile luteinizing hormone release in humans. J Clin Endocrinol Metab. 1981;52:583–85.

70. Snowden E, Khan-Dawood FS, Dawood MY. The effect of naloxone on endogenous opioid regulation of pituitary gonadotropins and prolactin during the menstrual cycle. J Clin Endocrinol Metab. 1984;59:298–302.

71. Shoupe D, Montz FJ, Lobo RA. The effects of estrogen and progesterone on endogenous opioid activity in oophorectomized women. J Clin Endocrinol Metab. 1985;60:178–83.

72. Wardlaw SL, Wehrenberg WB, Ferin M, et al. Effect of sex steroids on β-endorphin in hypophyseal portal blood. J Clin Endocrinol Metab. 1982;55:877–87.

73. Kesner JS, Kaufman JM, Wilson RC, et al. The effect of morphine on the electrophysiologic activity of the hypothalamic luteinizing hormone-releasing hormone pulse generator

in the rhesus monkey. Neuroendocrinology. 1986;43:686–88.

74. Seifer DB, Collins RL. Current concepts of β-endorphin physiology in female reproductive dysfunction. Fertil Steril. 1990 (in Press).

75. Amico JA, Seif SM, Robinson AG. Elevation of oxytocin and the oxytocin-associated neurophysin in the plasma of normal women during midcycle. J Clin Endocrinol Metab. 1981;53:1229–32.

76. Kaplan SA. The ovary and female sexual maturation. In: Rosenfield RL, ed. Clinical pediatric and adolescent endocrinology. Philadelphia: W. B. Saunders, 1982:217–68.

77. Wildt L, Marshall G, Knobil E. Experimental induction of puberty in the infantile rhesus monkey. Science. 1980;207:1373–75.

78. Marshall, JC, Kelch RP. Low dose pulsatile gonadotropin-releasing hormone in anorexia nervosa: a model of human pubertal development. J Clin Endocrinol Metab. 1979;49:712–18.

79. Wilson ME, Gordon TP, Collins DC: Ontogeny of luteinizing hormone secretion and first ovulation in seasonal breeding rhesus monkeys. Endocrinology. 1986;118:293–301.

80. Frisch RE. Body fat, menarche and reproductive ability. Semin Reprod Endocrinol. 1985;3:45.

81. Harris DA, Vanvleit G, Egli CA, et al. Somatomedin-C in normal puberty before and after treatment with a potent luteinizing hormone-releasing hormone agonist. J Clin Endocrinol Metab. 1985;61:152–59.

82. Mansfield MJ, Rudlin CR, Crigler JF Jr, et al. Changes in growth and serum growth hormone and plasma somatomedin-C levels during suppression of gonadal sex steroid secretion in girls with central precocious puberty. J Clin Endocrinol Metab. 1988;66:3–9.

83. Boyar R, Finkelstein J, Roffwarg H, et al. Synchronization of augmented luteinizing hormone secretion with sleep during puberty. N Engl J Med. 1972;287:582–86.

84. Burstein S, Schaff-Blass E, Blass J, et al. The changing ratio of bioactive to immunoreactive luteinizing hormone (LH) through puberty principally reflects changing radioimmunoassay dose response characteristics. J Clin Endocrinol Metab. 1985;61:508–13.

85. Blankstein J, Mashrach S, Lunenfeld B. Regulation of the female reproductive system. In: Blankstein J, Mashrach S, Lunenfeld B, eds. Ovulation induction and in vitro fertilization. Chicago: Mosby-Year Book, 1986:7–45.

86. Healy D, Hodgen G. The endocrinology of the human endometrium. Ob/Gyn Surv. 1983;38:509.

2
Ovarian Physiology and In Vitro Fertilization

GARY D. HODGEN

In discussing principles of ovarian physiology, ovulation induction, as applied during enhanced follicular recruitment during in vitro fertilization (IVF) therapies, serves as a perfect illustrative model. In developing a strategy for a descriptive linkage between ovarian physiology and IVF as it is applied in 1990, it is imperative to review briefly the chronology of ovarian management in IVF therapy.

First, we recall that Edwards and Steptoe tried both the natural cycle and various regimens for ovarian stimulation without success prior to 1978. These early failures in IVF attempts dissuaded them from the complications of such stimulated cycles. Thus, they had returned to the natural ovarian/menstrual cycle at the time that Louise Brown was conceived in the autumn of 1977.

The limitation of collecting just one oocyte, at best, put a heavy emphasis on tedious monitoring of the physiology of the woman's natural ovarian physiology. The combination of improved ultrasound technology, rapid urinary LH surge test kits, rapid serum estrogen assays, and good laparoscopic skills made the task effective, although it was expensive in terms of labor intensity.

The next era in the early and mid-1980s pitted clomiphene citrate and/or gonadotropin therapy against the natural cycle in terms of IVF efficacy. Literally hundreds of experimental regimens were investigated, often without persuasive outcomes because of poor study design, too few results, or empiricism over statistical validity of claimed advantages. However, there can be little doubt that ovarian physiology, as affected by exogenous gonadotropin therapy, has provided the single largest improvement in in-vitro fertilization results because of the availability of many eggs for fertilization and, in turn, more embryos for transfer to the uterus.

More recently, investigations on management of ovarian physiology for IVF have centered on the adjunctive use of GnRH analogs with FSH/LH regimens. Because agonistic analogs were clinically available first, they have progressed further to date. However, the antagonist analogs are now approaching clinical utility, promising greater convenience for both patients and the medical teams providing IVF therapy. This course of investigation is likely to continue into the 1990s but may be replaced by oocyte maturation in vitro at some point in the coming decade.

What follows is my account of the basic ovarian physiology on which clinical IVF therapy was developed. Even so, there is still so much to be learned.

Physiological Basis

Over the past 15 years, we have studied basic mechanisms of ovarian function in the primate menstrual cycle. As previously reviewed, these investigations were directed at understanding follicular growth and atresia,[1] corpus luteum (CL) function,[2,3] ovum maturation,[4] and the initiation of ovulatory men-

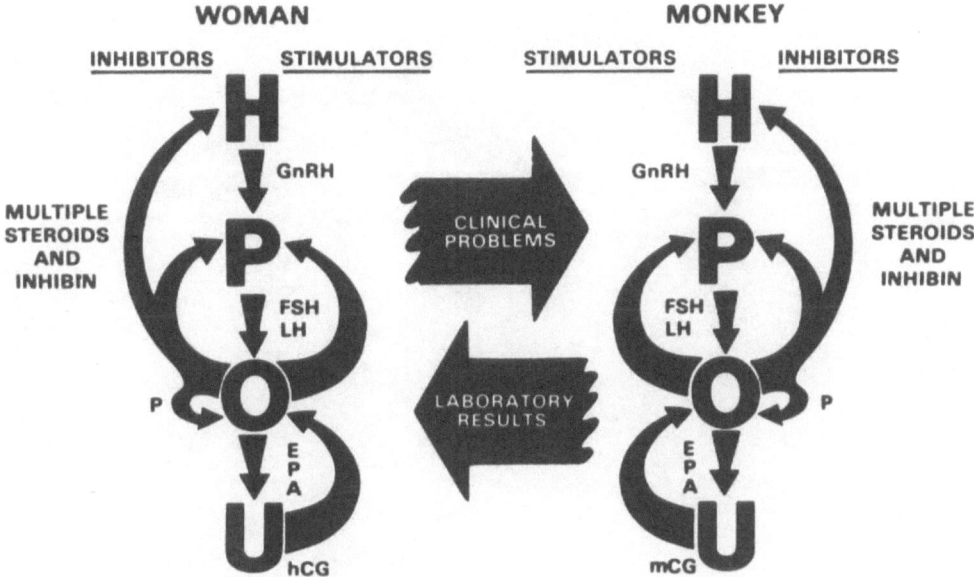

FIGURE 2-1. The ovarian/menstrual cycle. Extensive mimicry of the human HPOU axis in monkeys allows effective use of these surrogate primates when ethical and legal constraints limit direct clinical investigation.

strual cycles after menarche and the post-partum hiatus.[5] In this chapter, it is our challenge to convey the relevance of that research to the practitioner of reproductive medicine, especially the physician providing endocrine infertility treatment, with the expectation that these new findings may enrich existing skills and knowledge in clinical care.[6]

The principal advantages in employing nonhuman primate models for research lie in (1) their extensive mimicry of many fundamental properties (anatomic, functional, and temporal) of the human hypothalamic–pituitary–ovarian–uterine (HPOU) axis; (2) freedom to pursue aggressive protocols having the capacity to resolve questions about the reproductive process, thereby accelerating and guiding the course of subsequent clinical research; and (3) freedom from inherent moral constraints on direct clinical investigation. Prevailing ethical and legal standards restrict the design and conduct of studies on many of the foremost endocrine infertility problems confronting the clinician, and quite appropriately, our concern for individual patient welfare supersedes the quest for new understanding.

That there are obvious limitations in the use of these surrogate primates (rhesus and cynomolgus monkeys) must be realized. Respect for these limitations is shown in their selective application in the laboratory, followed by conservative interpretation and use of the results toward the resolution of clinical problems (Fig. 2-1).

Because many recent advances reflect the results of parallel clinical and laboratory studies, this review builds on previous texts[1-5] in discussing the dominant ovarian follicle of the natural cycle or folliculogenesis during ovulation induction in in vitro fertilization–embryo transfer therapy (IVF-ET).

The Natural Ovarian/Menstrual Cycle

The specialized gonadal stroma of the growing preovulatory follicle and its successor, the corpus luteum, establish and maintain the changing hormonal milieu that nurtures the ovum through maturation, fertilization, and the initial stages of embryogenesis. In-

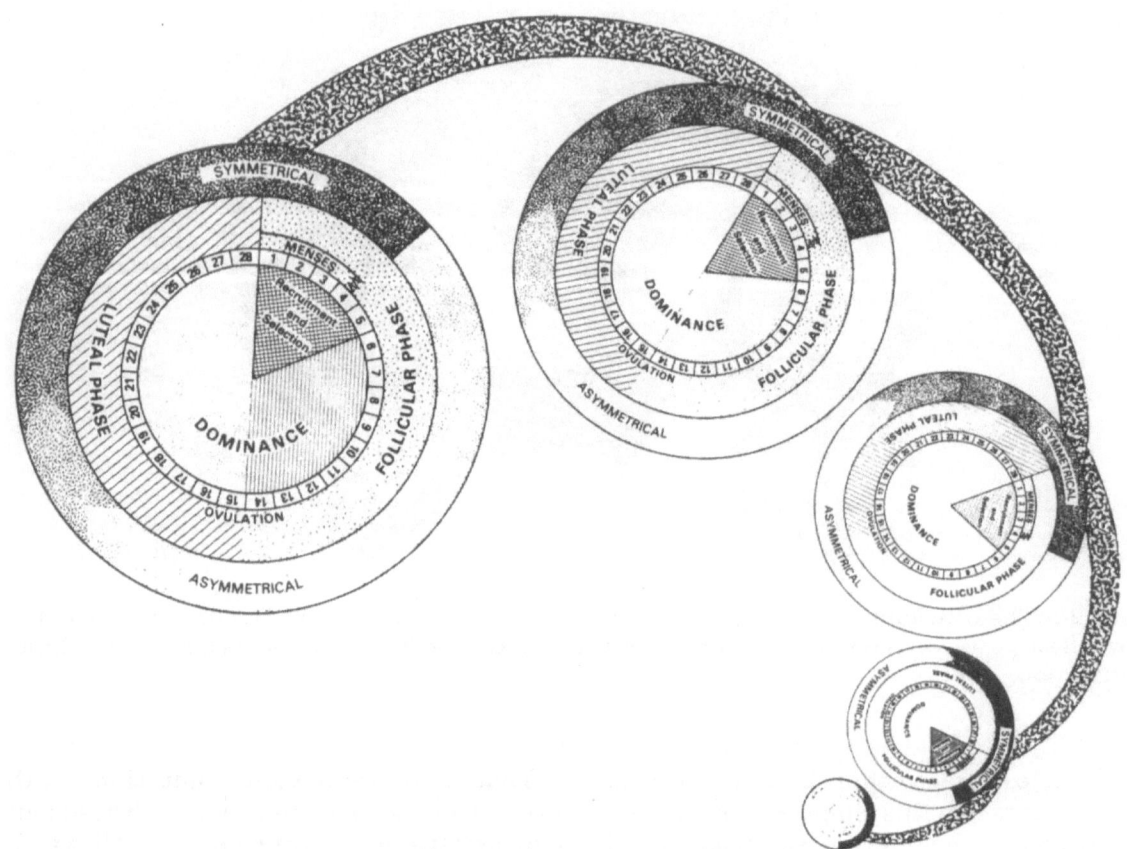

FIGURE 2-2. Conceptualization of the primate ovarian/menstrual cycle. From ref. 1, with permission, © by The Endocrine Society.

deed, it is the ovarian cycle that temporally modulates hypothalamic–pituitary function through both negative and positive feedback on gonadotropin release as well as orchestration of uterine proliferative and secretory phases of the menstrual cycle (Fig. 2-2). It is no wonder that the sequelae to aberrancies during folliculogenesis (spontaneous or induced) include abnormalities of the cervical mucus (CM), the endometrium, circulating gonadotropins, the corpus luteum, and even the ovum. Accordingly, fertility in the female depends most fundamentally on a background of intraovarian processes that account for timely follicular growth culminating in ovulation of a healthy fertilizable oocyte, as well as its subsequent nurturing.

Whereas many follicles may begin this developmental course in each ovarian/men-

strual cycle, typically only a single follicle sustains its inherent gametogenic potential; all others succumb to atresia, finally having forfeited their latency (Fig. 2-3). Of course, provision of more gonadotropins in stimulated or induced cycles by clomiphene citrate (CC) or human menopausal gonadotropin (hMG) or both will violate the normal monovular quota. On a controlled basis, this outcome may be desirable in order to facilitate IVF-ET. Even so, the attendant risk is to have impaired (qualitatively) the normality of the growing follicles and the sequelae of the ovarian/menstrual cycle, requisite for establishing a viable pregnancy. Moreover, aspiration of the preovulatory follicle to accomplish ovum collection is necessarily associated with removal of some follicular fluid and granulosa cells. These constituents

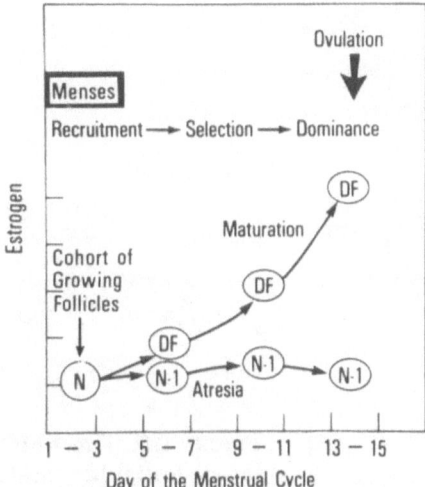

FIGURE 2-3. Time course for recruitment, selection, and ovulation of the dominant ovarian follicle, with onset of atresia among other follicles of the cohort.

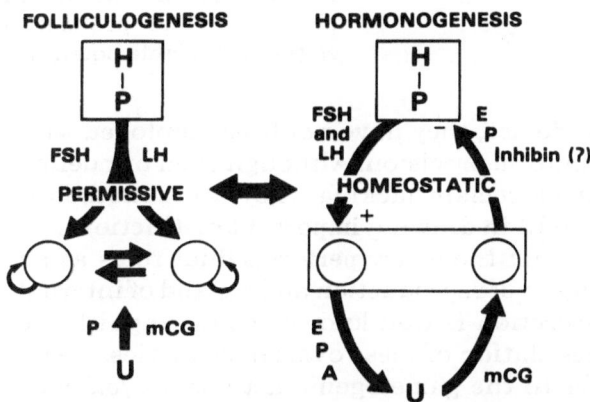

FIGURE 2-4. The primate ovarian menstrual cycle. A proposed two-tier mechanism involving both intraovarian and extraovarian regulation of folliculogenesis. Ovarian (follicular) factors acting directly on the ovaries against a background of permissive gonadotropic support are hypothesized to be the primary regulators of follicle selection dominance. From ref. 7, with permission.

of the intrafollicular milieu surely participate in ovum maturation, engendering the ovum's fertilizable status in the final hours of the preovulatory gonadotropin surges.

We have hypothesized (1) that the precise regulation of follicle growth and selection is

accomplished primarily by specific ovarian factors that act directly on the ovaries and (2) that gonadotropins, at tonic levels, are merely permissive to folliculogenesis.[7] We envisage a two-tier ovarian mechanism (Fig. 2-4). At the first tier, specific ovarian factors govern the progressive winnowing of the cohort of developing follicles down to the size of the species-characteristic ovulatory quota each cycle. Some factors may act within the ovary of origin as intraovarian regulators; other ovarian factors may be secreted and circulate to the opposite ovary to act as extraovarian signals (but of ovarian origin). Together, they regulate the culling out or inhibit the maturation of supernumerary growing follicles. This first tier of the proposed ovarian mechanism, which precisely regulates follicle selection (cohort size), is operative, however, only when circulating gonadotropins are above minimal tonic levels and near the tonic "set point."

At the second tier, ovarian hormones (steroidal and nonsteroidal) inhibit gonadotropin secretion in a negative feedback fashion to constrain circulating gonadotropin levels to an appropriate range around the tonic set point. If gonadotropin levels are too far below the tonic set point, folliculogenesis will be arrested as a result of inadequate stimulation. Contrariwise, if circulating gonadotropin levels are too far above the tonic set point, first-tier ovarian mechanisms, ordinarily at work to regulate the size of the ovulatory quota, are impaired or inactivated; in such instances superovulation occurs. That is, we propose that the emergence of multiple follicles on both ovaries after administration of exogenous gonadotropins to monkeys or women is not only the result of augmenting the availability of gonadotropins per se but also an indirect result of overriding first-tier ovarian mechanisms of follicle selection (Fig. 2-5).

Clearly, as exploited by several well-known bioassays for gonadotropins, both follicle-stimulating hormone (FSH) and luteinizing hormone (LH) can have graded, dose-dependent effects on the ovary. However, in the physiological setting of the menstrual cycle, we find it more useful to consider that the

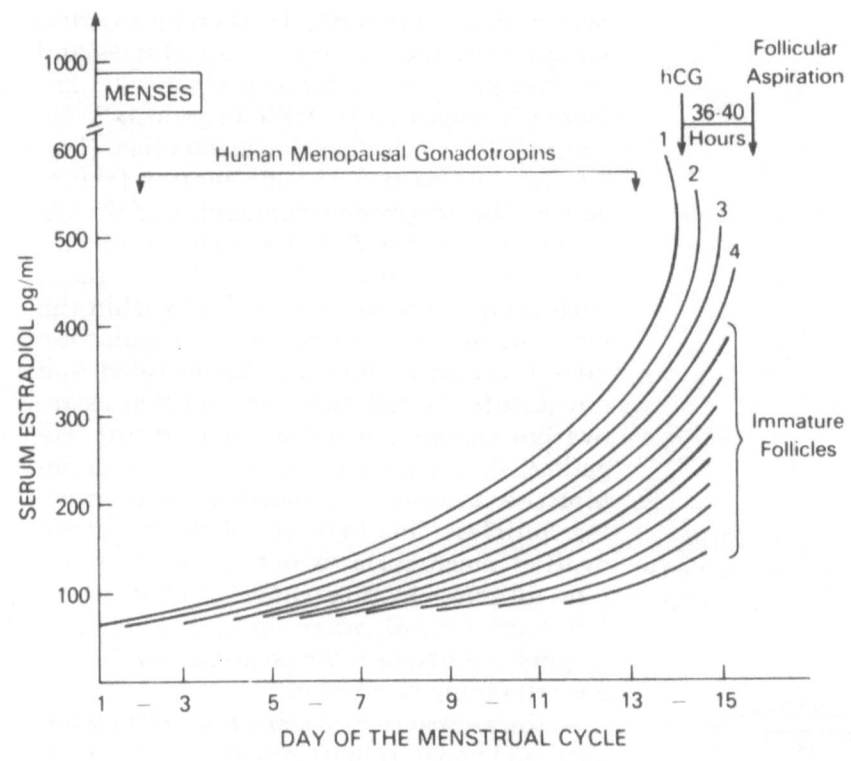

FIGURE 2-5. The hMG-stimulated follicular maturation overrides selection of a single dominant follicle in the natural cycle. Note that only a few follicles can be regarded as developing (quasi)synchronously. If hCG is given too late, the most advanced follicles may yield postmature eggs of low viable potential.

folliculogenic actions of gonadotropins (principally FSH) are permissive at tonic levels and that the steroidogenic actions of gonadotropins (principally LH) are graded. If FSH at tonic levels is actually permissive to folliculogenesis, the graded effects observed may be attributable to supraphysiological (supratonic) levels. Graded actions of gonadotropins on steroidogenesis [and perhaps on "inhibin" secretion(s) as well; see below] are necessary for the second tier of the ovarian mechanism to constrain circulating gonadotropins near the tonic set point, so that first-tier mechanisms of follicle selection are effective. Evidence that these two activity tiers are dissociated in some circumstances is presented below. More direct evidence for this hypothesis must come from future studies.

Terminology

Before considering how we arrived at this hypothesis, we shall explain some important terms. They are not new, but, although in wide use, they have not been employed with uniform precision. Although even our definitions remain lacking, they are nonetheless useful in drawing important distinctions.

That the ovary performs dual roles as an organ of reproduction and a gland of internal secretion is well known. To distinguish the regulation of these ovarian activities, we refer to the gametogenic activity as *folliculogenesis* and to the secretory activity as *hormonogenesis* (see Fig. 2-4). Extraovarian or intraovarian factors that directly influence the ovary's gametogenic role have a folliculogenic action or elicit a folliculogenic response. Although some readers may balk at the introduction of a term such as *hormonogenesis*, it is used here because we find current nomenclature inadequate. Since, in our scheme, some ovarian secretions may act locally within the ovary in a paracrine (or perhaps even an autocrine) fashion, they are not, in the strictest sense, endocrine. In addition, since some ovarian hormones secreted into the circulation may be nonsteroidal ("inhibins"), *steroidogenesis* is too restric-

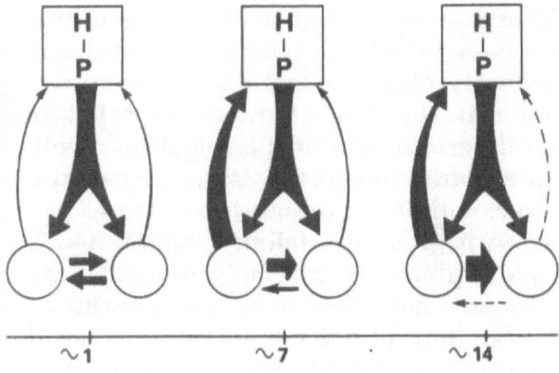

FIGURE 2-6. Hypothetical scheme depicting the relationships between the regulation of the ovary's gametogenic and secretory activities by extraovarian and intraovarian factors. From ref. 7, with permission.

tive. Consequently we use the term *hormonogenesis* to encompass all nature and manner of such ovarian secretions (Fig. 2-6).

During each cycle primordial follicles depart from the resting pool and begin a well-characterized pattern of growth and development.[8,9] Groups of (quasi)synchronously growing follicles are called *cohorts*. In the same or some subsequent cycle, a few members (or only one) of one cohort continue

to develop and escape atresia, until they become preovulatory graafian follicles, ultimately providing the species-characteristic ovulatory quota of eggs. Schwartz has aptly termed this pattern the "trajectory of follicle growth."[10] Extending the trajectory metaphor into our hypothesis outlined above, we see gonadotropins as providing the "thrust" and ovarian factors the "guidance" along the trajectory, not unlike some surface-launched missile (Fig. 2-7). Clearly, without continued "thrust" in excess of the guidance system's design, the accuracy and precision of the course are compromised.[7]

We use the term *recruitment* (Fig. 2-8) to indicate that a follicle has entered on the growth trajectory. Thus, under this definition, recruitment includes the entry of primordial follicles onto the trajectory without excluding the reentry of more mature follicles that may have been transiently at rest. Pedersen's studies in mice have generally been interpreted to mean that, once a follicle leaves the resting primordial pool, it must continue to mature or succumb to atresia—that is, it does not again enter the resting phase.[11] Whether or not this is the case for primates is unknown; hence the broader definition is being used here. Since follicles at various preantral stages of development were

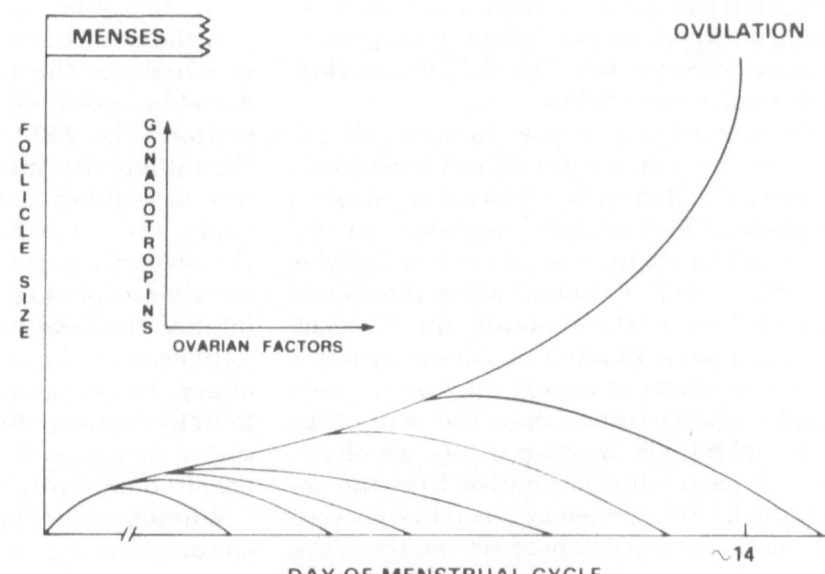

FIGURE 2-7. Proposed relationship between gonadotropins and ovarian factors in regulating maturation or atresia along the so-called trajectory of follicle growth. From ref. 7, with permission.

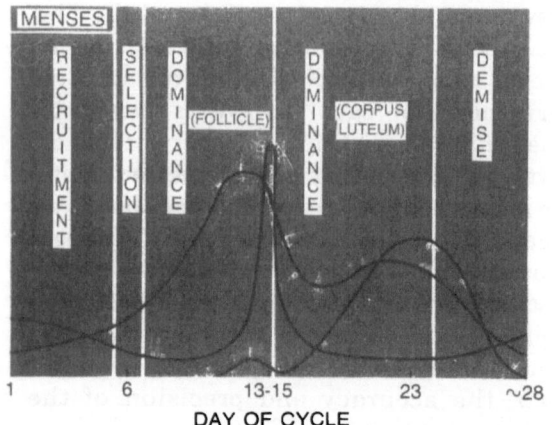

FIGURE 2-8. The terms used to describe the sequence of principal ovarian events during follicular maturation and CL function are temporally defined in the menstrual cycle. The curves depict idealized (stereotypical) patterns of E_2, pituitary gonadotropins, and P in peripheral circulation.

observed in ovaries of hypophysectomized rats and rabbits,[12] recruitment of primordial follicles is not wholly dependent on gonadotropins but may only be enhanced by these hormones.[13] Growing follicles are vulnerable to atresia and may depart from the trajectory at any point. Thus, although it is an obligatory step, recruitment does not guarantee ovulation. That recruitment is a necessary but not sufficient condition for ovulation is particularly important when one interprets results of experiments employing exogenous gonadotropins to stimulate follicle development, as discussed below.

The term *selection* is used here to indicate the final winnowing of the cohort (via atresia of "excess" follicles) down to a size equal to the species-characteristic ovulatory quota. That is, when the number of healthy follicles (i.e., with ovulatory potential) in the cohort equals the size of the ovulatory quota, selection is complete. Implicit in this definition is the notion that the cohort may be the regulated variable rather than the fate of an individual follicle. In other words, which follicles, in particular, are culled from the cohort may be determined by a random process that continues until cohort size matches the ovulatory quota, in contrast to a deterministic process in which specific follicles are individually chosen according to some unknown criteria. The character (stochastic versus deterministic) of the selection mechanism remains uncertain. What is certain, however, is that the process operates in primates with great precision; a spontaneous multiple ovulation is extremely atypical. Like recruitment, selection does not guarantee ovulation, but given its greater temporal proximity to ovulation, selection may, with high probability, be expected to be followed by ovulation in a typical cycle. Evidence will be presented that selection is begun and is completed only during the cycle in which ovulation occurs. In contrast, the time of recruitment and, thus, the total length (duration) of the trajectory are unknown. On the basis of findings discussed below, the duration of the trajectory in macaques and women appears to be not less than about 2 weeks.

Clearly, the ovulatory quota in higher primates is generally unity. Hence, although actual cohort size as a function of day of cycle is unknown, the possibility of a "cohort of one" even as early as recruitment is not excluded. Even if this were true, cohort remains a meaningful construct, and it is still useful to consider recruitment and selection as distinct processes.

Although we are anticipating facts not yet in evidence, the term *dominance* is introduced here to limit our lexicography to this section (Fig. 2-8). As we demonstrate later, the follicle destined to ovulate plays a key role in regulating the size of the ovulatory quota, at least in monkeys. This is, the follicle selected for ovulation is functionally (not merely morphologically) dominant, since it inhibits the development of other competing follicles on both ovaries. As a necessary corollary, the dominant follicle (i.e., the sole follicle destined to ovulate) somehow continues to thrive in a milieu it has made inhospitable for others.

Whether this capacity to thrive under such circumstances results from a unique ability of the dominant follicle that is newly acquired or from a preexisting ability originally shared by the entire cohort but retained only by the dominant follicle is unclear. That is, does the survival of the dominant follicle depend on a process of acquisition or of retention of metabolic properties to resist atresia? Underpinning this issue is how the dominant follicle actually exerts its eminence. How is it spared from the very inhibition it imposes on others? As one mechanism, we hypothesize that the dominant follicle secretes a substance we call "*selectron*," which acts directly on the ovaries to inhibit the development of potentially competing follicles. The motivation for this hypothesis is developed in more detail below. As we have shown, the selected follicle becomes dominant about a week before ovulation. Consequently, it must maintain its dominance during this interval. Unresolved is whether the mechanism(s) by which the follicle *attains* dominance are the same as the mechanism(s) by which the follicle *maintains* dominance. Unresolved as well is the precise temporal relationship between selection and dominance.[7]

Gonadotropic Stimulation of the Ovarian Cycle: Blockade of the Preovulatory LH Surge

Administration of human menopausal gonadotropin (hMG) preparations to ovulatory monkeys, either an FSH–LH combination (Fig. 2-9)[14] or "pure" FSH (Fig. 2-10),[15] produces the familiar bilateral ovarian hyperstimulation with attendant supraphysiological rises in circulating estradiol. Despite these raised estrogen levels, the monkeys fail to manifest a timely gonadotropin response to estrogen-positive feedback; that is, usually these normal, intact, cycling primates do not have the expected midcycle-like LH surges despite escalating concentrations of serum estradiol that usually exceed 400 pg/mL during 12 days of FSH therapy.[16] Also, we have noted that there are no spontaneous

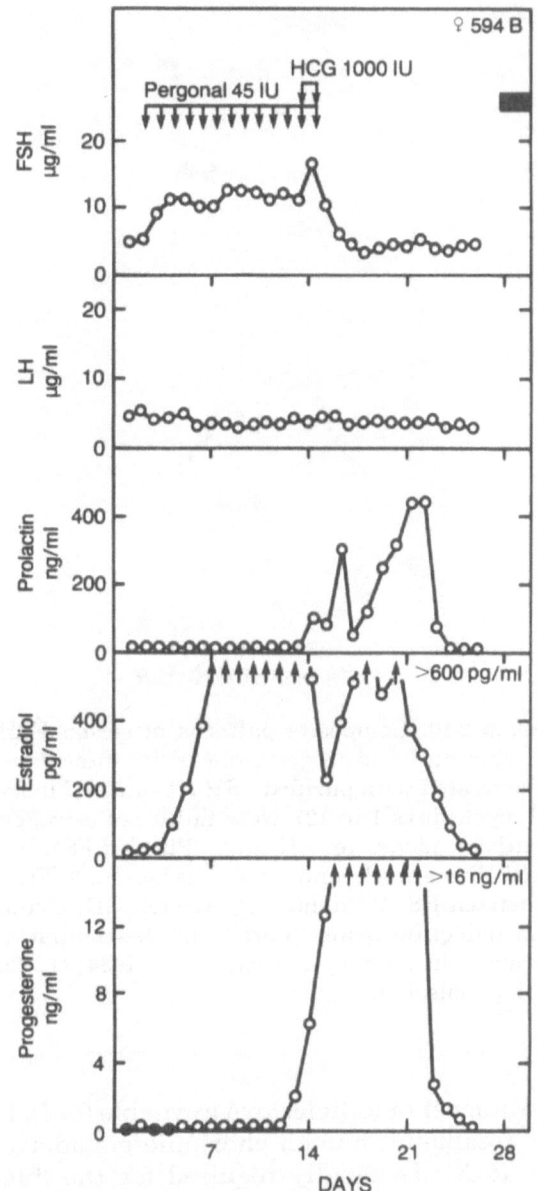

FIGURE 2-9. Appearance of hMG-induced ovarian hyperstimulation in a postpartum, nonnursing monkey. Note absence of an endogenous LH surge and the induction of hyperprolactinemia. From ref. 14, with permission of Butterworth Publishers.

LH surges when hMG-induced ovarian hyperstimulation occurs in postpartum monkeys. These observations fit with the frequent clinical finding that when endocrinologically normal patients are given hMG to increase

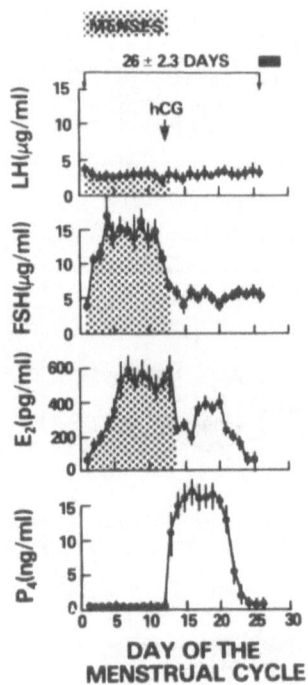

FIGURE 2-10. Composite patterns of serum FSH, LH, estradiol, and progesterone in five intact monkeys treated with purified FSH (25 or 50 IU daily, IM, cycle days 1 to 12). Note failure of estrogen-positive feedback for LH surge. Purified FSH was Urofollitropin (Serono Laboratories, Inc.). From Schenken RS, Williams RF, Hodgen GD: Ovulation induction using "pure" follicle-stimulating hormone in monkeys. *Fertil Steril* 1984;41:629, with permission.

the number of follicles/ova available for IVF-ET treatment, human chorionic gonadotropin (hCG) is usually required for the final maturation of the follicles.[17] These women seldom have spontaneous LH–FSH surges, even though circulating estradiol levels exceed 300 pg/mL for several days.[18]

Why is the surge mode of LH secretion not operational? Perhaps excessive secretion of one of more inhibitors of ovarian origin is driven uncontrollably by unrelenting (exogenous) FSH stimulation, thereby blocking the expected LH surges otherwise induced by estrogen positive feedback on the hypothalamic–pituitary unit. Indeed, we have reported[19] that pretreating monkeys with

charcoal-extracted porcine follicular fluid prevents both the FSH and LH surges after a conventional estrogen challenge in the follicular phase (Fig. 2-11). Similarly, it was shown that acute release of FSH and LH induced by gonadotropin-releasing hormone (GnRH) was blunted when castrated monkeys were pretreated with a porcine follicular fluid extract.[20]

Next, we asked whether the ovaries undergoing exogenous stimulation with purified FSH were obligatory for this blockade of the spontaneous LH surge, or was the inhibition mediated by a "short-loop" feedback of FSH. Administration of FSH (12 days) to long-term ovariectomized monkeys did not inhibit responses to an estradiol benzoate challenge; typical midcycle-like gonadotropin surges were observed. Accordingly, the occurrence of estrogen-induced FSH–LH surges in FSH-treated castrated monkeys shows that among intact monkeys the ovaries (hyperstimulated) surely do participate in the blockade of estrogen-positive feedback during exogenous gonadotropin therapy. Furthermore, with hMG medication, blockade of the LH surge probably develops as a result of the actions of its FSH component.[15]

With regard to hCG injections to replace the blocked LH surge, we have shown disparate effects of hCG during the late follicular phase of the primate ovarian cycle.[21] More specifically, if the estrogen-induced surges of FSH and LH had been initiated, ovarian function was unaffected by hCG. In contrast, hCG given before incipient gonadotropin surges led to anovulation lasting 4 to 6 weeks and sometimes disruption of the tonic FSH secretion (Fig. 2-12). Indeed, these findings may indicate some potential risks of premature administration of hCG to women during induced follicular maturation. Inappropriately timed (precocious) administration of hCG may actually preclude the objective, namely, to provide fertilizable oocytes and a milieu in which to nurture the embryo(s) through a normal luteal phase while achieving a fertile menstrual cycle.

As illustrated in Fig. 2-5, hMG treatment will sustain the concurrent development of

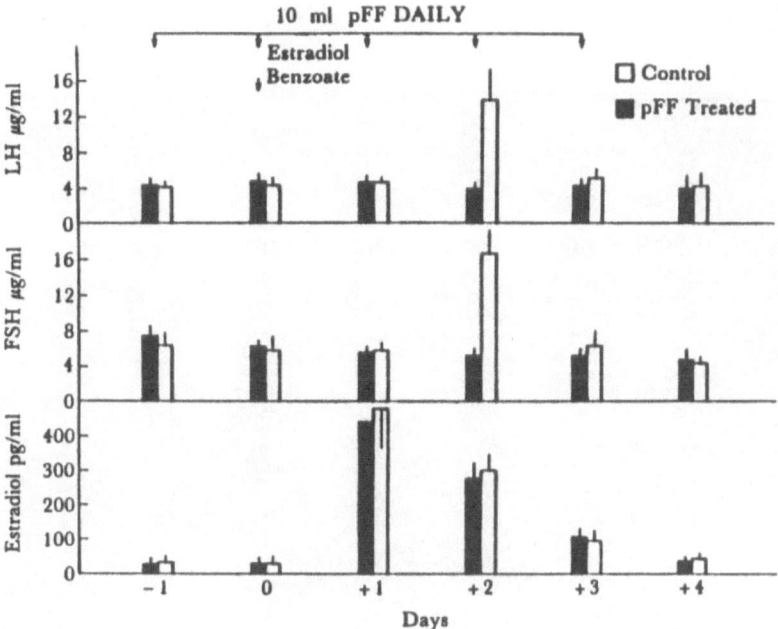

FIGURE 2-11. Serum concentrations of LH, FSH, and E_2 in early follicular-phase rhesus monkeys receiving an E_2 benzoate challenge (50 μg/kg) with or without pFF (extract of porcine follicular fluid/inhibin) treatment. Values shown are mean $\pm$ SE ($N = 5$ each).

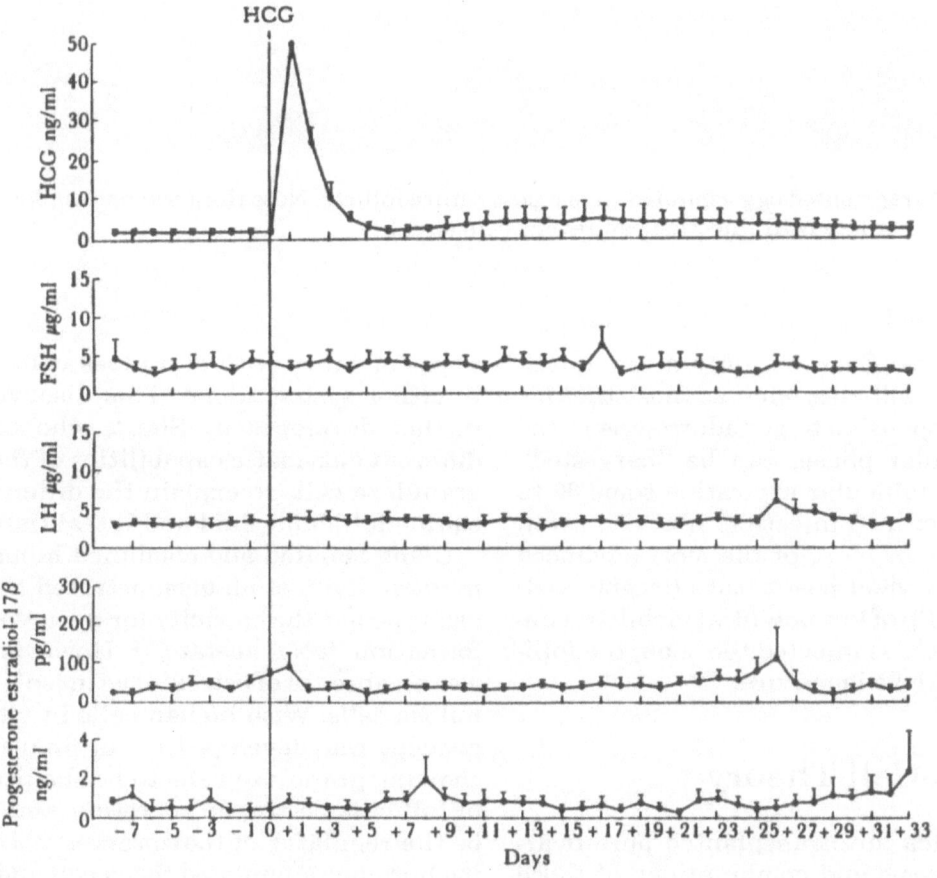

FIGURE 2-12. Peripheral serum concentration of hCG, FSH, LH, 17-β-estradiol, and progesterone in monkeys treated during the periovulatory interval with 1,000 IU of hCG. Hormone concentrations did not deviate from tonic levels.

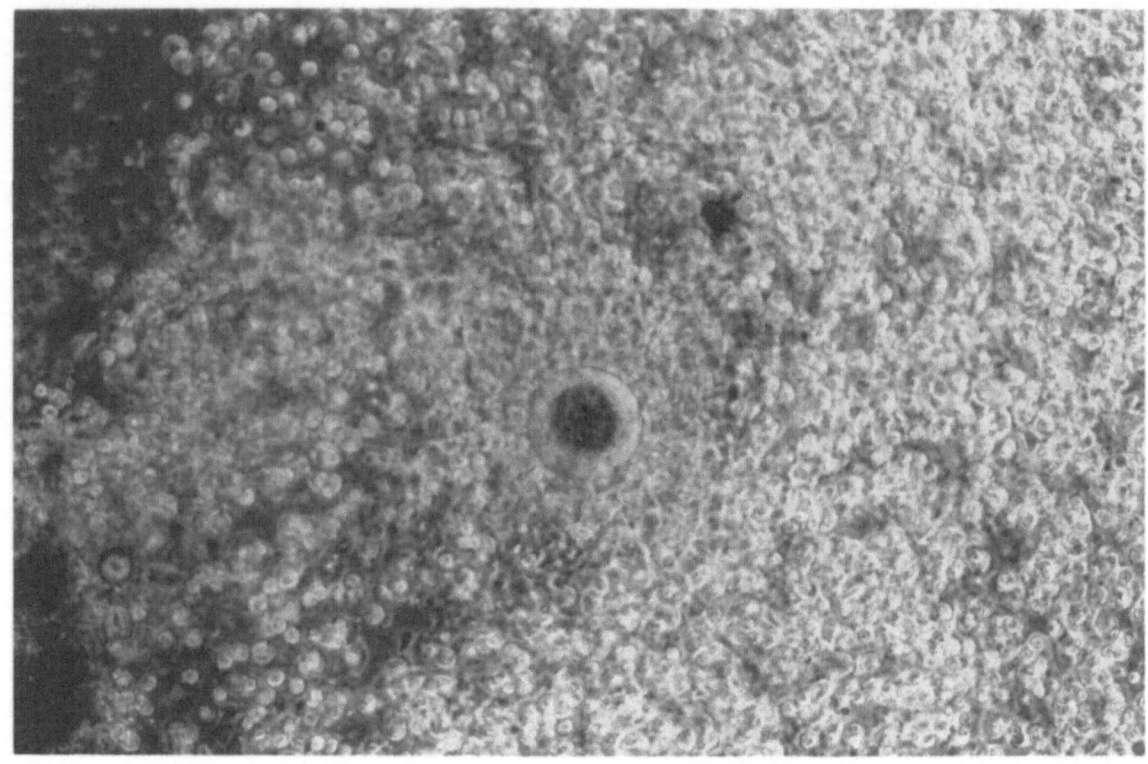

FIGURE 2-13. A fragmented egg aspirated from a postmature follicle. Note the darkened ooplasm. Delay of the LH surge or late hCG injection can reduce ovum quality.

many follicles. Even so, only a few quasi-synchronous follicles, such as those that begin to be responsive to gonadotropins in the early follicular phase, can be "harvested" together by follicular aspiration some 36 to 40 hours after hCG injection. If hCG is given too late, one or more of the most advanced follicles may yield postmature (fragmented) eggs (Fig. 2-13) of low potential viability; conversely, if hCG is injected too soon, the follicles/eggs may be immature.[16,21]

The Two-Cell Theory

In 1959, Falck autotransplanted pure ovarian cell systems and combinations of those cells into spayed rats.[22] He found that estrogen secretion was obtained when theca cells were combined with granulosa cells but not in either system alone. This discovery was further developed by Short, who proposed different enzymatic capabilities of theca and granulosa cells to explain the differences in equine follicular fluid and luteal tissue.[23]

Using isolated and combined human cells in vitro, Ryan et al. demonstrated that each cell type has the capacity for de novo steroid formation from acetate.[24] However, there was an absence of estradiol with isolated granulosa cells. With human cells in vitro, this concept was developed to its final form by showing granulosa cells to be the prime site of follicular estrogen secretion and FSH to be the regulator of that process.[25] Luteinizing hormone stimulated theca cell androgens, and FSH stimulated aromatization of those androgens to estrogen by granulosa cells.

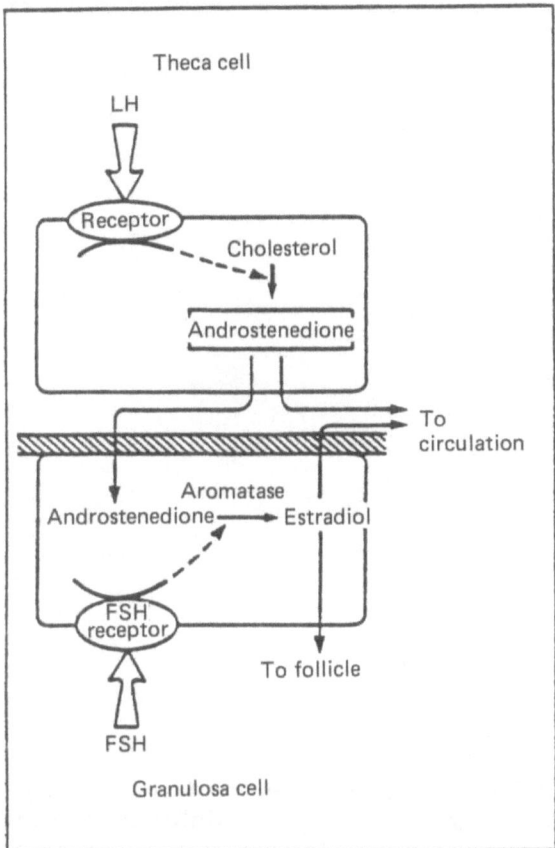

Theca cell

LH

Receptor

Cholesterol

Androstenedione

To circulation

Aromatase
Androstenedione ⟶ Estradiol

FSH receptor

To follicle

FSH

Granulosa cell

FIGURE 2-14. The two-cell theory. Schematic representation of a theca cell and a granulosa cell with LH and FSH receptors, respectively. Androgens are produced by the theca and are then converted to estrogens by the granulosa.

Therefore, a two-cell, two-gonadotropin theory of control and performance of estrogen biosynthesis was complete (Fig. 2-14).

Ovulation Induction

The above principles were influential on researchers working to develop ovulation induction agents. The two-cell theory proposed the coequal importance of FSH and LH. When tested at an empirical 50:50 ratio of FSH to LH, it was found that urinary gonadotropins had improved efficacy over the FSH derivatives of human pituitary used initially.[26-28]

Success rates in achieving ovulation in the entire spectrum of anovulatory disorders of a supraovarian origin were excellent. Furthermore, variability of response and higher than natural pregnancy loss rates were attributed to the underlying pathophysiological disorders in the patients.[29]

With the advent of IVF-ET treatment came the first large experience with administering ovulation induction agents to women who were otherwise endocrinologically normal. In the attempt to achieve multiple follicular stimulation to enhance oocyte recovery and the probability of fertilization, it became apparent that these otherwise normally cycling women showed striking differences in ovarian response to gonadotropin therapy.[17] In 390 cycles stimulated by hMG in Norfolk, Virginia, 107 distinct patterns of estradiol rise were distinguished (H. W. Jones and G. S. Jones, personal communication). Moreover, these response types tend toward a consistent pattern from cycle to cycle, thus suggesting a constancy of physiological status as opposed to a random response. With this background, we began seeking ways of reducing individual variability of responses to gonadotropin therapy based on understanding the physiologic origin(s) of that variability.

Clinical experience over the last 25 years has shown that it is often easier to manage gonadotropin therapy in severely hypogonadotropic patients than in those presenting anovulation of other etiologies. This realization has prompted other attempts at inducing a transient hypogonadotropic state in individuals undergoing ovulation induction, with the goal of achieving more uniform responses and fewer therapeutic complications for greater ultimate efficacy. Jones et al. attempted pretreatment with synthetic steroids to suppress the pituitary over a 2-month interval prior to gonadotropin therapy.[30] Fleming et al. pretreated patients with a GnRH agonist before administering exogenous gonadotropin.[32] Why have such strategies not been adopted more widely?

The above approaches have notable dis-

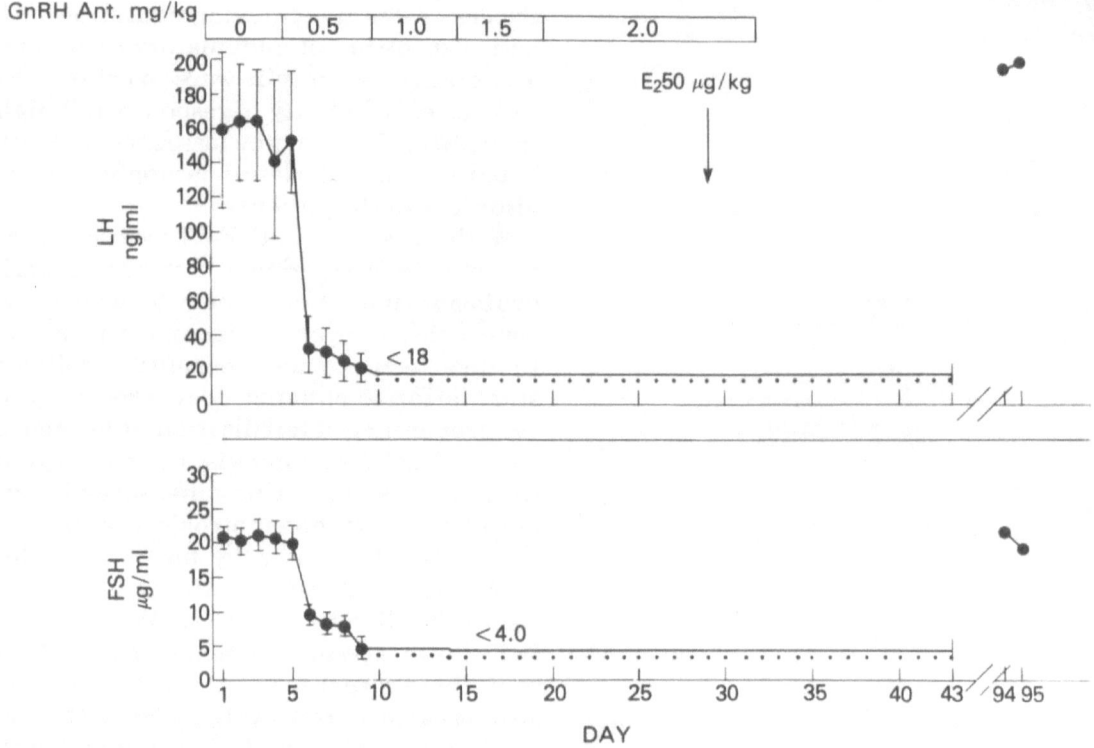

FIGURE 2-15. Plasma LH and FSH values (mean ±SEM) in three long-term castrated female monkeys treated with GnRH antagonist [(Ac-pClPhe[1], pClDPhe[2], DTryp[3], DArg[6], DAla[10])-GnRH HCl] in increasing doses producing suppression of FSH and LH levels in serum to or below the limits of assay detection. Subjects did not respond to an estrogen challenge test. Note full recovery of gonadotropin secretion by 2 months after cessation of treatment. From Kenigsberg D, Littman BA, Hodgen GD: Medical hypophysectomy: I. Dose-response using a gonodotropin-releasing hormone antagonist. *Fertil Steril* 1984;42:112–115, with permission.

advantages: (1) progestins are thought to inhibit folliculogenesis in the primate ovary directly[1]; also, exogenous progestins modify the milieu of the uterine endometrium, cervix, and fallopian tubes prematurely, during the proliferative phase; (2) GnRH *agonists* actually enhance gonadotropin and estradiol secretion for the initial 10 to 14 days of treatment, before a state of pituitary suppression is attained.[32,33] In contrast, the GnRH *antagonist* used in the present study only diminishes FSH and LH levels without concurrent elevations of ovarian steroid secretion (Fig. 2-15). Although GnRH or its analogues may influence the ovaries directly in rodents,[34] persuasive evidence obtained in women and monkeys argues against a direct

action of these synthetic decapeptides in the primate ovary.[35,36]

Accordingly, we set out to determine whether a GnRH antagonist would reduce individual variation in response to gonadotropin therapy through diminished functions of the hypothalamus and pituitary.[37] In monkeys, with a strategy that employed a 17-day pretreatment with a potent GnRH antagonist followed by concurrent treatment with the GnRH antagonist plus exogenous gonadotropin therapy, either FSH and LH in equal portions or FSH alone, the following was demonstrated (Fig. 2-16).

Pretreatment with the GnRH antagonist increased the homogeneity of ovarian estradiol (E_2) secretion during exogenous gonado-

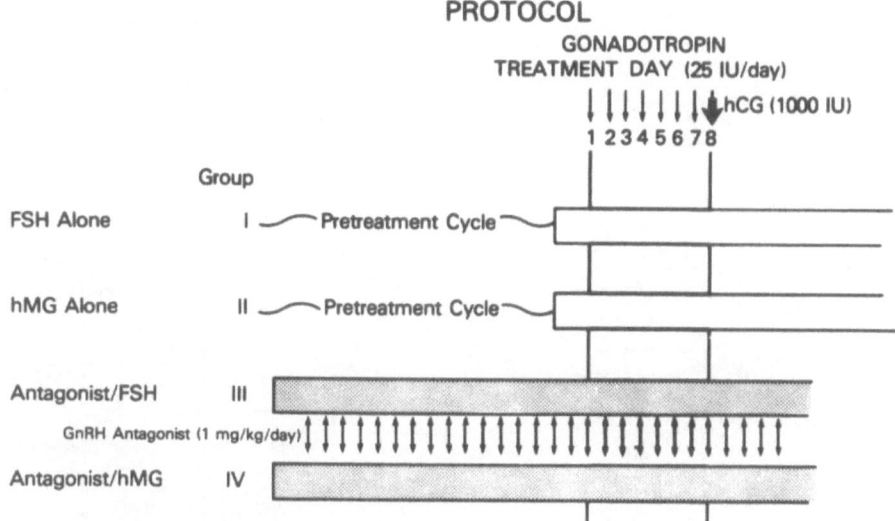

FIGURE 2-16. Protocol for previously normal ovulatory monkeys, groups I to IV. All subjects entered study on cycle day 3. Groups I and II received no pretreatment with GnRH antagonist; therefore, gonadotropin treatment day 1 corresponds to cycle day 3. Groups III and IV received pretreatment and concurrent treatment with the GnRH antagonist beginning on cycle day 3. For an interval of 17 days (cycle days 3 to 18) pretreatment with GnRH antagonist was given alone. While GnRH antagonist therapy is continued, gonadotropin treatment day 1 corresponds to cycle day 19. In all groups FSH or hMG (25 IU/day) was given for 7 consecutive days followed by hCG, 1,000 IU, on the eighth day. Thus, days are normalized and referred to as "gonadotropin treatment days 1–8" in all groups. See Fig. 2-17. From ref. 38, with permission.

tropin therapy among responsive females as compared to non-GnRH antagonist, gonadotropin-responsive subjects (Fig. 2-17). This constraint on individuality of responders by the GnRH antagonist suggests that an important part of the source of individual variation in response to gonadotropin therapy is supraovarian; that is, our findings indicate that hypothalamic–pituitary functions contribute substantially to the variability of ovarian response during gonadotropin treatment.

Further, there was nearly even distribution of nonresponder monkeys irrespective of whether the GnRH antagonist was given. Thus, the source of relative resistance among nonresponders may derive from the ovaries themselves, as opposed to factors contributed by supraovarian components that might be influenced by the GnRH antagonist. Whether this relative refractoriness to exogenous stimulation in some females is at the receptor or the humoral level remains to be determined.

It should be appreciated that, unlike the clinical situation, the fixed protocols employed here did not allow the nonresponders to receive more exogenous gonadotropin or the high responders to receive less exogenous gonadotropin than others in the study; comparison of like-treatment individuals in all groups was thus permitted. In all likelihood, even greater conformity of subject response could be obtained with daily gonadotropin dose adjustments.

Another important finding in these experiments concerns the comparison of the different exogenous gonadotropin preparations. Here, "pure" urinary FSH was compared to a mixture of urinary FSH and LH (hMG) of even proportions. Regardless of whether GnRH antagonist was added, there was equal responsiveness in monkeys treated with FSH alone and those given hMG. In contrast, stud-

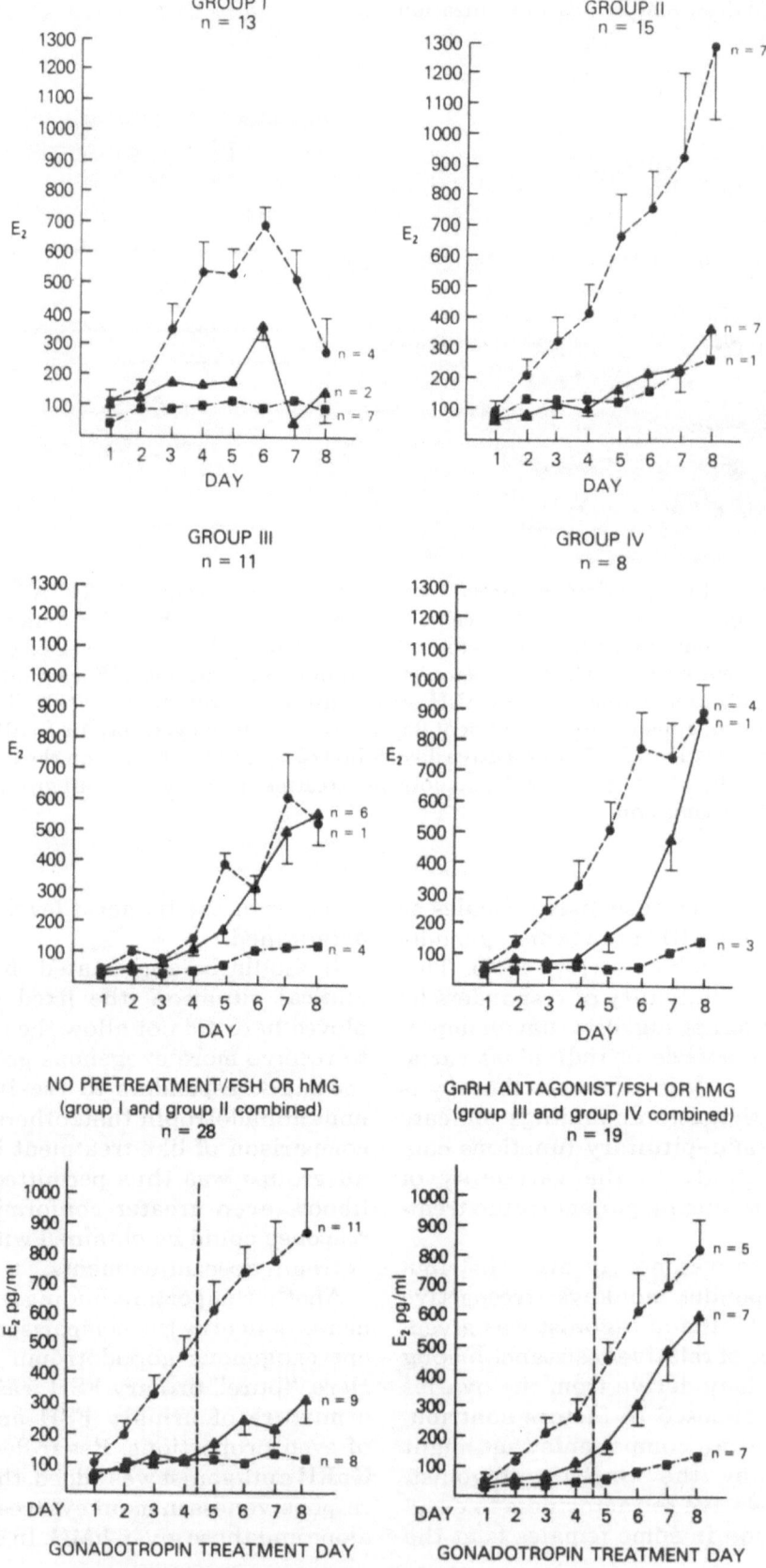

GROUP I
n = 13

GROUP II
n = 15

GROUP III
n = 11

GROUP IV
n = 8

NO PRETREATMENT/FSH OR hMG
(group I and group II combined)
n = 28

GnRH ANTAGONIST/FSH OR hMG
(group III and group IV combined)
n = 19

GONADOTROPIN TREATMENT DAY

GONADOTROPIN TREATMENT DAY

FIGURE 2-18. GnRH antagonist [(Ac-pClPhe[1], pClDPhe[2], DTryp[3], DArg[6], DAla[10])-GnRH HCl] followed by FSH therapy in intact cycling monkeys. Note suppression of endogenous gonadotropin secretion and ovarian responsiveness to FSH treatments, as indicated by elevations of estradiol (E_2) in serum. From ref. 38, with permission.

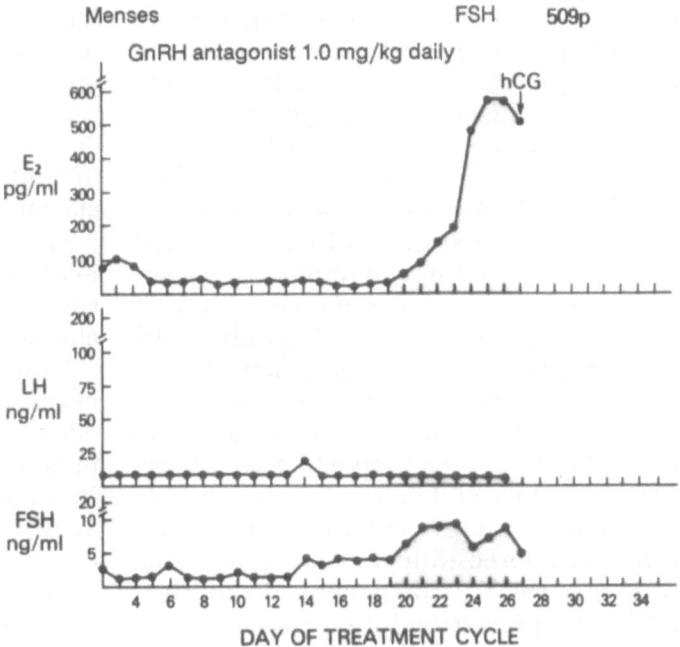

ies in humans using pituitary FSH preparations for ovulation induction indicated lower E_2 responses when FSH was administered alone, compared to urinary preparations containing both FSH and LH.[26–28] These older studies could be interpreted as supporting evidence of the two-cell theory; LH was deficient. Alternatively, the results may have been influenced by the shorter circulatory half-life of pituitary FSH compared to the longer-acting FSH entities extracted from postmenopausal urine.[38]

In these primate experiments we have also shown that "pure" FSH of urinary origin is capable of stimulating ovarian E_2 secretion at a level not dissimilar from that obtained by the same dose of a urinary hMG preparation containing an equal ratio of FSH to LH. Furthermore, we have demonstrated un-

diminished ovarian estradiol production when "pure" FSH was administered in the presence of a GnRH antagonist that maintained a relative hypogonadotropic state, that is, essentially no endogenous gonadotropin secretion (Fig. 2-18). This does not necessarily negate the two-cell therapy of ovarian steroidogenesis; however, it does open to question the previous assumptions about the relative importance of FSH and LH. In the primate ovarian cycle, it seems that FSH is of far greater significance.

Early Progesterone Rise

Recent studies have described a rise of plasma progesterone up to 12 hours prior to initiation of the LH surge in the normal human

---

FIGURE 2-17. Panels (A–D) represent serum E_2 levels (mean $\pm$ SEM). (A) Group I ($n = 13$) received "pure" FSH. (B) Group II ($n = 11$) received hMG (FSH and LH). (C) Group III ($n = 11$) received pretreatment and concurrent treatment with GnRH antagonist and "pure" FSH. (D) Group IV ($n = 8$) was treated with GnRH antagonist plus hMG (see Fig. 2-16 for protocol). Subjects were divided into fast responders, slow responders, and nonresponders on gonadotropin treatment days 1 to 8 (•, fast responder; ▲, slow responder; ■, nonresponder). Bottom panels represent the composite of (E) Groups I and II ($n = 28$) versus (F) Groups III and IV ($n = 19$), i.e., those that did not receive and those that did receive pretreatment and concurrent treatment with the GnRH antagonist. From ref. 38, with permission.

menstrual cycle.[39] That this progesterone elevation occurs in the absence of perceptible changes in the endogenous LH pulse amplitude or frequency may implicate an independent intraovarian mechanism that begins to shift ovarian steroidogenesis and secretion toward progesterone, even before initiation of the LH surge. Collins et al. used monkeys in an attempt to mimic the hyperstimulation seen among some patients who show a marked sensitivity to the hMG (FSH and LH) preparation.[40] These patients have a very early and sustained rise in serum estradiol levels. Of 16 monkeys achieving an estradiol level of 1,000 pg/mL, five had serum progesterone values of 2 to 8 ng/mL as much as 1 week prior to an LH surge. This finding has yet to be explored in humans, but it is suggested that the LH component of the hMG might cause premature luteinization.

Two monkeys treated with "pure" FSH in the presence of the GnRH antagonist, with barely detectable LH in plasma, also had serum progesterone elevations as much as 4 days prior to hMG treatment and without an endogenous LH surge.[37] This observation may fit with a growing body of evidence that steroidogenic shifts to progesterone can be initiated by intraovarian events, thereby usurping onset of the LH surge as the initiator of these events.

Future Considerations

The new experiences gained from familiarity with IVF-ET procedures have led to a reexamination of the physiology of the ovary and preimplantation embryo. The previously described experiments with ovulation induction suggest that newer gonadotropin preparations, with a greater emphases on FSH, could improve the quality of ovarian stimulation. Adjunctive treatments, as with a GnRH antagonists, offer hope that greater control and efficiency can be gained in ovulation induction by reducing the confounding problem of individual variation in response to treatment with gonadotropins.

A recrudescence of interest in intraovar-

ian factors that affect the growth of follicles locally and feedback on the hypothalamic–pituitary axis distally has developed. In the setting of treating infertility, a greater understanding of the mechanisms involved in follicular–oocyte well-being will enhance the efficiency of IVF-ET therapies. Of equal importance is the potential for inhibition of follicular maturation and LH surges for contraceptive therapy by way of previously uncharacterized ovarian factors.

Now that follicular fluid, oocytes, and embryos are being observed with great frequency, this scrutiny can provide a better understanding of the impact of oocyte quality on early embryonic normality or abnormality. This has far-reaching implications in cytogenetics for both prenatal embryonic diagnosis and DNA therapy in the future. I expect that by the mid-1990s, fully one-half of the couples seeking in vitro fertilization therapy will not be infertile. Instead, they will be asking for genetic diagnosis of the preembryo in order to avoid confrontation with therapeutic abortion because of sickle-cell anemia, β-thalassemia, cystic fibrosis, Tay–Sachs, Huntington's chorea, or other single-gene defects for which the structure of the human genome is known. Thus, in vitro fertilization will likely serve embryo biopsy, DNA amplification, genomic evaluation, and selective embryo transfer. Accordingly, the impact of ovarian physiology on in vitro fertilization therapy will likely be felt directly for at least another decade.

References

1. diZerega GS, Hodgen GD. Folliculogenesis in the primate ovarian cycle. Endocr Rev. 1981;2:27–49.
2. diZerega GS, Hodgen GD. Initiation of asymmetrical ovarian estradiol secretion in the primate ovarian cycle after luteectomy. Endocrinology. 1981;108:1233–36.
3. diZerega GS, Hodgen GD. Luteal phase dysfunction infertility: a sequel to aberrant folliculogenesis. Fertil Steril. 1981;35:489–99.
4. Hodgen GD. In vitro fertilization and alternatives. JAMA. 1981;246:590–97.
5. Williams RF, Hodgen GD. Initiation of the pri-

mate ovarian cycle with emphasis on perime-
narchial and postpartum events. In: Greep
RO, ed. Reproductive physiology, Vol IV.
Baltimore: University Park Press, 1983:1–55.

6. Hodgen GD. The dominant ovarian follicle.
Fertil Steril. 1982;38:281–300.

7. Goodman AL, Hodgen GD. The ovarian triad
of the primate menstrual cycle. Recent Prog
Horm Res. 1983;39:1–73.

8. Brambell FWR. Ovarian changes. In: Parkes
AS, ed. Marshall's physiology of reproduction, Vol. I, Part 1. New York: Longman,
1956:397–542.

9. Clayton RN, Huhtaniemi IT. Absence of gonadotropin-releasing hormone receptors in human gonadal tissue. Nature. 1982;299:56–59.

10. Schwartz NB. The role of FSH and LH and
of their antibodies on follicle growth and on
ovulation. Biol Reprod. 1974;10:236–72.

11. Pedersen T. Follicle kinetics in the ovary
of the cyclic mouse. Acta Endocrinol.
1970;64:304–23.

12. Hertz R, Hisaw FL. Effects of follicle-stimulating and luteinizing pituitary extracts on the
ovaries of the infantile and juvenile rabbit. Am
J Physiol. 1934;108:1–15.

13. Lunenfeld B, Kraiem Z, Eshkol A. Structure
and function of the growing follicle. Clin Obstet Gynecol. 1976;3:27–42.

14. Goodman AL, Hodgen GD. Postpartum patterns of circulating FSH, LH, prolactin, estradiol and progesterone in nonsuckling cynomolgus monkeys. Steroids. 1978;31:731–744.

15. Schenken RS, Hodgen GD. FSH induced ovarian hyperstimulation in monkeys: blockade
of the LH surge. J Clin Endocrinol Metab.
1983;57:50–55.

16. Hodgen GD. Oocyte transfer and fertilization
in vivo. In: Crosignani P, ed. In vitro fertilization and embryo transfer. Serono Symp.
1983;47:126–38.

17. Garcia JE, Jones GS, Acosta AA, et al. Human
menopausal gonadotropin/human chorionic
gonadotropin follicular maturation for oocyte
aspiration: Phase II, 1981. Fertil Steril.
1983;39:174–79.

18. Laufer N, DeCherney AH, Hazeltine FP, et al.
The use of hi-dose human menopausal gonadotropin in an in vitro fertilization program. Fertil Steril. 1983;40:734–41.

19. Channing CP, Anderson LD, Hoover DJ, et
al. Inhibitory effects of porcine follicular fluid
upon monkey serum FSH levels and follicular
maturation. Biol Reprod. 1981;25:885–903.

20. Rettori V, Siler-Khodr TM, Pauerstein CJ, et
al. Effects of porcine follicular fluid on gonadotropin concentrations in rhesus monkeys. J
Clin Endocrinol Metab. 1982;54:500–03.

21. Williams RF, Hodgen GD. Disparate effects of
human chorionic gonadotropin during the late
follicular phase in monkeys: normal ovulation,
follicular atresia, ovarian acyclicity, and hypersecretion of follicle stimulating hormone.
Fertil Steril. 1980;33:64–68.

22. Falck B. Site of production of estrogen in rat
ovary as studied in micro-transplants. Acta
Physiol Scand. 1959;47:Suppl 163–69.

23. Short RV. Steroids in the follicular fluid and
the corpus luteum on the mare. A "two-cell
type" theory of ovarian steroid synthesis. J
Endocrinol. 1962;24:59–63.

24. Ryan KJ, Petro Z, Kaiser J. Steroid formation
by isolated and recombined ovarian granulosa
and theca cells. J Clin Endocrinol Metab.
1968;28:355–58.

25. Moon YS, Tsang BK, Simpson C, et al. 17-β-
estradiol biosynthesis in cultured granulosa
and theca cells of human ovarian follicles:
stimulation by follicle-stimulating hormone.
J Clin Endocrinol Metab. 1978;47:263–67.

26. Berger MJ, Taymor ML, Karam K, et al. The
relative roles of exogenous and endogenous
FSH and LH in human follicular maturation and ovulation induction. Fertil Steril.
1972;23:783–90.

27. Jacobson A, Marshall JR. Ovulatory response
rate with human menopausal gonadotropins
of varying FSH–LH ratios. Fertil Steril.
1969;20:171–75.

28. Jewelewicz R, Warren M, Dyrenfurth I, et al.
Physiological studies with purified human pituitary FSH LH–FSH. J Clin Endocrinol Metab. 1971;32:688–91.

29. Ben-Rafael Z, Dor J, Mashiach S, et al. Abortion rate in pregnancies following ovulation
induced by human menopausal gonadotropin/
human gonadotropin. Fertil Steril.
1983;39:157–61.

30. Jones GS, Ruehsen MDM, Johanson AJ, et al.
Elucidation of normal ovarian physiology by
exogenous gonadotropin stimulation following steroid pituitary suppression. Fertil Steril.
1969;20:14–34.

31. Fleming R, Adam AH, Barlow DH, et al. A new
systematic treatment for infertile women with
abnormal hormone profiles. Br J Obstet Gynaecol. 1982;89:80–83.

32. Schmidt-Gollwitzer M, Hardt W, Schmidt-

Gollwitzer K, et al. Influence of the LH–RH analog buserelin on cyclic ovarian function and on the endometrium. A new approach to fertility control? Contraception. 1981;23:187–95.

33. Werlin LB, Hodgen GD. Gonadotropin-releasing hormone agonist suppresses ovulation, menses and endometriosis in monkeys: an individualized, intermittent regimen. J Clin Endocrinol Metab. 1983;56:844–48.

34. Richards JS. Maturation of ovarian follicles: actions and interactions of pituitary and ovarian hormones in follicular cell differentiation. Physiol Rev. 1980;60:51–89.

35. Asch RH, Van Sickle MV, Rettori V, et al. Absence of LH–RH binding sites in corpora lutea from rhesus monkeys (*Macaca mulatta*). J Clin Endocrinol Metab. 1981;53:215–17.

36. Harrison RJ, Weir BJ. Structure of the mammalian ovary. In: Zuckerman S, Weir BJ, eds. The ovary, Vol. 1, Second edition. New York: Academic Press, 1977:113–218.

37. Kenigsberg D, Littman BA, Williams RF, et al. Medical hypophysectomy: II. Variability of ovarian response to exogenous gonadotropins. Fertil Steril. 1984;42:116–26.

38. Mancuso S, Dell'Acqua S, Donini P, et al. Disappearance rate, urinary excretion and effect on ovarian steroidogenesis of highly purified urinary FSH, administration to a hypophysectomized women. In: Bettendort G, Insler V, eds. Clinical application of human gonadotropins. Stuttgart: Thieme, 1970:151–59.

39. Hoff JD, Quigley ME, Yen SSC. Hormonal dynamics at midcycle: a reevaluation. J Clin Endocrinol Metab. 1983;57:792–96.

40. Collins RL, Williams RF, Hodgen GD. Endocrine consequences of prolonged ovarian hyperstimulation: hyperprolactinemia, follicular atresia and premature luteinization. Fertil Steril. 1984;42:436–45.

3
Anovulation

Bryan Cowan

Chronic Anovulation

Chronic anovulation is manifested clinically as amenorrhea or menstrual irregularity. Disruption in the integrated function of the hypothalamic – pituitary – ovarian – endometrial axis can occur endogenously [within the hypothalamic–pituitary–ovarian (HPO) axis], or perturbation can arise from peripheral endocrine dysfunctions. In general, dysfunctions of the hypothalamic–pituitary system occur secondary to psychogenic causes or develop as a result of structural defects or lesions within the central nervous system, as peripheral endocrine disorders that induce menstrual disturbances attenuate the proper cyclic sex steroid signals to the responding elements of the HPO axis.

Historically, great significance has been assigned to the difference between primary and secondary amenorrhea. Although the incidence of genetic and anatomic abnormalities is higher in patients with primary amenorrhea, the distinction between primary and secondary forms can be misleading. Most authors no longer emphasize the distinction, since these terms represent an arbitrary assignment of a diagnosis based on the presence or absence of menarche. It is probably more appropriate to assess the developmental maturation of secondary sex characteristics and the pathophysiological changes that give rise to the symptoms of anovulation/amenorrhea.

The criteria for diagnosis of amenorrhea are satisfied when a woman who previously had experienced regular menses has absence of menstruation for 3 months or more or when menarche has not occurred by the age of 16 years regardless of the stage of secondary sexual development. The clinician treating women with amenorrhea thus has the task of properly classifying and appropriately treating the various causes of amenorrhea. The pathophysiological causes of amenorrhea may be grouped into CNS lesions or dysfunction, anatomic causes, gonadal failure, or chronic anovulation syndrome. Fortunately a few appropriate tests of endocrine function combined with proper clinical interpretation are all that is necessary to diagnose virtually all causes of amenorrhea/anovulation.

Control of the self-regulated ovarian menstrual cycle is entrained in the "ovarian clock" conceptualized by Yen.[1] In this model, nonlinear feedback of incremental estradiol is generated over a well-defined time course. The two principal sources of circulating estrogen are gonadal estrogens and extragonadal conversion of estrogen precursors. In the ovary, *gonadotropin-dependent*[2] cyclic estrogen production (Fig. 3-1) is mediated by granulosa cell responses to FSH in which androgens (androstenedione and testosterone) are converted to estrogens (estrone and estradiol). *Extraglandular gonadotropin-independent*[3] conversion of androgens to estrogens (Fig. 3-2) provides a second and steady-state mechanism for estrogen production. The pre-

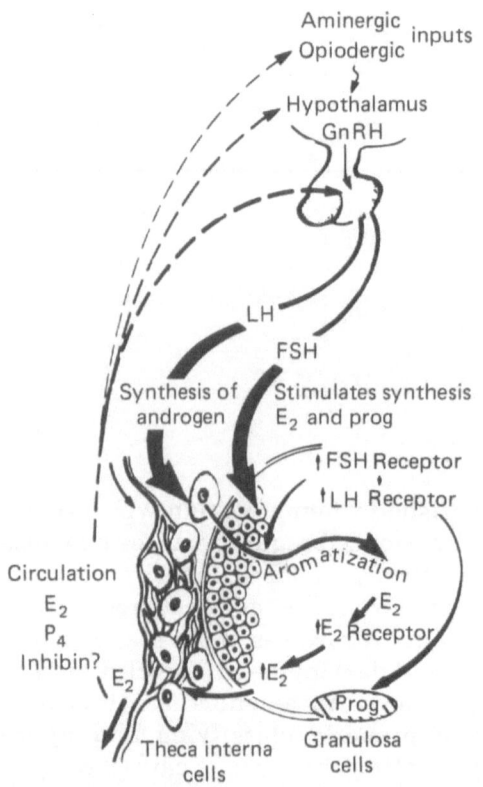

FIGURE 3-1. Gonadotropin–ovarian interaction and regulation of follicular maturation and steroidogenesis. E_2, estradiol; prog, progesterone. Reproduced with permission from Yen SSC, Jaffe RB (eds): *Reproductive Endocrinology*. Philadelphia: W. B Saunders, 1986, p 205.

dominant estrogen produced by peripheral conversion of androgens is estrone (E_1). Although the precise role of extraglandular conversion of androgens to estrogens is not clear, this event may be a mechanism to allow high concentrations of estrogens to exist locally in target tissues without the need for delivering high concentrations of the hormone to the systemic circulation. The E_1/E_2 ratio is often used to compare the relative contributions of extraglandular (E_1) and ovarian (E_2) estrogen to the circulation. High E_1/E_2 ratios (>1) are associated with excess extraglandular conversion of androgens and anovulation. Although the E_1/E_2 ratio is infrequently applied clinically, the concept helps describe the genesis of peripheral endocrine dysfunction that produces anovulation.

In addition to estrogens, androgens significantly affect the ability of the HPO axis to respond properly to feedback signals. In women there are two sources of circulating androgens. *Gonadotropin-stimulated ovarian stroma* produces primarily androstenedione and testosterone, while *corticotropin (ACTH)-stimulated adrenal zona reticularis* produces androstenedione, testosterone, DHEA, and DHEAS. The most biologically important androgen produced by these two organs is testosterone. The ovary[4] produces 25% of the circulating testosterone, 25% more is contributed by the adrenal glands,[5] and a final 50% is derived from peripheral metabolism of testosterone precursors (Fig. 3-3). The principal testosterone (T) precursor

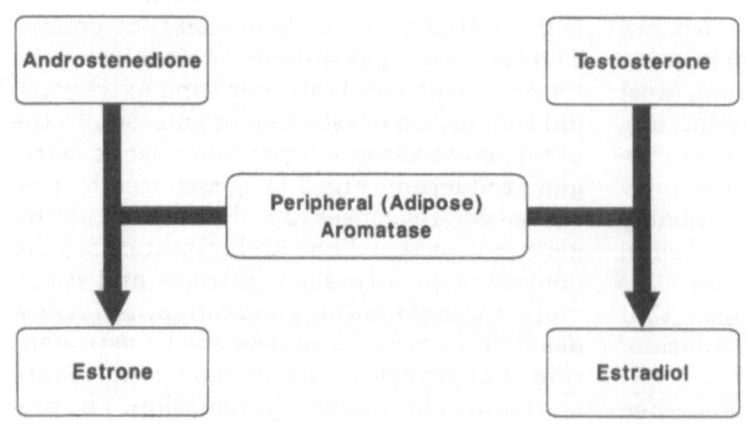

FIGURE 3-2. Peripheral conversion of androgens (androstenedione, testosterone) to their respective estrogens (estrone, estradiol) by peripheral (adipose) aromatase.

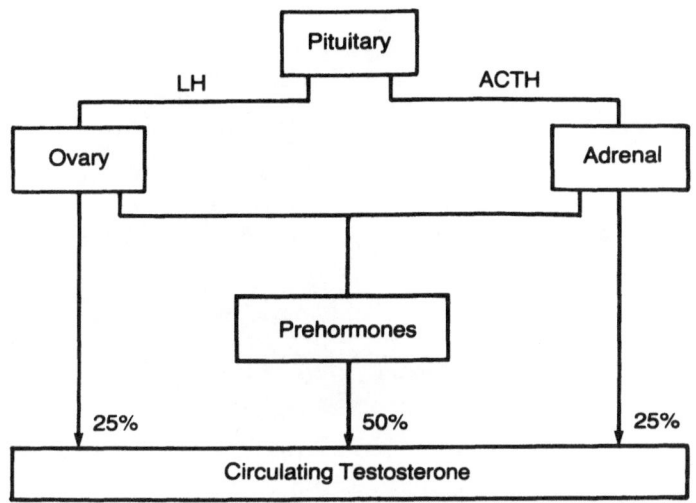

FIGURE 3-3. Origin of testosterone in normal women. LH, luteinizing hormone; ACTH, adrenocorticotropin.

is androstenedione, which is transformed to T at several sites.[6]

Although estradiol and testosterone are important mediators of HPO responses, hormone-binding globulins unquestionably modulate the peripheral hormone effects of these steroids.[7-9] In general, specific binding globulins exist for all biologically potent hormones, and the bulk of steroid hormones that circulate in the plasma are bound by proteins. Sex hormone-binding globulin (SHBG) (Table 3-1), also named testosterone-estradiol-binding globulin (TeBG), has a high affinity for testosterone, estradiol, and 5α-dihydrotestosterone. In addition to the specific steroid-binding protein SHBG, albumin plays a major role in binding sex steroids. This action of albumin is particularly important for

TABLE 3-1. Characteristics of sex hormone-binding globulin (SHBG)

1. Molecular weight 90,000
2. Synthesized in the liver
3. Binds T, E$_2$, 5α-DHT with high affinity
4. Synthesis decreased by:
   - Progestins
   - Glucocorticoids
   - Androgens
   - Hypothyroidism
5. Synthesis increased by:
   - Estrogens
   - Hyperthyroidism

estradiol, since approximately 60% of the circulating hormone is bound to albumin, 40% is bound to SHBG, and only 2% of estradiol is free in circulation (Fig. 3-4). The SHBG-bound steroids are generally not available for target tissue binding and action,[10] thus establishing SHBG as the most important regulator of peripheral hormone effect. In contrast, albumin-bound sex steroids are biologically active and must be considered available for both peripheral metabolism and peripheral end-organ action.

Adult women have about twice the plasma concentration of SHBG as adult men, principally because hepatic production of SHBG is promoted by estrogen but inhibited by androgen. Potent synthetic progestins,[11] glucocorticoids,[12] growth hormone excess,[13] and thyroxin deficiency[11] also lower SHBG. On the other hand, hyperthyroidism, from either endogenous or exogenous sources, is associated with a marked elevation in SHBG. Thus, the level of circulating SHBG must be considered a major controlling factor in the balance between biologically active androgens and estrogens. This relationship represents an important factor in the interpretation of circulating hormonal levels and biological action at target tissues.

An algorithm for the diagnostic evaluation of women with anovulation/amenorrhea is illustrated in Fig. 3-5. All algorithms pro-

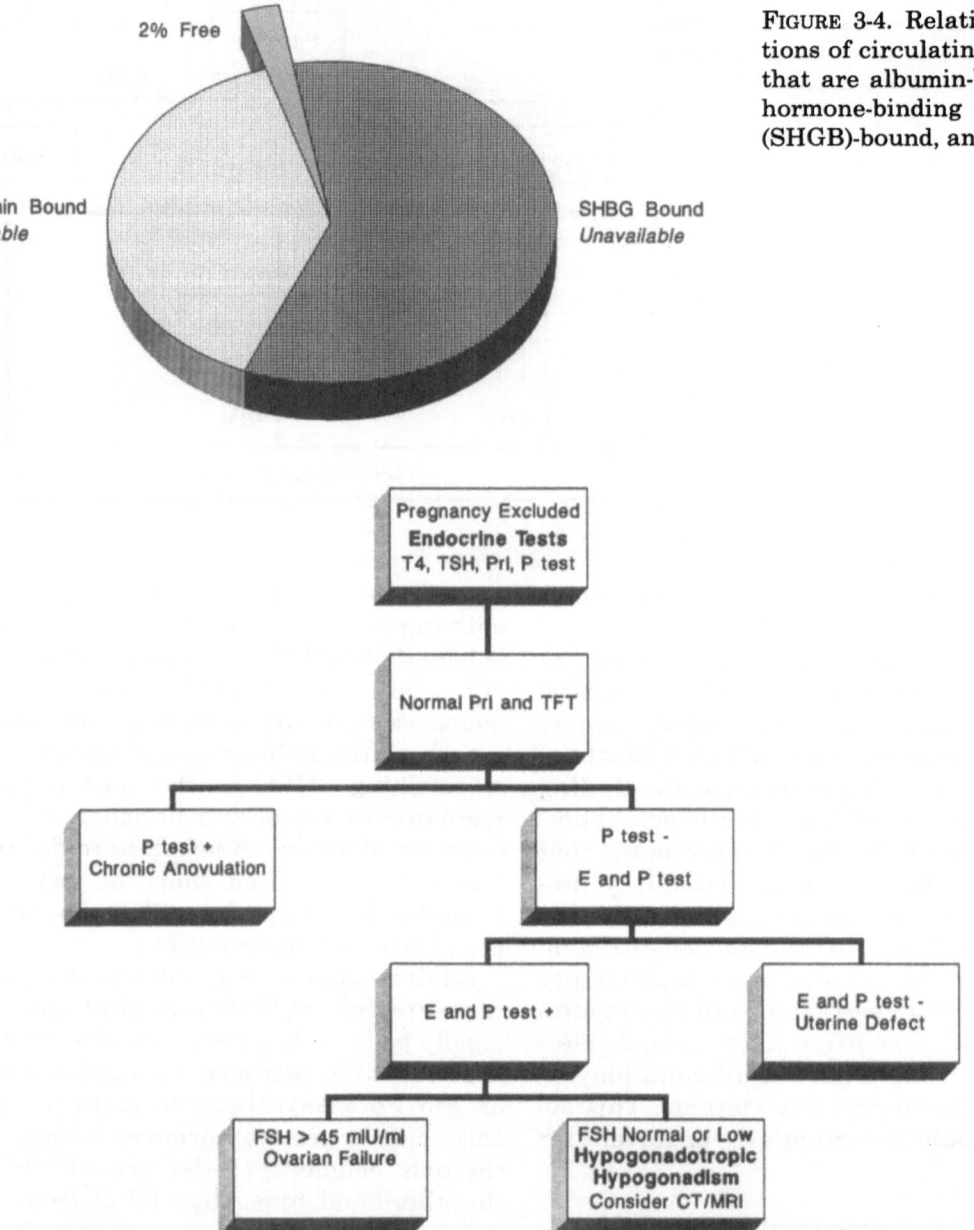

FIGURE 3-4. Relative proportions of circulating estradiol that are albumin-bound, sex hormone-binding globulin (SHGB)-bound, and free.

FIGURE 3-5. Algorithm for the evaluation of women with amenorrhea. P test, progestin withdrawal; E & P test, estrogen-stimulated progestin withdrawal; PRL, prolactin; TFT, thyroid function test.

posed for the evaluation of anovulatory women consider the same elements, but there can be variability in the order in which some tests are performed. Since the most common cause of secondary amenorrhea is pregnancy, it is important to make this diagnosis prior to any further evaluation. Currently both serum and urine kit assays employ the β subunit

method for detection with high sensitivity (10 to 25 mIU/mL). The cost of the test is low compared to other hormonal assessments. In our program, all patients with a negative pregnancy test who fulfill the criteria of amenorrhea are initially evaluated by measuring serum prolactin, thyroxin (T_4), thyroid-stimulating hormone (TSH), and gonadotropins (FSH, LH). Additionally, a progestin withdrawal test (P test) is initiated at that visit. Our progestin withdrawal test employs 10 mg of medroxyprogesterone acetate for 7 days. The rationale for this approach is that hormone testing early in the evaluation avoids ambiguous results induced by hormone administration and considerably reduces the time interval from the initial evaluation to discriminate diagnosis.

Interpretation of the Amenorrhea Evaluation

Prolactin

The purpose of the prolactin measurement is to exclude hyperprolactinemia as a cause of amenorrhea.[14] Hyperprolactinemia is a common occurrence that affects approximately 35% of all women with the anovulation/amenorrhea syndrome.[15] Its detection is significant since approximately 40% of patients[16] with hyperprolactinemia have pituitary adenoma, and treatment of anovulation/amenorrhea in women with hyperprolactinemia usually requires unique drugs or surgery (Chapter 9).

Thyroid Function

Thyroid dysfunction causes anovulation/amenorrhea in approximately 2% to 5% of these patients.[17] The most common thyroid dysfunction presenting with anovulation/amenorrhea is hypothyroidism. Hyperthyroidism is typically associated with a hypermetabolism that is usually expressed as hypermenorrhea or polymenorrhea. An elevated T_4 level associated with a normal TSH level would indicate hyperthyroidism, and elevated TSH with low normal or subnormal T_4 levels would indicate primary hypothyroidism.

Progestin Withdrawal

The progestin withdrawal test determines the estrogen status of the patient. The test is interpreted as positive (and hence the patient is considered "estrogenized") if uterine bleeding occurs 2 to 14 days after discontinuing the medication. Occasionally the progestin is administered concomitantly with an LH surge (or initiates the LH surge), and bleeding can be delayed for 14 days. Spotting is considered to indicate a positive test, but this alone should not be interpreted as a reassuring sign that no other endocrine dysfunction is present.

Gonadotropins

Gonadotropin measurements establish the functional capacity of the ovary. The criterion that establishes ovarian failure is an FSH level >45 mIU/mL. Approximately 40% of patients with polycystic ovarian syndrome (PCO) will demonstrate abnormally high LH,[18] but FSH will be low.

Estrogen-Stimulated Progestin Withdrawal

This test determines the presence or absence of a responsive endometrium in combination with a competent outflow tract. It is performed after a negative progestin withdrawal test. We use 2.5 mg of conjugated estrogens for 25 days and add medroxyprogesterone (10 mg) on days 16 to 25. Menstrual flow at the end of the test confirms the presence of both a hormonally responsive endometrium and an outflow tract. The failure of this test suggests an unresponsive or absent endometrium (e.g., Asherman's syndrome or hysterectomy), an obstructed outflow tract (e.g., Mullerian defects or cervical lesions), or pregnancy (remember to test for pregnancy prior to drug administration).

Classifications of Anovulation

The relative frequencies of the causes of amenorrhea/anovulation in women who present for evaluation are dependent somewhat on practice patterns but are distributed in our population as shown in Table 3-2. Chronic anovulation is by far the most common etiology of disrupted HPO function, but hy-

TABLE 3-2. Amenorrhea/anovulation

1. Hyperprolactinemia	35%
2. Thyroid dysfunction	2%
3. Chronic anovulation	50%
4. Ovarian failure	5%
5. Hypogonadotropic hypogonadism	5%
6. Uterine defect	3%

perprolactinemia affects a significant group as well. The remaining causes of ovulation failure collectively make up less than 15% (uterine defect excluded) of patients evaluated in our clinics.

Chronic Anovulation

Seven defects of peripheral endocrine function may influence circulating estrogen/androgen concentrations and result in aberrant feedback signals to the HPO axis (Table 3-3). Polycystic ovarian syndrome (PCO) is

TABLE 3-3. Classification of anovulation

Chronic anovulation
a. Polycystic ovarian syndrome (PCO)
b. Congenital adrenal hyperplasia
    (classic and adult-onset)
c. Hormone-secreting tumors (ovary or adrenal)
d. Hyperadrenalism (Cushing's syndrome)
e. Aging (increased aromatase enzyme)
f. Obesity (increased converting enzyme)
g. Thyroid dysfunction (SHBG alterations)

TABLE 3-4. Frequency of clinical manifestations of proven cases of polycystic ovary syndrome ($N = 1,079$)[a]

	Fequency (%)	
	Mean	Range
Obesity	41	16–49
Hirsutism	69	17–83
Virilization	21	0–28
Amenorrhea	51	15–77
Infertility	74	35–94
Functional bleeding	29	6–65
Biphasic basal temperature	15	12–40
Corpus luteum at operation	22	0–71

[a] From Goldzieher, JW, Green JA: *J Clin Endocrinol Metab* 1962;22:325, © by the Endocrine Society.

the most common cause of chronic anovulation. The term polycystic ovarian disease or polycystic ovarian syndrome emphasizes the heterogeneity of this entity (Table 3-4),[19] since ovulatory failure, infertility, hirsutism, obesity, and bilateral polycystic ovaries are not unique to PCO. A variety of endocrine dysfunctions of diverse etiologic origin, including Cushing's syndrome, congenital adrenal hyperplasia, virilizing ovarian and adrenal tumors, hyperprolactinemia, and thyroid dysfunction can present with the clinical manifestations associated with PCO.

Although hyperandrogenism in PCO is well established, the issue of its source (adrenal versus ovarian) has been the subject of several studies. Direct adrenal and/or ovarian vein catheterization studies[20] suggest that PCO patients have a *combined* adrenal and ovarian origin for androgen excess. Furthermore, selective "medical ovariectomy" with GnRH agonist[21] has been used as a probe to determine the contributions of ovarian and adrenal androgens to this syndrome. After suppression of ovarian function with GnRH agonist, measurements of peripheral androgens revealed that ovarian hormones (androstenedione, testosterone, and 17-hydroxyprogesterone) were reduced to castrate levels, whereas adrenal hormones (DHEA and DHEA sulfate) were unaffected. Thus, biglandular excess production of both ovarian and adrenal androgens contributes to the overall androgen excess present in PCO.

Secretion of excessive amounts of androgen and its subsequent conversion to estrogen constitute the basis for chronic anovulation in PCO. Relatively constant levels of estrogen are reflected mainly by chronically elevated levels of estrone (rather than estradiol) derived from extraglandular conversion of androstenedione. This tonically elevated estrogen environment provides acyclic feedback and inappropriate secretion of LH and FSH by the hypothalamic–pituitary system. Patients with PCO typically demonstrate inappropriately elevated blood LH concentrations with relatively constant or low FSH levels, and the LH/FSH ratio is usually greater than 3. The disparity between LH and FSH

TABLE 3-5. Disparity of LH and FSH secretion in women with PCO

1. The negative feedback inhibition of both estradiol and estrone is greater on FSH than on LH.
2. FSH release is relatively insensitive to GnRH stimulation.
3. A multicystic ovary in PCO patients may secrete significant amounts of follicular inhibin (an inhibitor of FSH release), which further inhibits the release of FSH.

secretion in patients with PCO can be explained by greater estrogen suppression of FSH than LH, insensitivity of FSH release to GnRH, and the existence of other ovarian regulations of pituitary function (Table 3-5).

In addition to abnormal androgen/estrogen metabolism, PCO is associated with peripheral resistance to insulin and glucose intolerance.[22-24] Both obese and nonobese women demonstrate a positive correlation between hyperinsulinemia and hyperandrogenism, implying that androgen excess may somehow mediate peripheral insulin resistance. A unique type of extreme insulin resistance in this syndrome is manifested by obesity, significant androgen excess, amenorrhea, bilateral polycystic ovaries, and acanthosis nigricans. The insulin resistance in these women is related to two types of insulin receptor abnormalities: reduction of the number of insulin receptors (type A) or the presence of autoantibodies to the insulin receptor (type B). However, type A and type B defects in glucose receptor action do not appear to be related exclusively to androgen excess, since normalization of androgens in these syndromes does not alter hyperinsulinemia and progression of acanthosis nigricans.

The pathophysiology of chronic anovulation producing PCO[1] can be summarized by the events described in Fig. 3-6. Here the genesis of PCO is not related to an inherent defect in the HPO axis but rather is initiated and then sustained by elevated circulating androgens from any source. Increased androgen production leads to increased acyclic peripheral estrogen formation. Peripheral

estrogen preferentially inhibits pituitary FSH secretion and establishes a high LH/FSH ratio that sustains acyclic nonincremental estrogen feedback on the HPO axis. Luteinizing hormone stimulation of the ovarian stroma cells with associated excess secretion of ovarian androgens then follows. Excess production of adrenal and ovarian androgens reduces SHBG production, and this alteration further augments the biological activity of circulating androgens. Additionally, the increased availability of circulating androgens for end-organ action makes them more available for peripheral conversion to estrogen. Thus, elevated androgens induce an acyclic steady state of estrogen production that perpetuates chronic anovulation. Ovarian changes such as inadequate follicular maturation and increased follicular atresia are secondary events that occur from both inadequate FSH and excess LH stimulation to the follicle.

Other conditions that can mimic PCO include congenital adrenal hyperplasia (CAH) (classic and adult-onset), androgen- or estrogen-secreting tumors of the ovary and adrenal, hyperadrenalism of Cushing's syndrome, and thyroid dysfunction. The clinician must

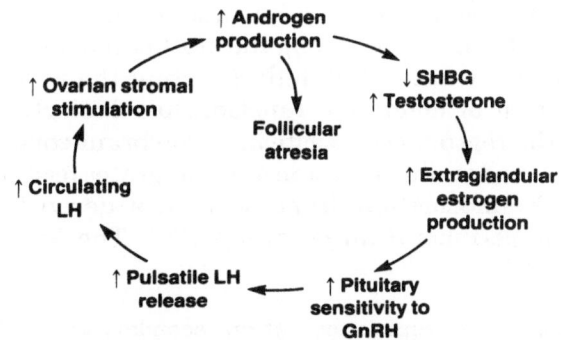

FIGURE 3-6. Anovulation and polycystic ovary syndrome. Increased androgen production from either adrenal or ovarian sources leads to steady-state excess ovarian androgen production. From Yen SSC, Jaffe RB (eds): *Reproductive Endocrinology: Physiology, Pathophysiology, and Clinical Management*. Philadelphia: W. B. Saunders, 1986, p 461 and Yen SSC, et al: *In* James VHT et al (eds): The Endocrine Function of the Human Ovary. New York: Academic Press, 1976, pp 373–385

also consider that aging in women (as well as men) is associated with a two- to fourfold increase in extraglandular estrone formation (increased aromatase activity) and that obese women have excessive converting tissue (adipose tissue). Furthermore, the conversion of androgens to estrogens is uniquely modulated by thyroid dysfunction in that SHBG is preferentially increased in hyperthyroidism but conversely reduced in hypothyroidism.

Anovulation Caused by CNS–Hypothalamic–Pituitary Dysfunction

Anovulation or amenorrhea secondary to CNS dysfunction can occur from either aberrations of CNS–hypothalamic function or from structural or developmental defects of the hypothalamic–pituitary axis. Factors responsible for chronic anovulation resulting from dysfunction of the hypothalamic–pituitary unit are presented in Table 3-6.

Aberrations of CNS–Hypothalamic Interaction

Emotional states influence menstrual and reproductive function in humans. Psychological influences are among the most potent and prevalent natural stimuli affecting the regulation of endocrine function, particularly of the reproductive system.[25] The brain controls endocrine secretion and integrates feedback information from hormones derived from peripheral target organs.[26,27] The *lim-*

TABLE 3-6. Chronic anovulation secondary to dysfunction of the hypothalamic–pituitary unit

1. Aberration of hypothalamus
   a. Pseudocyesis
   b. Anorexia nervosa
   c. Stress or nutritional anovulation
2. Pituitary defects
   a. Hypothalamic lesions (reduced GnRH)
   b. Kallmann's syndrome (isolated GnRH deficiency)
   c. Sheehan's syndrome
   d. Pituitary or stalk tumors

bic system is recognized as a crucial linkage between behavioral stimuli and the inner communication with the endocrine and autonomic nervous system. The functional state of the hypothalamus is thus inseparably related to the pattern of neural activity in the limbic circuit. Physical, emotional, and social stresses activate the sympathetic nervous system and stimulate pituitary release of stress hormones (prolactin, growth hormone, and ACTH). Central to this response to stress is the release of CRF from the hypothalamus. When delivered to the portal circulation, CRF stimulates ACTH and β-endorphin release by the anterior pituitary. The subsequent acute release of cortisol affects the immune system and mood and may regulate enzymatic activity for the biosynthesis of catecholamines. The elevated cortisol levels provide negative feedback for the secretion of ACTH, and thus chronic activation of the CRF–ACTH–adrenal axis from repeated stressful stimuli may ultimately induce down-regulation of this axis.

Pseudocyesis[28,29] represents the classic example of willful or emotional alteration of reproductive function. This syndrome of "phantom pregnancy" has been recognized since ancient times. In women affected with pseudocyesis, there is hypersecretion of prolactin and pituitary LH. Circulating estradiol and progesterone levels are increased, and the elevated levels of prolactin and LH are high enough to maintain luteal function and galactorrhea in affected women. It is postulated that reduced tone of the hypothalamic–pituitary axis is responsible for the hypersecretion of both prolactin and LH in this syndrome. Such patients demonstrate dramatic responses to GnRH and increased sensitivity to dopamine suppression.

Anorexia nervosa represents another extraordinary psychogenic reproductive disorder. The salient features of anorexia nervosa are summarized in Table 3-7. Physical symptoms include hypothermia, hypotension, and amenorrhea. Several specific hypothalamic abnormalities have been described in this syndrome and include amenorrhea, reduced frequency and amplitude of LH pulses, abnor-

TABLE 3-7. Features of anorexia nervosa

1. Adolescent girls
2. Obsession with dieting
3. Morbid fear of losing control over body weight and body image
4. Amenorrhea
5. High achievement with intense and commonly obsessive–compulsive behavior
6. Distorted self-perception
7. Family history of sexual abuse with a domineering and/or insensitive parent

mal thermoregulation, abnormal pituitary response to GnRH and TRH, and hypersecretion of cortisol.[30-32] Paradoxically, hypersecretion of adrenal cortisol is associated with suppression of adrenal androgen secretion.[33,34]

Psychogenic amenorrhea (functional hypothalamic amenorrhea) represents one of the most common types of amenorrhea. In contrast to adolescent girls with anorexia nervosa, psychogenic amenorrhea tends to affect adult women. Affected women tend to be unmarried, engaged in intellectual occupations, report stressful life events, often consume sedatives or hypnotic drugs, practice weight control, and have a history of previous menstrual irregularities.[35] Substantial evidence indicates an impairment of the hypothalamic GnRH pulse generator as the underlying cause of pituitary–ovarian inactivity in women with hypothalamic amenorrhea.[36] In general the frequency and amplitude of GnRH pulses are diminished, and ovarian activity virtually ceases. In essence the entire HPO system functionally regresses to the prepubertal state. Under these conditions, progesterone withdrawal bleeding does not occur, and treatment with clomiphene citrate for ovulation induction is usually not efficacious. Spontaneous reversal of hypothalamic amenorrhea following appropriate counseling or life changes provides strong evidence for a psychogenic cause of this disorder.

Exercise-related menstrual dysfunction is occurring more frequently in association with a rapid increase in the popularity of physical exercise during the past decade.[37-39] The type, duration, and intensity of exercise as well as the body composition and stress factors of individual participants are confounding factors to be considered in assessing exercise-related amenorrhea. Most women with exercise-induced amenorrhea participate in strenuous competition-type sports such as running, swimming, ballet dancing, and field events. The incidence is much higher in high-intensity runners and ballet dancers than in swimmers and joggers. This difference is mostly attributable to the relatively high percentage of body fat among swimmers compared to the reduced body fat among runners and ballet dancers.

Hypothalamic Pituitary Dysfunction

Hypogonadotropic hypogonadism associated with anosmia was described by Kallmann and associates in 1944.[40] Uniquely, Kallmann's syndrome occurs more frequently in males than in females. Levels of circulating LH and FSH are usually undetectable, although low-normal values are occasionally found.[41] Puberty is delayed, and on physical examination patients typically express eunuchoid proportions. This syndrome is often transmitted as an autosomal dominant trait but may also occur sporadically.[42] Anatomic evidence supports partial or complete agenesis of the olfactory apparatus, which produces anosmia and defective neuronal control of GnRH release.

Pituitary tumors occur frequently and may be detectable in as many as 10% of normal patients. However, endocrinologically active tumors or structural tumors that compromise the HPO axis occur rarely. Hypersecreting pituitary adenomas secrete ACTH, growth hormone, prolactin, TSH, FSH, LH, and β-endorphin. Additionally, endocrinologically inactive tumors may be detectable on CT scans. Pituitary tumors account for approximately 10% of clinically significant intracranial neoplasms.

Craniopharyngioma is the most important hormonally inactive tumor and arises from embryological remnants of Rathke's pouch. This neoplasm accounts for only 3% of intracranial tumors, but because it develops along the anterior surface of the infundibulum of the pituitary stalk, it commonly interferes with hypothalamic–pituitary endocrine function.[43,44] Craniopharyngiomas are more common in men than women, and occur with the highest incidence in the second decade. The most common presenting features are visual impairment (70%) or headache (50%), but dynamic pituitary testing will demonstrate some degree of hypopituitarism in almost all cases. Growth hormone and gonadotropin deficiency are invariably seen in association with this tumor.

Other neoplastic processes that produce hypothalamic hypopituitarism include germinoma, glioma, Hand–Schuller–Christian disease, midline dermoid cysts and teratoma, endodermal sinus tumor, tuberculosis, sarcoidosis, and metastatic disease. In addition to primary neoplastic processes, metastatic disease may also affect the pituitary and produce amenorrhea. Occasionally, the empty sella syndrome is seen in association with defective hypothalamic–pituitary function, but usually women with an empty sella show no endocrine impairment.

Acquired hypopituitarism may result from surgical or radiological ablation or may occur as a result of infarction from a large pituitary tumor, granulomatous lesions, or postpartum hypotension (Sheehan's syndrome).[45] Panhypopituitarism is expressed by amenorrhea, hair loss, fatigue, and hypotension. With hypothalamic releasing hormone challenge, degrees of pituitary hypofunction can be detected for TRH, gonadotropins, ACTH, and growth hormone. Evidence of prolactin deficiency is uniquely associated only with Sheehan's syndrome.

References

1. Yen SSC. Chronic anovulation caused by peripheral endocrine disorders. In: Yen SSC, Jaffe RB, eds. Reproductive endocrinology physiology, pathophysiology, and clinical management. Philadelphia: W. B. Saunders, 1986:441–49.
2. Hillier SG, Reichert LE Jr, Van Hall EV. Control of preovulatory follicular estrogen biosynthesis in the human ovary. J Clin Endocrinol Metab. 1981;52:847–56.
3. Rebard R, Judd HL, Yen SSC. Characterization of the inappropriate gonadotropin secretion in polycystic ovary syndrome. J Clin Invest. 1976;57:1320–29.
4. Horton R, Tait JF. Androstenedione production and interconversion rates measured in peripheral blood and studies on the possible site of its conversion to testosterone. J Clin Invest. 1966;45:301–13.
5. Kirschner MA, Zucker IR, Jesperson DL. Ovarian and adrenal vein catheterization studies in women with idiopathic hirsutism. In: James VHT, Serio M, Guisti G, eds. The endocrine function of the ovary. New York: Academic Press, 1976:443–56.
6. Bardin CW, Lipsett MB. Testosterone and androstenedione blood production rates in normal women with idiopathic hirsutism or polycystic ovaries. J Clin Invest. 1967;46:891–902.
7. Igball MJ, Johnson MW. Purification and characterization of human sex hormone binding globulin. J Steroid Biochem. 1979;10:535–40.
8. Longcope C, Williams KIH. The metabolism of estrogens in normal women after pulse injections of ³H-estradiol and ³H-estrone. J Clin Endocrinol Metab. 1974;38:602–07.
9. Rosenfield RL, Moll GW Jr, The role of proteins in the distribution of plasma androgens and estradiol. In: Moinatti CG, Martini L, James BHT, eds. Androgenization in women. New York: Raven Press, 1983:25–45.
10. Pardridge WM. Transport of protein-bound hormones into tissues in vivo. Endocr Rev. 1981;2:103–23.
11. Anderson DC. Sex hormone-binding globulin. Clin Endocrinol. 1974;3:69–96.
12. Vermeulen A, Verdonck L, VanderStraetin M, et al. Capacity of the testosterone-binding globulin in human plasma and influence of specific binding of testosterone on its metabolic clearance rate. J Clin Endocrinol Metab. 1969;29:1470–80.
13. DeMoor P, Heyns W, Bouillion R. Growth hormone and the steroid binding B-globulin of human plasma. J Steroid Biochem. 1972;3:593–600.
14. Crosignani PG, Ferrari C, Malinverni A, et al. Effect of central nervous system dopaminergic

activation on prolactin secretion in man: evidence for a common central defect in hyperprolactinemic patients with and without radiological signs of pituitary tumors. J Clin Endocrinol Metab. 1980; 51: 1068–73.

15. Pepperell RJ. Prolactin and reproduction. Fertil Steril. 1981; 35: 267–74.

16. Kleinberg DL, Noel GL, Frantz AG. Galactorrhea: a study of 235 cases, including 48 with pituitary tumor. N Engl J Med. 1977; 296: 589–600.

17. Rogers J. Menstruation and systemic disease (continued). N Engl J Med. 1958; 259: 721–27.

18. Yen SSC, Vela P, Rankin J. Inappropriate secretion of follicle-stimulating hormone and luteinizing hormone in polycystic ovarian disease. J Clin Endocrinol Metab. 1970; 30: 435–42.

19. Goldzieher JW, Green JA. The polycystic ovary. I. Clinical and histologic features. J Clin Endocrinol Metab. 1962; 22: 325–38.

20. Kirschner MA, Jacobs JB. Combined ovarian and adrenal vein catheterization to determine the site(s) of androgen overproduction in hirsute women. J Clin Endocrinol Metab. 1971; 33: 199–209.

21. Chang RJ, Laufer LR, Meldrum DR, et al. Steroid secretion in polycystic ovarian disease after ovarian suppression by a long-acting gonadotropin-releasing hormone agonist. J Clin Endocrinol Metab. 1983; 56: 897–903.

22. Burghen GA, Givens JR, Kitabchi AE. Correlation of hyperandrogenism with hyperinsulinism in polycystic ovarian disease. J Clin Endocrinol Metab. 1980; 50: 113–16.

23. Chang RJ, Nakamura RM, Judd HL, et al. Insulin resistance in non-obese patients with polycystic ovarian disease. J Clin Endocrinol Metab. 1983; 57: 356–59.

24. Taylor SI, Dons RF, Hernandez R, et al. Insulin resistance associated with androgen excess in women with autoantibodies to the insulin receptor. Ann Intern Med. 1982; 92: 851–55.

25. Axelrod J, Reisine TD. Stress hormones: their interaction and regulation. Science. 1984; 224: 452–59.

26. Knobil E. On the control of gonadotropin secretion in the rhesus monkey. Recent Prog Horm Res. 1974; 30: 1–46.

27. Swanson LW, Mogenson GJ. Neural mechanisms for the functional coupling of autonomic, endocrine, and somatomotor responses in adaptive behavior. Brain Res Rev. 1981; 3: 1–34.

28. Yen SSC, Rebar RW, Quesenberry W. Pituitary function in pseudocyesis. J Clin Endocrinol Metab. 1976; 43: 132–36.

29. Zarate A, Canales ES, Soria J, et al. Gonadotropin and prolactin secretion in human pseudocyesis: effect of synthetic luteinizing hormone-releasing hormone (LH-RH) and thyrotropin releasing hormone (TRH). Ann Endocrinol. 1974; 35: 445–50.

30. Vigersky RA, Loriaux DL, Andersen AE, et al. Delayed pituitary hormone response to LRF and TRF in patients with anorexia nervosa and with secondary amenorrhea associated with simple weight loss. J Clin Endocrinol Metab. 1976; 43: 487–96.

31. Travaglini P, Peccoz-Beck P, Ferrari C, et al. Some aspects of hypothalamic–pituitary function in patients with anorexia nervosa. Acta Endocrinol. 1976; 81: 252–62.

32. Beumont PJV, George GCW, Pimpstone BL, et al. Body weight and the pituitary response to hypothalamic releasing hormones in patients with anorexia nervosa. J Clin Endocrinol Metab. 1976; 43: 487–96.

33. Boyar RM, Hellman LD, Roffwarg H, et al. Cortisol secretion and metabolism in anorexia nervosa. N Engl J Med. 1977; 296: 190–93.

34. Doerr P, Fichter M, Pirke KM, et al. Relationship between weight gain and hypothalamic pituitary adrenal function in patients with anorexia nervosa. J Steroid Biochem. 1980; 13: 529–37.

35. Fries H, Nillius SJ, Patterson F. Epidemiology of secondary amenorrhea: II. A retrospective evaluation of etiology with special regard to psychogenic factors and weight loss. Am J Obstet Gynecol. 1974; 118: 473–79.

36. Yen SSC, Rebar R, Vandenberg G, et al. Pituitary gonadotropin responsiveness to synthetic LRF in subjects with normal and abnormal hypothalamic–pituitary–gonadal axis. J Reprod Fertil. (Suppl) 1973; 20: 137–61.

37. Cumming DC, Rebar RW. Exercise and reproductive function in women. Am J Int Med. 1983; 4: 113–25.

38. Frisch RE, Wyshak G, Vincent L. Delayed menarche and amenorrhea in ballet dancers . N Engl J Med. 1980; 303: 17–19.

39. Feicht CB, Johnson TS, Martin BJ, et al. Secondary amenorrhea in athletes. Lancet. 1978; 2: 1145–46.

40. Kallmann FJ, Schoenfeld WA, Barrera SE. The genetic aspects of primary eunuchoidism. Am J Ment Defic. 1944; 48: 203–36.

41. Lieblich JM, Rogol AD, White BJ, et al. Syn-

drome of anosmia with hypogonadotropic hypogonadism. Am J Med. 1982;73:506–19.

42. Santen RJ, Paulsen CA. Hypogonadotropic eunuchoidism: I. clinical study of the mode of inheritance. J Clin Endocrinol Metab. 1973;36:47–54.

43. Jenkins JS, Gilbert J, Ang V. Hypothalamic–pituitary function in patients with cranio-

pharyngiomas. J Clin Endocrinol Metab. 1976;43:394–99.

44. Hoff JT, Patterson RH Jr. Craniopharyngiomas in children and adults. J Neurosurg. 1972;36:299–302.

45. Sheehan HL. Simmond's disease due to postpartum necrosis of the anterior pituitary. Q J Med. 1939;8:277–309.

4
Diagnosis of Ovulation and the Role of Ultrasound in Monitoring the Follicular Response

Cynthia Miles Austin

Ultrasonography was introduced for use in obstetrics and gynecology in the 1960s. Initially the technique was applied primarily for evaluation of pregnancy and of pelvic masses. The capability of ultrasound to allow visual assessment of the functional anatomy of the female pelvis has, however, led to its growing role in the diagnosis and management of female infertility. Information provided by standard laboratory and clinical techniques, including basal body temperature charts, assessment of cervical mucus, serum estrogen and progesterone levels, and endometrial biopsy, is useful, but it is also indirect and often subjective. Over the past 5 years, experience with ultrasonographic evaluation of ovarian function, both normal and pathological, has greatly expanded. Diagnostic ultrasound can provide information that approximates a surgical assessment of reproductive anatomy without the expense and risks of a surgical procedure. Ultrasound can also be utilized repetitively throughout a single ovulatory cycle, providing dynamic information regarding ovarian function in a safe, convenient, noninvasive, and, when properly applied, cost-effective manner.

Equipment

Gynecologic ultrasonography is standardly performed using a real-time B-mode scanner. Real-time ultrasonography allows continuous imaging as the transducer is moved over the body surface. Although a static scanner may be adequate for ovarian examination, real-time B-mode scanning provides the best assessment of three-dimensional pelvic anatomy. In addition, the ability to identify motion can be useful for differentiating ovarian cysts from loops of bowel or vascular structures scanned in cross section. The linear array transducer, which is commonly use for obstetrical ultrasonography, is, because of the shape of transducer, of limited use for examination of the pelvis, particularly the ovaries. However, the phase array (sector) or the curvilinear probe facilitates visualization of laterally placed pelvic organs, particularly the ovaries. Scanning can be done abdominally using the distended bladder as an acoustic window or transvaginally using a specially designed transducer.

During abdominal scanning, the distended bladder facilitates imaging of the reproductive organs by displacing the small bowel and omentum out of the pelvis and by providing an acoustical window through which sound waves are readily transmitted. Generally, a 3.5-MHz transducer provides optimal imaging in the average gynecologic patient. However, as transducer frequency is increased, axial resolution is increased, but tissue penetration is reduced. Therefore, a higher-frequency transducer is advantageous for examining very thin or pediatric patients, whereas examination of obese patients requires the use of a lower-frequency transducer, on the order of 2.5 MHz.

Increasingly, transvaginal ultrasound examination is replacing the transabdominal approach for examination of nonpregnant and early pregnant reproductive organs. Specifically designed probes that can be inserted comfortably into the vagina are available from a large number of companies. The transvaginal approach is particularly useful for examination of the ovaries since in most patients they are located within centimeters of the vaginal apex. Because the pelvis is viewed through the vaginal fornices, a full bladder is unnecessary. It is generally preferable that the patient empty her bladder immediately prior to the examination in order to avoid displacing the ovaries out of the pelvis. A higher-frequency transducer can be used because of the close proximity of the transducer to the pelvic structures. These features of the transvaginal ultrasound transducer allow the creation of an image with improved resolution and reproducibility as compared with transabdominal imaging. The advantage of transvaginal over transabdominal scanning is particularly apparent among obese patients and those with extensive pelvic adhesions, because it avoids the excessive fatty tissue and/or dense scar tissue that interferes with penetration of the abdominal wall by the ultrasonic waves.

In addition to using the appropriate equipment, it is imperative that the ultrasonographer be well acquainted with the use of the particular machine. Failure to adjust the controls properly will invariably lead to poor imaging and incorrect clinical assessment.

Patient Examination

Transabdominal Pelvic Ultrasonography

Patient preparation requires the presence of a full bladder. With the bladder used as a sonolucent window, the vagina, cervix, and uterus can be identified as midline structures. The axis of the body of the uterus and the endometrial cavity may vary in the right-to-left and anterior-to-posterior positions. The relative positioning of the uterine cavity and cervical canal can be accurately assessed by

ultrasonographic examination. The ovaries can be found lying lateral to the uterus. The ovaries of women with a history of pelvic surgical procedures are not uncommonly found in somewhat aberrant locations, such as at the level of the uterine cornua. The ovaries of women with a history of extensive adhesion formation tend to be fixed but in relatively normal anatomic location. Using the transabdominal approach enables the examiner to image the pelvis in the true transverse and sagittal planes. The resolution with which the ovaries and cystic structures contained therein can be visualized by the transabdominal approach is dependent on the capabilities of the probe and ultrasound machine in use as well as the body habitus of the patient being examined. Examination of the obese patient is particularly difficult because penetration of the abdominal wall by the ultrasound waves is retarded by the excessive subcutaneous tissue.

Transvaginal Pelvic Ultrasonography

Transvaginal ultrasonography is well adapted to imaging of pelvic anatomy, especially the ovaries, in virtually all women. It is particularly useful for examination of obese patients or those with dense pelvic adhesions, in whom adequate tissue penetration for transabdominal imaging is difficult to achieve. A specifically designed transducer covered with a sterile condom should be used. A small amount of conducting jelly is placed in the condom before covering the transducer to create a film between the condom and transducer head. It is preferable to use water as a lubricant for insertion of the probe, since many lubricating gels are spermicidal and may potentially interfere with fertility.

Vaginal probes are slender and can be easily inserted into the vagina of even the postmenopausal patient without discomfort. The patient's bladder should be empty or nearly empty for optimal vaginal scanning. Elimination of the need for a full bladder makes transvaginal ultrasound examinations significantly more comfortable than transabdominal scans. Although issues of patient embarrassment may initially be of some concern to the occasional patient, virtually all patients accept the procedure, and most prefer it to abdominal scanning.

Scanning is performed through the vaginal fornices. Because the pelvic structures are in close proximity to the head of the transducer, a high-frequency probe is used. Examiners who are accustomed to transabdominal ultrasonography may initially find themselves somewhat disoriented when beginning to do transvaginal scanning. The orientation of the vaginal probe relative to the pelvic anatomy is not unlike that of the standard bimanual pelvic examination. The true sagittal plane can be achieved only in the direct midline. Thereafter, when scanning laterally, the two-dimensional image cuts tangentially across the pelvis. The true transverse plane is never visualized using the transvaginal approach. Instead, the patient is imaged in coronal planes.

The examination is initiated by identifying the uterus, with the bladder, if visible, anteriorly and the cul de sac posteriorly. The adnexal structures can then be identified by scanning laterally. Usually the ovaries can be found lying within several centimeters of the vaginal apex.

Whether an abdominal or a vaginal approach is used to examine the pelvis, appropriate interpretation of the two-dimensional images formed requires a good understanding of pelvic anatomy coupled with awareness of the positioning of the transducer during the examination. Likewise, the individual interpreting the ultrasonographic findings must have a solid understanding of the dynamics of ovarian function as well as specific details of the patient's clinical history. It is for this reason that we feel that the reproductive gynecologist is an ideal ultrasonographer.

Monitoring Ovarian Function

The ovaries are dynamic organs, the functions of which are reflected in cyclic hormonal and anatomic changes. Ultrasonographic findings can be used to supplement the laboratory and clinical changes that are used traditionally in the management of female infertility to gain more detailed and accurate insight into the physiology and pathophysiology of ovarian function. The formation of ovarian cysts throughout the menstrual cycle is normal. Appropriate interpretation of the findings on ultrasound requires knowledge of the status of the patient's current cycle as well as an understanding of the normal ovarian changes that occur as the cycle progresses.

Folliculogenesis

Ovarian follicles are in a constant process of maturation and atresia, independent of gonadotropin stimulation. All follicles are predestined to become atretic unless rescued by follicle-stimulating hormone (FSH). Under the influence of FSH, an initial cohort of follicles is recruited from that pool of independently maturing follicles. By day 5 to 7, this cohort will become visible on ultrasound as small sonolucent cysts measuring approximately 5 to 8 mm. On day 8 to 10 the single dominant follicle that is destined to ovulate will become apparent when its growth exceeds that of the other follicles. In approximately 5% to 10% of spontaneous cycles, two dominant ovulatory follicles will develop. In as many as 80% of spontaneous cycles, one or two subordinate follicles will continue to undergo parallel but limited development, rarely exceeding a diameter of 14 mm.[1] Although these subordinate follicles are destined to become atretic, they are hormonally active and contribute to the overall hormonal milieu of the normal ovulatory cycle. The peak follicular diameter that corresponds to ovum maturity varies from individual to individual with an average range of 18 to 28 mm. Among repeated spontaneous cycles, however, the same woman tends to produce the same follicular size at ovum maturity.[1-8]

As the oocyte contained within matures, the dominant follicle pursues a linear rate of growth of approximately 1.5 to 3 mm each day. The peripheral estradiol level continues to rise as follicular maturation continues, demonstrating a positive correlation with dominant follicular diameter.[1,4-11] The dominant follicle(s) contributes approximately 95% of the circulating estradiol. Peripheral estradiol reaches a sustained peak, initiating the luteinizing hormone (LH) surge. The mean peak estradiol corresponding to a single dominant follicle is 324 pg/mL.[8] During the 36 hours following the onset of the LH surge and preceding ovum release, the follicle undergoes rapid exponential growth. Under the influence of LH, granulosa cells begin to luteinize and produce progesterone. Thecal tissue becomes hypervascular and edematous and begins to separate from the granulosa layer. These changes may be seen sonographically as a line of decreased contrast surrounding the follicle.[1-8] As the follicle approaches ovum release, an area of increased echogenicity can be identified in some patients; this is thought to represent the cumulus mass.[1] Midcycle surveillance of ovaries reveals that mittelschmerz is associated not with follicular rupture and escape of follicular contents but with the rapid expansion of the dominant follicle preceding ovulation. In 77% of women studied, the pain coincided with the onset of the LH surge. In 97% of patients the pain preceded follicular rupture.[1-12]

Ovulation and Corpus Luteum Formation

Although rapid growth of the follicle exceeding 3 mm in a 24-hour period is suggestive of impending ovulation, there are no specific signs that indicate that ovulation is about to take place. Sequential sonographic surveillance can confirm that follicular rupture has already occurred. Prior to ovulation, the follicle appears as a round to oval homogeneously sonolucent cyst. With ovulation, the previously well-defined follicular cyst may appear to have collapsed, forming an irregular cyst containing low-level echoes. Complete follicular emptying occurs over about 45 minutes.[13] Fluid is frequently found in the cul de sac. With follicular rupture and formation of the corpus luteum, the follicle is replaced by an irregular cyst with indistinct margins and nonhomogeneous echoes. This may gradually disappear over the next 4 to 5 days or may increase in size before disappearing. The corpus luteum cyst may persist for as long as a week into the next ovulatory cycle.[1,7,13-15]

Abnormal Ovarian Function

Abnormal Folliculogenesis

Serial sonographic examination during apparently normal menstrual cycles suggests that abnormal follicular development and/or ovulation may occur in as many as 4 out of 10 cycles. Asynchrony between estradiol peak, LH surge, and the growth and disappearance of ovarian follicles have been documented.[7,16-18] Varying degrees of follicular development have also been documented in women taking oral contraceptives who have missed a single pill as well as those who have taken their pills appropriately[19] (J. Evans, personal communication, 1988).

Luteinized unruptured follicle syndrome (LUFS) is a condition in which the follicle becomes luteinized without release of the ovum. It cannot be diagnosed by standard indirect methods of ovulation documentation including progesterone assay, endometrial biopsy, or basal body temperature charting. Sequential sonographic surveillance can, with a moderate degree of confidence, document the occurrence of LUFS. A normal pattern of follicular growth is observed until the LH surge. An echo-free cyst is observed that continues to grow in the absence of any signs of ovum release. As the granulosa becomes luteinized, the normal sharp-edged appearance of the follicle may be replaced by a gradual thickening to form a 4- to 7-mm gray margin.[20-22] Serial ultrasonographic examination must be performed during the time of ovulation in order to distinguish LUFS from a normal cystic corpus luteum. This pattern of abnormal follicular luteinization has been documented in some series as occurring in as many as 5% of cycles of fertile women and slightly more often, 9%, among women with infertility.[21,22] Whether or not this syndrome represents a significant cause of infertility remains controversial.

Polycystic Ovary Syndrome

Polycystic ovary syndrome (PCO) was first described in 1935 as a triad of clinical findings—obesity, hirsutism, and amenorrhea—occurring in association with a specific histological appearance on ovarian biopsy. Current thinking, however, defines PCO as occurring in a subset of chronically anovulatory women with essentially normal prolactin and gonadotropin levels. These women may or may not be obese, hirsute, or amenorrheic. They may or may not have histologically "polycystic" ovaries. The classically described polycystic ovary is not the cause but the result of years of chronic anovulation. The tiny cysts and thickened theca are the result of multiple atretic follicles that were never adequately "rescued" by FSH.

The ultrasonographic appearance of a classically polycystic ovary is that of a symmetrically enlarged ovary containing numerous small cysts. A number of studies, however, reveal that only a third of women with clinically diagnosed PCO will have polycystic appearing ovaries on ultrasound imaging. Conversely, 20% of normally ovulating women will, by ultrasound imaging, have polycystic ovaries.[23] Polycystic ovary syndrome is a diagnosis that can and should be made clinically.

Endometriosis

Ultrasonographic examination is of limited use in the diagnosis and staging of endometriosis. It can be useful to follow the progress of a patient with previously diagnosed endometriosis. Although endometrial implants cannot be visualized by pelvic ultrasound, endometriomas of modest size can. The ultrasonographic appearance of an endometrioma is not specific and may consist of any combination of solid and cystic components. The most common appearance is that of a symmetrical round or oval cyst with homogeneously increased echogenicity somewhat less than that of the uterus. Ultrasound alone cannot be used to exclude other clinical possibilities, including ovarian neoplasm. Information obtained by ultrasound must be interpreted in light of the clinical presentation.

Induced Ovarian Cycles

Clomiphene Citrate

Clomiphene citrate (CC) stimulates ovulation by binding to estrogen receptors and inducing increased endogenous secretion of pituitary gonadotropin. In 25% to 60% of CC cycles, the natural process for selection of a single dominant follicle is overridden, resulting in stimulation of multiple ovulatory follicles.[24,25] Follicular development can usually be seen by ultrasound by day 12 when clomiphene is started on cycle day 5. Although follicles may be recruited sequentially and be of differing sizes, in CC cycles, as in spontaneous cycles, they demonstrate a positive correlation between follicular growth and circulating estradiol levels. Maximum follicular diameter consistent with ovum maturity is 22 to 23 mm, similar to that seen in spontaneous cycles.[24-26]

Patients undergoing CC stimulation will usually have a spontaneous LH surge approximately 5 to 7 days after the completion of clomiphene therapy and will undergo spontaneous ovulation. Under certain circumstances, the physician may want to time ovulation more precisely by administering human chorionic gonadotropin (hCG), causing ovulation to occur approximately 36 hours later. In addition, some women taking CC undergo adequate follicular maturation but require administration of hCG to achieve ovulation. Although use of hCG during a CC cycle can clearly cause luteinization and secretion of ovarian progesterone, it is not clear that ovum release has occurred unless follicular rupture is confirmed by ultrasound. Until recently, hCG has empirically been administered 5 to 7 days after completion of CC therapy. If the hCG is given at any time other than at follicular maturity, inhibition of ovum release and atresia will occur. By using ovarian ultrasound examination to evaluate follicular size, hCG can be administered with improved accuracy to ensure ovum release. In

CC-stimulated cycles, hCG should be administered when the dominant follicle reaches a minimum of 18 to 20 mm in diameter. When this criterion is used, ovulation is expected to occur in 90% of cycles.[24-26]

Human Menopausal Gonadotropin

Ovarian stimulation with human menopausal gonadotropin (hMG) involves daily intramuscular administration of equal quantities of pituitary hormones FSH and LH (Pergonal, Serono Laboratories, Inc., Randolph, MA) and/or FSH alone (Metrodin, Serono Laboratories, Inc., Randolph, MA). In almost all gonadotropin-induced cycles, ovum release following follicular maturation requires the addition of hCG. Traditionally, ovulation induction with hMG has been managed by titrating the dose to the daily serum estradiol and administering hCG when the serum estradiol levels reaches 1,000 to 1,500 pg/mL. Experience with follicular ultrasound during hMG administration, however, reveals that follicular diameter as seen on ultrasound is a better indicator of ovum maturity than estradiol levels alone.[27-29] Multiple follicular development occurs in more than 80% of hMG-stimulated ovarian cycles. The follicular diameter that corresponds to ovum maturity is 15 to 18 mm, smaller than that usually seen in spontaneous cycles. Although serum estradiol levels demonstrate a positive correlation with follicular growth during the hMG cycle, the estradiol level that corresponds to follicular maturity depends on the number and diameter of the growing follicles. For example, a level of 400 pg/mL may correspond to two 18-mm follicles or to multiple smaller, less mature follicles. Administration of hCG before follicles have reached 15 mm induces luteinization but inhibits ovum release.

Risks of Ovulation Induction

Five percent of clomiphene-induced pregnancies and 10% of hMG induced pregnancies are multiple gestations. Almost all of the multiple gestations conceived on clomiphene will be twins, with rare triplets. Two thirds of multiple gestations conceived using hMG will be twins, and one third will be triplets. Only rarely will pregnancies in excess of triplets be encountered when patients are monitored appropriately. It has been suggested that ultrasound examination could be used to reduce the risk of multiple gestation by identifying those cycles in which multiple mature follicles have developed. Since multiple follicular development is seen in 80% of hMG cycles but the risk of multiple gestation is considerably less, it is clear that most multiple ovulations do not lead to multiple gestation. Withholding hCG or insemination will result in a lower pregnancy rate by eliminating many potentially productive cycles.[28-30] It is not our practice to withhold the chance of pregnancy in the presence of multiple follicular development.

Ovarian hyperstimulation is the most serious potential complication of ovulation induction. Mild cases are characterized by cystic ovarian enlargement, mild abdominal distension, and weight gain not in excess of 5 lb (2.25 kg). Mild hyperstimulation can be expected to occur in as many as 25% of all hMG cycles and only occasionally in CC cycles. Although ovaries will be tender and are at increased risk for torsion, no active intervention is necessary. It may, in fact, be cause for optimism, since mild hyperstimulation is more frequently encountered in pregnancy cycles.

Severe cases are potentially life-threatening. Severe hyperstimulation is associated with massively enlarged and fragile ovaries, ascites, pleural effusion, hemoconcentration, hypovolemia, oliguria, and electrolyte imbalance. If the potential for development of hyperstimulation is recognized during hMG stimulation, it can be prevented by withholding hCG. Ovarian ultrasonography in combination with serum estradiol levels can be utilized to reduce significantly the risk of serious hyperstimulation without significantly reducing the pregnancy rate. Estradiol levels should be substantiated by confirming adequate follicular development on ultrasound. Human chorionic gonadotropin should not be administered if the serum estradiol exceeds 400 pg/mL per follicle or when rapidly rising serum estradiol is found in the presence of multiple immature follicles. Regardless of the number or size of follicles, hCG should be withheld if the estradiol level is greater than 4,000 pg/mL. When hyperstimulation is suspected, ultrasound examination allows accurate assessment of ovarian enlargement and ascites with minimal risk of rupturing the fragile cystic ovaries.[30-33]

Ultrasonography and In Vitro Fertilization

Ultrasonography is used extensively by in vitro fertilization (IVF) programs to monitor ovarian stimulation and to perform ovum retrieval. During pharmacological ovarian stimulation, ultrasonographic examinations are performed on a regular basis to assess follicular number and diameter in order to assure presence of adequate numbers of mature follicles to justify ovum retrieval and to time hCG administration appropriately.

Ultrasound-guided ovum retrieval is rapidly gaining popularity, and in many IVF programs it has replaced laparoscopic ovum retrieval. Transvesicular, transurethral, and transvaginal routes have all been used successfully.[34-37] The advantages of ultrasound-guided retrieval are several. Ultrasound-guided needle aspiration allows access to follicles in patients with extensive pelvic adhesions that make the ovaries inaccessible to laparoscopic visualization. The procedure is performed by many programs with local anesthesia with or without sedation, thereby avoiding the risks and costs of general anesthesia and dramatically reducing postoperative morbidity. The elimination of the requirement for general anesthesia makes it possible to move the procedure out of the operating suite into a treatment room in the office setting, further reducing patient costs. Some clinicians have raised concerns regarding possible toxic effects of the local anesthetics on ova and embryos. This has not been substantiated by controlled study. To the contrary, some authors have suggested that avoiding general anesthesia may be beneficial.[38]

Evaluation of Abnormal Gestation

Women with a history of infertility are at risk for ectopic pregnancy. Ultrasonographic examination of the pelvis in combination with serum hCG determination can be valuable in the differential diagnosis of an abnormal gestation. Human chorionic gonadotropin is first detectable in the serum at about 1 week after ovulation and rises rapidly thereafter. The level should reach nearly 200 mIU/mL by the first missed menstrual period and greater than 6,000 mIU/mL by the fourth week after ovulation (6 weeks from the last menstrual period in a 28-day cycle). A gestational sac should become visible within the uterus by 5 weeks menstrual age on vaginal ultrasound scans and by 6 weeks on abdominal scans.

If the pregnancy is ectopic or an impending abortion, thickened decidua is often observed in the uterine cavity. Only rarely can an ectopic pregnancy be identified in the adnexa. If the serum hCG level is above 6,000 mIU/mL and there is a sac within the uterus, the chance that there is a simultaneous ectopic pregnancy is remote. If the serum hCG level is greater than 6,000 mIU/mL and there is no gestational sac seen within the uterus, laparoscopy is indicated to rule out an ectopic gestation. If the hCG level is less than 6,000 mIU/mL and there is no gestational sac seen within the uterus, the status of the pregnancy is uncertain.[39] In clinically suspicious situations, the rate at which the serum hCG is rising should be followed. If there is a healthy intrauterine pregnancy, the hCG level should approximately double every 2 to 3 days. If the rate of rise does not follow this pattern, an abnormal gestation should be suspected.

Conclusion

Ultrasonography is becoming an integral tool in the evaluation and management of female infertility. The morphological features of spontaneous and stimulated cycles continue to be studied and described. These reports provide insight into the possible subtle errors of folliculogenesis and ovulation that may contribute to infertility and that may be amenable to treatment. Ultrasonographic evaluation of follicular development, ovulation, and corpus luteum formation can improve the accuracy, safety, and efficacy of ovarian stimulation. In addition, vaginal ultrasonography has improved the efficiency of the IVF process.

References

1. Kerin J, Edmonds D, Warnes G, et al. Morphological and functional relations of Graafian follicle growth to ovulation in women using ultrasonic, laparoscopic, and biochemical measurements. Br J Obstet Gynaecol. 1981;88:81–90.
2. O'Herlihy C, DeCrespigny L, Lopata A, et al. Preovulatory follicular size: a comparison of ultrasound and laparoscopic measurement. Fertil Steril. 1980;34:24–26.
3. O'Herlihy C, Decrespigny L, Robinson H. Monitoring ovarian follicular development with real-time ultrasound. Br J Obstet Gynaecol. 1980;87:613–18.
4. Smith D, Picker R, Sinosich M, et al. Assessment of ovulation by ultrasound and estradiol levels during spontaneous and induced cycles. Fertil Steril. 1980;33:387–90.
5. Renaud R, Macler J, Dervain I, et al. Echographic study of follicular maturation and ovulation during the normal menstrual cycle. Fertil Steril. 1980;33:272–76.
6. Lemay A, Bastide A, Lambert R, et al. Prediction of human ovulation by rapid luteinizing hormone (LH) radioimmunoassay and ovarian ultrasonography. Fertil Steril. 1982;38:194–201.
7. Queenan J, O'Brien G, Bains L, et al. Ultrasound scanning of ovaries to detect ovulation in women. Fertil Steril. 1980;34:99–105.
8. Hackeloes B, Fleming R, Robinson H, et al. Correlation of ultrasonic and endocrine assessment of human follicular development. Am J Obstet Gynecol. 1979;135:122–28.
9. Bryce R, Shuter B, Sinosich M, et al. The value of ultrasound, gonadotropin, and estradiol measurements for precise ovulation prediction. Fertil Steril. 1982;37:42–45.
10. Baird D, Fraser I. Blood production and ovarian secretion rates of estradiol and estrone in women throughout the menstrual cycle. J Clin Endocrinol Metab. 1974;38:1009–17.
11. Buttery B, Trounson A, McMaster R, et al. Evaluation of diagnostic ultrasound as a parameter of follicular development in an in vitro fertilization program. Fertil Steril. 1983;39:458–63.
12. Marinho A, Sallam H, Goessen L, et al. Real time pelvic ultrasonography during the periovulatory period of patients attending an artificial insemination clinic. Fertil Steril. 1982;37:633–38.
13. DeCrespigny L, O'Herlihy C, Robinson H. Ultrasonic observation of the mechanism of human ovulation. Am J Obstet Gynecol. 1981;139:636–39.
14. Wetzels L, Hoogland H. Relation between ultrasonographic evidence of ovulation and hormonal parameters: luteinizing hormone surge and initial progesterone rise. Fertil Steril. 1982;37:336–41.
15. Fleischer A, Rodier J, James A. Sonographic monitoring of ovarian follicular development. J Clin Ultrasound. 1981;9:275–80.
16. Polan M, Totora M, Caldwell B, et al. Abnormal ovarian cycles as diagnosed by ultrasound and serum estradiol levels. Fertil Steril. 1982;37:342–47.
17. Geisthovel F, Skubsch U, Zabel G, et al. Ultrasonographic and hormonal studies in physiologic and insufficient menstrual cycles. Fertil Steril. 1983;39:277–83.
18. Doody MC, Gibbon WE, Buttram VC. Linear regression analysis of ultrasound follicular growth series: evidence of an abnormality of follicular growth in endometriosis patients. Fertil Steril. 1988;49:47–51.
19. Killick S, Eyong E, Elstein M. Ovarian follicular development in oral contraceptive cycles. Fertil Steril. 1987;48:409–13.
20. Ying Y-K, Daly DC, Randolph JF, et al. Ultrasonographic monitoring of follicular growth for luteal phase defects. Fertil Steril. 1987;48:433–36.
21. Hamilton C, Wetzels L, Evan J, et al. Follicle growth curves and hormonal patterns in pa-

tients with the luteinized unruptured follicle syndrome. Fertil Steril. 1985;43:541–48.

22. Daley D, Soto-Albers C, Walter C, et al. Ultra-sonographic assessment of luteinized unruptured follicle syndrome in unexplained infertility. Fertil Steril. 1985;43:62–65.

23. Orsini L, Venturoli S, Lorusso R, et al: Ultra-sonic findings in polycystic ovarian disease. Fertil Steril. 1985;43:709–14.

24. O'Herlihy C, Robinson H. Ultrasound timing of human chorionic gonadotropin administration in clomiphene stimulated cycles. Obstet Gynecol. 1982;59:40–45.

25. Vargyas J, Marrs R, Kletzky O, et al. Correlation of ultrasonic measurement of ovarian follicle size and serum estradiol levels in ovulatory patients following clomiphene citrate for in vitro fertilization. Am J Obstet Gynecol. 1982;144:569–73.

26. Leerentuead R, VanGent I, DerStoep M, et al. Ultrasonographic assessment of Graafian follicle growth under monofollicular and multi-follicular conditions in clomiphene citrate stimulated cycles. Fertil Steril. 1985;43:565–69.

27. Mantzavinos T, Garcia J, Jones H. Ultrasound measurement of ovarian follicle stimulated by human gonadotropins for oocyte recovery and in vitro fertilization. Fertil Steril. 1983;40:461–65.

28. Seibel M, McArdle C, Thompson I, et al. The role of ultrasound in ovulation induction: a critical appraisal. Fertil Steril. 1983;36:573–77.

29. Haning R, Austin C, Kuzma D, et al. Ultrasound evaluation of estrogen monitoring for induction of ovulation with menotropins. Fertil Steril. 1982;37:627–32.

30. Cabau A, Bessis R. Monitoring of ovulation induction with human menopausal gonadotropin and human chorionic gonadotropin by ultrasound. Fertil Steril. 1981;36:178–82.

31. Bryce R, Pickert R, Saunders D. Ultrasound in gonadotropin therapy: a better predictor of ovarian hyperstimulation? Aust NZ J Obstet Gyneaecol. 1981;21:237–39.

32. McArdle C, Seibel M, Hann I, et al. The diagnosis of ovarian hyperstimulation (OHS): the impact of ultrasound. Fertil Steril. 1981;39:464–67.

33. Haning R, Austin C, Carlson I, et al. Plasma estradiol is superior to ultrasound and urinary estriol glucuronide as a predictor of ovarian hyperstimulation during induction of ovulation with menotropins. Fertil Steril. 1983;40:31–36.

34. Lenz S, Lauritsen J. Ultrasonically guided percutaneous aspiration of human follicles under local anesthesia: a new method of collecting oocytes for in vitro fertilization. Fertil Steril. 1982;38:673–77.

35. Wickland M, Nilsson L, Hansson R, et al. Collection of human oocytes by the use of sonography. Fertil Steril. 1983;39:603–08.

36. Gleicher N, Grieberg J, Fullan N, et al. Egg retrieval for in vitro fertilization by sono-graphically controlled vaginal culdecentesis. Lancet. 1983;2:508–09.

37. Seifer DB, Collins RL, Paushter DM, et al. Follicular aspiration: a comparison of an ultrasonic endovaginal transducer with fixed needle guide and other retrieval methods. Fertil steril. 1988;49:462–67.

38. Lavy G, Restrepo-Candelo H, Diamond M, et al. Laparoscopic and transvaginal ova recovery: the effect on ova quality. Fertil Steril. 1988;49:1002–06.

39. Kadar N, Devore G, Romero R. Discriminatory hCG zone: its use in the sonographic evaluation for ectopic pregnancy. Obstet Gynecol. 1981;58:156–61.

5
Use of Clomiphene Citrate for Ovulation Induction

JOSEF BLANKSTEIN

Clomiphene Citrate

Clomiphene citrate (CC) is a nonsteroidal triphenylethylene compound currently used as the first choice of treatment for induction of ovulation in anovulatory or oligoovulatory women. It is suitable in cases in which endogenous gonadotropin secretion is desirable for induction of ovulation. Structurally, it is related to the potent synthetic estrogen diethylstilbestrol. At the recommended doses in humans, CC is an antiestrogen. Although the exact mechanism of action of an antiestrogen is not yet clear, CC binds to multiple target organs through the estrogen receptor machinery (i.e., it competes with estrogens for the receptor binding sites). The threshold of the antiestrogen effects of CC varies among tissue sites and depends on individual tissue estrogen receptor concentrations.

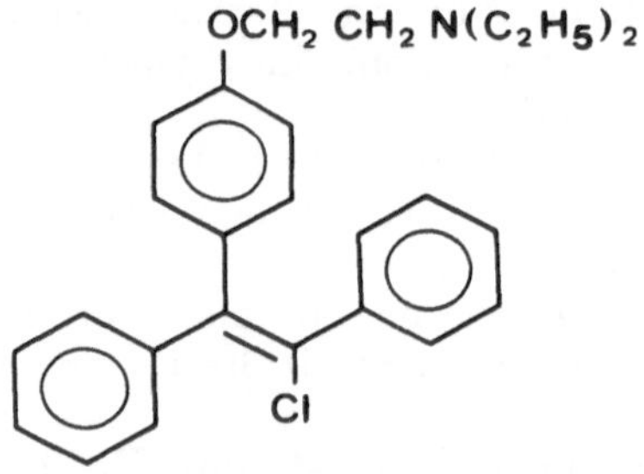

Mode of Action

The stereoscopic configuration of CC is sufficiently similar to that of β-estradiol to compete with it for available estrogen receptor sites in all estrogen-dependent target cells such as the hypothalamus, pituitary, ovary, uterus, and cervical glands (Fig. 5-1).

The mode of action of CC in the induction of ovulation may be tentatively described as follows. "Blinded" by CC molecules occupying the estrogen receptor sites, the hypothalamus and pituitary are unable to perceive

$$OCH_2\ CH_2\ N(C_2H_5)_2$$

clomiphene

FIGURE 5-1. Chemical structure of clomiphene citrate.

correctly the real level of estrogens in the blood. A false message of insufficient estrogen concentration is registered and acted on, resulting in exaggerated secretion of FSH and LH. When CC is administered, there is an early rise in pituitary gonadotropins that is higher and more sustained for LH than FSH.[1,2] The ovarian follicles, in the presence of increased LH levels, produce more estrogens than are synthesized in normal cycles. The estrogen biosynthesis continues to increase markedly after cessation of CC ingestion until a maximum is reached the day before the preovulatory LH surge. Estrogens enhance the pituitary response to pulsatile GnRH from the hypothalamus and increase ovarian sensitivity to gonadotropins. Highly sensitized preovulatory follicles exposed to exaggerated gonadotropic stimulation are thus induced to ovulate. The occupation of hypothalamic estrogen receptors by CC is a time-limited process of rather short duration. A fair chance exists that, by the time ovarian follicles that are stimulated by the CC-induced gonadotropin elevation reach the preovulatory stage, the hypothalamus is already free of CC influence and ready to perceive the correct steroid signal. From this moment on, the events are regulated and controlled by the endogenous feedback mechanisms within the hypothalamic–pituitary–ovarian (HPO) axis.

Metabolism of Clomiphene Citrate

Studies with ^{14}C-labeled CC have indicated that it is readily absorbed after oral administration and is excreted mainly in the feces.[3] The half-life for the administered radioactivity in an oral tracer dose is 5 days. However, the drug is still present in the feces up to 6 weeks after administration, and thus enterohepatic recycling is suspected. Recently, a simple radioreceptor assay suitable for simultaneously measuring CC and active metabolites demonstrated that ligands reached maximal concentration 4 to 5 hours after a single dose of CC was administered, and declined with a half-life of 4.5 to 10 hours. In patients receiving CC on day 5 to day 9 in the cycle, ligands are still present on day 14 in the cycle and in some patients on day 22 of the cycle, but no ligands were detected 60 days after CC treatment[4] (Fig. 5-2).

Antiestrogenic Effects on the Cervix and Endometrium

The antiestrogenic effect of CC may exert an adverse effect on the uterus and the cervix. This detrimental effect, caused by the drug's

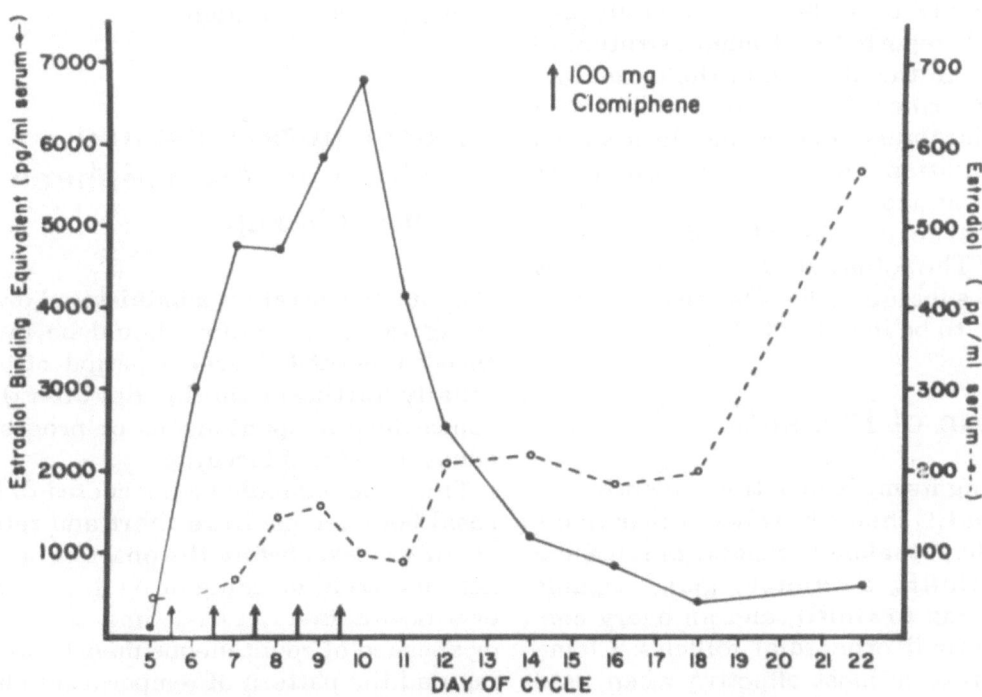

FIGURE 5-2. Serum concentration of estradiol binding equivalent (essentially CC) (●---●) and E_2 (o---o) in an anovulatory menstruating patient during and after 5 days of CC administration (100 mg/day). Each data point represents the mean ± standard error of the mean. From Geier et al.,[4] reproduced with permission of the publisher, The American Fertility Society.

competition for estrogen receptors, is claimed to be one factor responsible for the discrepancy between the ovulation rate (85%) and the pregnancy rate (43%) of women receiving CC treatment.[5] Most investigators report decreased secretion of mucus from the cervical glands caused by antiestrogenic agents such as CC or tamoxifen citrate. The antiestrogenic effect on the cervical mucus, when present, is expressed by a decreased amount of mucus, spinnbarkeit, and ferning, which occurs despite the relatively high levels of estrogens in the circulation. In many patients given CC, the cervical mucus does not exhibit any depressed effects. To understand this phenomenon, we must remember that the antiestrogen effect on the hypothalamus will result in elevated circulating FSH and LH levels. The elevated gonadotropin levels may cause multifollicular development, which, in turn, enhances estrogen production. The elevated estrogen levels, 5 to 10 times higher than in normal cycles, sometimes mask the antiestrogen effect of CC and tamoxifen citrate in the cervix and uterus.[6] Eden et al. reported that administration of CC results in the absence of the normal increase in uterine volume and an inhibition of endometrial thickening around the assumed time of ovulation. This recent study proposes that the antiestrogen effect of CC may inhibit the normal cyclic growth of the endometrium.[7] The potential adverse affect of this finding on subsequent fertility and implantation needs to be investigated.

Selection of Patients

Considering its mode of action, an antiestrogen such as CC should be effective in patients having a hypothalamus capable of releasing pulsatile GnRH, a pituitary gland capable of responding to GnRH, and an ovary containing normal primordial follicles. Clomiphene citrate is most effective when used in patients with hypothalamic–pituitary dysfunction. These patients lack the proper regulation within the HPO axis, but they have some endogenous GnRH secretion and estra-

diol production. These infertile women probably have irregularities in the pulsatile secretion of GnRH, even though they do have fluctuating, detectable levels of gonadotropins and estrogens. They present with various types of menstrual disorders and anovulatory cycles, such as oligomenorrhea, regular or irregular cycles with absent or infrequent ovulation, luteal-phase deficiencies, polycystic ovarian disease (PCO), or amenorrhea with endogenous estrogenic activity. Women with hypothalamic pituitary failure with absent endogenous GnRH and estrogens are generally not responsive to CC.

Age, per se, is not a selection criteria for treatment, since arbitrary limits can wrongly influence treatment decisions in some patients. Ovarian responsiveness, especially in women older than 35, can be predicted on the basis of gonadotropin response to CC stimulation. An augmented FSH response to CC (compared to LH response) was found to be associated with a diminished ovarian reserve, probably because of a reduced capacity of the ovary to secrete inhibin.[8]

Treatment Schema and Monitoring of Clomiphene Citrate Therapy

Clomiphene citrate is administered orally in 50-mg tablets. Therapy should be initiated with 50 mg of CC over a period of 5 days, usually starting on the fifth day after the first appearance of spontaneous or progestin-induced menstrual bleeding.

The patient should be instructed to keep a basal body temperature chart and return in about 4 weeks, before the onset of or during her menstrual bleeding or by day 35, whichever occurs first. At that time, the presence or absence of spontaneous menstrual bleeding and the pattern of temperature changes will suggest whether ovulation has been successfully induced. If ovulation has not occurred, another withdrawal period is induced, and the CC is increased to 100 mg a day, days

5 through 9. The dosage of CC is increased by 50 mg per month each month until ovulation appears to be occurring based on temperature chart and spontaneous menstrual bleeding. If ovulation has occurred, the CC dose should be repeated and should not be increased. In each cycle prior to reinstitution of CC, whether or not ovulation is occurring, a bimanual pelvic examination must be done to exclude ovarian cyst formation. Clomiphene-citrate-induced ovarian cysts resolve spontaneously as long as additional CC is not administered during the subsequent cycle.

Once ovulation appears to be occurring, a premenstrual endometrial biopsy should be done to insure that there is an adequate luteal phase with a receptive endometrium. In addition, a postcoital test (generally scheduled on cycle day 15 or 16 or timed based on ultrasound findings) is performed to ensure that the antiestrogenic effect of CC has not adversely affected the quantity and quality of the cervical mucus. If the mucus has been adversely affected, then ethinyl estradiol, 20 μg, is added from days 9 through 16.

If a woman is ovulating normally and spontaneously, the administration of CC will not increase her fertility. In fact, the antiestrogenic effects of CC on the cervical mucus and endometrium may actually reduce her fertility. Despite the above concerns, Fisch et al.[9] have recently shown that there might be some beneficial effect of treatment with CC in couples with unexplained infertility. However, more prospective experimental studies are needed to prove its effectiveness.

Once an ovulatory dosage of CC has been achieved, postcoital test results are adequate, and an endometrial biopsy indicates normal luteal function, there is a relative contraindication to increase the dose of CC.

Patients who do not respond even to 150 mg of CC or who do not become pregnant with the "ovulating" dose of CC within six treatment cycles should be considered for combination therapies of CC plus hCG. Only if these treatments have failed should patients be considered for gonadotropin therapy.

Moreover, if conception does not occur within four to six ovulatory cycles, other infertility factors should also be excluded. The usual recommendation is that hMG therapy should be considered if conception does not occur within 12 cycles (in the absence of other infertility factors). Recent data suggest switching to hMG even earlier, perhaps at 6 months, with CC conception failure. These same data suggest an accumulation of CC within certain target tissues, such as cervical mucus glands.[10] Therefore, it is quite reasonable to consider changing to hMG at 6 months in patients with CC conception failure whose infertility evaluation is otherwise negative (see Chapter 8).

Clomiphene Citrate and hCG

Whenever the endogenous feedback mechanism responsible for the preovulatory LH surge is not properly activated, the midcycle LH peak may consequently be entirely absent, inadequate, or ill-timed, and hCG should be administered to induce ovulation. Since failure to ovulate on treatment with CC is most commonly caused by failure of folliculogenesis, i.e., an absent ovarian response to an appropriate rise in serum FSH,[11,12] it is not surprising that the pregnancy rate of the CC/hCG regimen has been found disappointing by some authors. To determine when to initiate hCG administration, O'Herlihy[13] used ultrasound scanning to detect the presence of a mature follicle. With this method, he achieved 14 ovulations from 21 previously nonovulatory women. Four of the seven who did not conceive were found by laparoscopy to have endometriosis.

It appears that ultrasound scanning may allow for more precise timing and delivery of hCG and thus produce some improvement in the ovulation rate and pregnancy rate. Premature administration of hCG is deleterious to the developing follicle. If one has the facilities, it might be beneficial to time the hCG administration by ultrasound scanning. In such cases, supplementation of CC therapy with properly timed hCG administration may result in ovulation in these resistant cases.

Clomiphene and hMG

The rationale of CC followed by hMG is to use the former to increase FSH in the initial phase (recruitment and selection) and then to maintain adequate FSH levels by administration of hMG during the follicular growth phase. This method has found wide acceptance in in-vitro fertilization programs and some acceptance in "clomiphene failure" patients prior to putting them through an hMG protocol.

March et al.[14] claimed that by using the combined CC–hMG protocol in normogonadotropic patients, he could reduce the necessary hMG requirement by 50%. Kistner[15] found a pregnancy rate of 28%, and Robertson[16] reported a pregnancy rate of 49%. It is interesting to note that this latter group demonstrated a high level of hyperstimulation, as evidenced by two triplets and three quadruplets in their series. The relatively high multiple-follicular growth rate in Robertson's series has been utilized effectively in in-vitro fertilization programs where the main aim is to obtain a multiplicity of eggs. However, in ovulation induction programs, these findings have negative impact, since one wishes to refrain from excessive multiple follicular development to prevent ovarian hyperstimulation with the development of multiple ovarian cysts and/or multiple pregnancies.

The CC–hMG treatment scheme is as follows: on the fifth through ninth days after induced or spontaneous bleeding, the normogonadotropic patient receives 100 mg of CC daily. From the eighth day onwards hMG is administered. The patient is carefully monitored by estrogen determination and ultrasound visualization of the growing follicle(s). This will help to determine if and when the ovulatory dose of hCG should be administered and to prevent hyperstimulation and multiple pregnancies. When estrogen reaches preovulatory levels in the presence of one or two mature follicles, 10,000 IU of hCG is administered.

Complications of Clomiphene Therapy

Complications of clomiphene therapy may be roughly divided into two groups: (1) untoward effects of ovarian stimulation and induction of ovulation and (2) side effects of the drug itself (Table 5-1). The incidence of severe hyperstimulation syndrome is very rare following clomiphene administration. Ovarian enlargement accompanied by some abdominal pain is, however, quite frequently encountered. Kistner,[17] reviewing treatment records of 5,836 patients treated with clomiphene, found ovarian enlargement in 13.8% of all cases. However, when short-course therapy (not exceeding 7 days) was used, the incidence of ovarian enlargement was reduced to 5.4% in single-course therapy and to 7.8% in multiple-course therapy. Murray[18] encountered painful ovarian enlargement in only two women among the 328 treated with 100–200 mg of CC daily for 4 days. It should be noted that the sensitivity of the ovary may vary from cycle to cycle and that the occurrence of hyperstimulation does not necessarily mean that the ovary will overreact to subsequent treatment cycles. Since the reaction of any patient to clomiphene is unpredictable, it is always advisable to begin with the lowest dose (50 mg daily) and then to increase it gradually in subsequent cycles. Ovarian cysts developing after clomiphene treatment usually resolve spontaneously within a few weeks. During this period clo-

TABLE 5-1. Complications of clomiphene citrate therapy

Ovarian enlargement	14.0%
Abdominal discomfort	8.0%
Hot flashes	10.0%
Nausea, vomiting	2.0%
Breast discomfort	2.0%
Visual disturbance	1.6%
Abnormal uterine bleeding	0.5%
Urticarial dermatitis	0.5%
Weight gain	0.4%
Reversible hair loss	0.3%

miphene should not be administered. One has to remember that combined treatment with clomiphene and hMG may be associated with severe ovarian hyperstimulation syndrome.

Apart from the complications directly related to ovarian stimulation, several side effects of CC due arising from the pharmacological action of the drug on various tissues and organs have been observed. Hot flashes are quite common, appearing in about 10% of the patients. Although resembling those observed during menopause, hot flashes caused by clomiphene are probably not related to the antiestrogenic effect of the drug, since they are not ameliorated by concomitant administration of estrogen. Nausea, vomiting, and breast discomfort occur in about 2% of patients and may be attributed to the relative hyperestrogenism caused by clomiphene. Mild visual disturbances are noted in 1.6%, skin reactions such as dermatitis or urticaria in 0.6%, and reversible hair loss in 0.4%. All of the above side effects are reversible and disappear several days after cessation of clomiphene ingestion.

Is Clomiphene Citrate Teratogenic?

Various studies on large series of patients who delivered after CC treatment do not report a significantly elevated malformation rate. Kurachi[19] compared the malformation rate among the 931 infants born after CC treatment with that of 30,033 infants born with no treatment at the same time of the study. He found no significant differences between groups in the incidence or types of malformation. Since in about two-thirds of DES-exposed offspring some cervical or uterine anomalies have been noted, and since CC is structurally related to DES, CC should be carefully avoided if pregnancy is suspected.

One has to realize that CC and/or metabolites present in blood of patients may affect the metabolism of estrogen-sensitive tissues such as follicular development, cervical gland secretion, and the endometrium preparation

for nidation.[10] Because at ovulation and after nidation elevated amounts of endogenous estrogens are present, it could be assumed that the amounts of CC and/or metabolites present at that time will in most cases not be sufficient to displace the estrogens so as to endanger the oocyte or latter estrogen-sensitive tissues during embryogenesis. Furthermore, regarding the similarity of the CC and DES molecules and the association between intrauterine exposure of the developing fetus to DES and the later occurrence of uterine, cervical, and vaginal anomalies, it is encouraging that no association with CC and/or its metabolites has been found. Final conclusions implicating CC with abnormal cervical development or other defects on organs arising from the Mullerian ducts will have to be delayed until surveys on postpubertal offspring following CC therapy have been concluded.

References

1. Jones GS, Wentz AC, Rosenwaks Z, et al. Dynamic testing of the hypothalamic–pituitary function in abnormalities of ovulation. Am J Obstet Gynecol. 1977;129:760–76.
2. Wu CH: Plasma hormones in clomiphene citrate therapy. Obstet Gynecol. 1977;49:443–48.
3. Schreiber E, Johnson JE, Plotz EJ, et al. Studies with ^{14}C labelled clomiphene citrate. Clin Res. 1966;14:287–89.
4. Geier A, Lunenfeld B, Pariente C, et al. Estrogen receptor binding material in blood of patients after clomiphene citrate administration: determination by a radioreceptor assay. Fertil Steril. 1987;47:778–84.
5. Gysler M, March CM, Mishell DR. A decade's experience with an individualized clomiphene treatment regimen including its effect on the post-coital test. Fertil Steril. 1982;37:161–67.
6. Tepper R, Lunenfeld B, Shalev J, et al. The effect of clomiphene citrate and tamoxifen on the cervical mucus. Acta Obstet Gynecol Scand. 1988;67:311–14.
7. Eden JA, Place J, Carter GD, et al. The effect of clomiphene citrate on follicular phase increase in endometrial thickness and uterine volume. Obstet Gynecol. 1989;73:187–90.

8. Navot D, Rosenwaks Z, Margalioth EJ Prognostic assessment of female fecundity. Lancet. 1987;8560:645–47.

9. Fisch P, Casper RF, Brown SE, et al. Unexplained infertility: evaluation of treatment with clomiphene citrate and human chorionic gonadotropin. Fertil Steril. 1989;51:5:828–33.

10. Mikkelson TJ, Kroboth PD, Cameron WJ, et al. Single-dose pharmacokinetics of clomiphene citrate in normal volunteers. Fertil Steril. 1986;46:392–96.

10. Jacobs HS. Polycystic ovaries and polycystic ovary syndrome. Gynecol Endocrinol. 1987;1:113–31.

12. Polson DW, Kiddy DS, Mason HD, et al. Induction of ovulation with clomiphene citrate in women with polycystic ovary syndrome: the difference between responders and nonresponders. Fertil Steril. 1989;51:30–34.

13. O'Herlihy C, Pepperell RJ, Robinson M. Ultrasound timing of hCG administration in clomiphene stimulated cycles. Obstet Gynecol. 1982;59:40–45.

14. March CM, Tredway DR, Mishell DR. Effect of clomiphene citrate upon amount and duration of human menopausal gonadotropin therapy. Am J Obstet Gynecol 1976;125:699.

15. Kistner RW. Sequential use of clomiphene citrate and human menopausal gonadotropin in ovulation induction. Fertil Steril. 1976;27:72.

16. Robertson S, Birrel W, Grant A. Fewer multiple pregnancies using clomiphene/human gonadotropin sequence. Fertil Steril. 1977;28:294.

17. Kistner RW. Induction of ovulation with clomiphene citrate, In: Behrman SG, Kistner RW, eds. Progress in infertility. Boston: Little, Brown, 1975:509–36.

18. Murray M, Osmond-Clark F. Pregnancy results following treatment with clomiphene citrate. J Obstet Gynaecol Br Commonw. 1971;78:1108.

19. Kurachi K, Aono T, Minagawa J, et al. Congenital malformations of newborn infants after clomiphene induced ovulation. Fertil Steril. 1983;40:187–89.

6
Recent Progress in Gonadotropin Therapy

ROBERT L. COLLINS

Since the induction of ovulation with human pituitary gonadotropins (hPG) was first achieved in 1958,[1] exogenous gonadotropin therapy has been successful in anovulatory infertile women. Ovulation induction using exogenous gonadotropins can be achieved in amenorrheic women with functional ovarian tissue.[2-5] Women with chronic anovulation who fail to ovulate with clomiphene citrate, either alone or with human chorionic gonadotropin (hCG), can also be candidates for treatment.[6-8]

Human menopausal gonadotropin (hMG) is a purified gonadotropin preparation extracted from the urine of postmenopausal women and containing equal amounts of luteinizing hormone (LH) and follicle-stimulating hormone (FSH). This urine extract of hMG (Pergonal, Serono Laboratories) was approved by the Federal Drug Administration for marketing in 1970.

Initially, functional disorders of the pituitary gland causing amenorrhea were successfully treated with exogenous gonadotropins. Now indications for treatment include other types of chronic anovulation,[9,10] luteal-phase defects, cervical factor,[11-13] and idiopathic (unexplained) infertility.[14,15] Exogenous gonadotropins have also been given to normal women to improve follicular stimulation and oocyte harvesting during assisted reproductive technologies.[16-19]

The intramuscular administration of hMG bypasses the pituitary gland, thereby allowing ovulation induction in hypophysectomized women. Early therapeutic trials with human gonadotropins were conducted with both human pituitary gonadotropins (hPG), containing mixtures of FSH and LH in varying proportions derived from pituitaries obtained at autopsy, and hMG. The seemingly unlimited supply of postmenopausal human urine and the limited supply of human pituitaries combined to make hMG the commercially available drug for induction of ovulation.

Historical Overview

The recognition in the mid 1920s that the male and female reproductive systems were under the functional control of the anterior hypophysis continues to be a major endocrinological milestone.[20,21] Significant historic milestones leading to the clinical use of human menopausal gonadotropin were reviewed by Swartz and Jewelewicz.[21] These accomplishments[21-28] are summarized in Table 6-1.

In 1954, Lunenfeld and others demonstrated that kaolin extracts from pooled menopausal urine contained FSH and LH activity in comparable amounts.[25,26] These urinary extracts prevented Leydig cell atrophy and retained complete spermatogenesis in hypophysectomized rats. It was also shown that these extracts were capable of inducing follicular growth and the production of corpora

TABLE 6-1. Historical milestones

Date	Author	Milestone
1927	Smith[22]	Proved gonadotropin-dependent ovarian function
1928	Zondek[20]	Proved gonadotropin-dependent ovarian function
1930	Cole[23]	Isolated pregnant mare gonadotropins
1945	Hamblen[24]	Induced ovulation in women using PMSG[a]
1954	Borth[25,26]	Proved equal urine FSH and LH activity
1958	Gemzell[1]	Induced ovulation with pituitary gonadotropins
1962	Lunenfeld[27]	Ovulation and pregnancy with hMG and hCG
1964	Donini[28]	Purified gonadotropins from menopausal urine

[a] PMSG, pregnant mare serum gonadotropin.

lutea in hypophysectomized rats. In 1958, Gemzell reported on the successful isolation of an FSH-like substance from human pituitary glands that successfully resulted in ovulation in three of five patients.[1] Later in 1961, Borth et al. showed that urinary extracts were successful in stimulating ovarian tissues in the human.[29] The latter discoveries led to the development of commercial preparations by pharmaceutical companies for clinical use.

Metabolism

The structures of FSH and LH have been determined and LH was recently synthesized using recombinant DNA techniques. These glycoproteins have molecular weights of around 30,000, and they contain about 20% carbohydrate. Highly purified human FSH and LH have been prepared from human pituitaries and urine, and hCG has also been prepared from human pregnancy urine.

Purified preparations of human FSH, LH, and hCG injected intravenously into humans had serum half-lives of 183 to 193 minutes, 42 to 60 minutes, and 8 hours respectively.[30] The higher carbohydrate content of hCG is responsible for its significantly longer half-life, as the removal of sialic acid reduces its half-life when compared to LH, and bioavailability. A hybridized hCG compound has been used successfully to induce ovulation and ovum release in women receiving hMG initially.[31]

Folliculogenesis

Gonadotropins derived from pituitary glands or extracted from postmenopausal urine have identical stimulatory effects on the ovary and give similar results. They both contain varying quantities and ratios of FSH and LH. Current dogma suggests that both FSH and LH are required to stimulate folliculogenesis and result in ultimate ovulation. According to the two-cell theory, FSH is necessary for the recruitment of the follicles and stimulation of the granulosa cells and is most likely responsible for the selection of the dominant follicle.[32] Luteinizing hormone stimulates the thecal cells to produce androgens, which are subsequently aromatized to estrogens by granulosa cells under the influence of FSH stimulation. This synergistic action of FSH and LH results in rising estrogen levels within the follicular fluid. These estrogens in turn influence the rate of follicular growth and the differentiation of follicular cells through the stimulation of gonadotropin receptor synthesis. Ovulation results when appropriate physiological ratios of FSH and LH are secreted from the pituitary gland. The pituitary gland is dependent on the pulsatile delivery of gonadotropin-releasing hormone (GnRH) from the hypothalamus. Significant alterations of either pulsatile GnRH secretion or pituitary gonadotropin secretion patterns will result in anovulation. Abnormal gonadotropin pulsatility can cause excessive circulating LH, which will lead to elevated androgens and the creation of an androgenic milieu. This androgenic environment promotes follicular atresia and it is not conducive to normal folliculogenesis. This condition is most commonly seen in polycystic ovarian disease (PCO). Since most gonadotropic preparations contain varying ratios of FSH and LH, ovulation can be achieved in most circumstances.

The administration of hMG can override normal ovulatory mechanisms for ovarian folliculogenesis, as evidenced by the use of these agents in normogonadotropic women undergoing in vitro fertilization treatments. The timing of the administration of gonadotropins is critical. Significantly more follicles are recruited and selected if hMG is administered earlier in the follicular phase.[30,33] Therefore, the number of follicles recruited and selected is dependent on the timing of hMG administration and the FSH content of the gonadotropin preparation.[18,34]

Luteinizing hormone continues to determine the steroidogenic pattern and the final maturation of the dominant follicle. Subsequent ovulation is induced by a surge of spontaneous LH activity (after adequate exposure of the pituitary gland to estrogens) or by the administration of an LH-like material such as hCG. Since the occurrence of a spontaneous endogenous LH surge is infrequent during gonadotropin therapy,[35] two different exogenous gonadotropin preparations are usually required for successful induction of ovulation. Luteinizing hormone or hCG is necessary for ovulation to occur after hMG-induced follicular growth and, more importantly, for the maintenance of the corpus luteum.[36-43] The corpus luteum is dependent on continued LH or hCG support, and without the luteotropic effects of hCG or LH, a truncation of menstrual cycle length is observed. Short luteal-phase duration, premature menstruation, and early pregnancy wastage occur without the provision of continued luteotropic support. This codependency led to the now widely used combination of hMG and hCG for follicular stimulation.

The recent availability of a product containing essentially pure FSH (LH selectively removed) has led to new insights into the physiology of folliculogenesis. In contrast to current dogma, which suggest that both FSH and LH are equally important in inducing ovulation, "pure FSH" has been capable of inducing folliculogenesis in monkeys receiving a GnRH antagonist[44] and in women. Luteinizing hormone is still required for successful ovulation and the development and maintenance of the corpus luteum. However, this experiment[44] and others[34] demonstrate the relative unimportance of LH initially during folliculogenesis when compared to FSH.

Urinary extracts contain equal proportions of both LH and FSH; rarely, variations in bioavailability occur.[45] By using anti-hCG antibodies to cause adsorption of LH onto gel columns, a highly purified FSH fraction was eluted from extracts of hMG. This purified urinary FSH extract was not made available for clinical investigations until the late 1970s. For the first time patients with excessive LH levels and relatively deficient FSH states could theoretically be candidates for FSH therapy.

Pure FSH has been used successfully to induced ovulation in PCO,[46,47] in patients with chronic anovulation resistant to clomiphene citrate,[48] and occasionally in patients with gonadotropin deficiencies.[49] Initial clinical studies using the preparation showed that purified FSH preparations were not as useful in severe hypothalamic amenorrhea, as some LH activity (endogenous or exogenous) is critical for stromal production of androgenic precursors that are necessary for estrogen production. This is in contrast to the previously referenced study suggesting the relative unimportance of endogenous LH production.[44] However, anovulatory patients with endogenous gonadotropins, such as those with polycystic ovarian disease, had very adequate responses to the pituitary FSH preparations. The high endogenous levels of LH made it unnecessary to add more LH to the same degree as it is found in hMG. However, hCG was still required as an ovulatory trigger because the spontaneous endogenous LH surge was also noted to be an infrequent event in patients receiving FSH.[46]

Despite the limited clinical trials to date, some conclusions can be made. Pure FSH tends to be less efficient in inducing ovulation in patients without endogenous LH (hypothalamic amenorrhea), and exogenous LH is required for follicular maturation and ovum release. Patients with adequate LH in circulation respond to pure FSH; however, hyperstimulation appears to be of greater concern in these individuals. Ovarian hyperstimulation has been shown to occur with intermediate dosages of FSH, even without hCG.[46] Additional clinical trials and studies to refine the dosage and duration of FSH usage will enhance the effectiveness and safety of this preparation for the treatment of anovulation in patients with relative FSH deficiency and LH excess, as in conditions such as polycystic ovarian disease.

Patient Selection

Ideal candidates for ovulation induction with the combination of hMG and hCG have functional ovarian tissue but have low endogenous gonadotropin secretion patterns and are amenorrheic or anovulatory (Table 6-2). These types of patients (i.e., normoprolactinemic eugonadotropic anovulation or hypogonadotropic hypogonadism) are also candidates for pulsatile GnRH treatment (Chapter 7).[50,51]

All patients should undergo a basic infer-

TABLE 6-2. Clinical indications for hMG–hCG therapy

Hypothalamic amenorrhea
Hypogonadotropic hypogonadism
Anovulation (clomiphene citrate failure)
Luteal-phase defects
Cervical factor
Timing artificial insemination
Unexplained infertility
Follicular development during IVF[a]

---

[a] In vitro fertilization.

tility investigation and be screened to rule out other causes of infertility. Evaluations should exclude other causes of amenorrhea and anovulation treatable by other direct means, such as hyperprolactinemia. Patients with hyperprolactinemia, either idiopathic or secondary to small pituitary microadenomas, can be considered candidates for hMG–hCG therapy if they were unresponsive or intolerant to primary therapy, such as bromocriptine.[52-54]

Prior to treatment, it is necessary to document the presence of functional ovarian follicles. Women who are responsive to a progesterone challenge, who present clinically with severe oligomenorrhea or amenorrhea, are presumed to have endogenous estrogen secretion and, therefore, to have functioning follicles. Women with either primary or secondary amenorrhea who do not have uterine bleeding after progesterone administration are presumed to be estrogen deficient, and these patients should have further evaluation. Measurement of serum FSH level is indicated. Elevated FSH concentration (hypergonadotropic hypogonadism) is consistent with ovarian failure, and these women are usually not candidates for treatment with ovulatory drugs. There are rare instances where exogenous gonadotropins are reported to have induced ovulation in hypergonadotropic hypogonadal patients with suspected premature ovarian failure or resistant ovary syndrome (Savage syndrome).[55,56]

Pretreatment studies should include a semen analysis to verify that the male does not have severe oligospermia, azoospermia, or another gross abnormality. The uterine and tubal factors should be investigated by hysterosalpingogram (HSG) and/or hysteroscopy. Diagnostic laparoscopy with chromopertubation should be done prior to initiation of treatment to assess completely and possibly treat tubal and peritoneal factors. These pretreatment procedures will serve to insure that absolute factors do not exist and multiple causes of infertility are not present. Although multifactorial infertility is not a contraindication to treatment, the chance for successful conception is reduced in such patients, and the couple should be afforded a realistic prognosis based on accurate information.

Extensive counseling of the couple regarding side effects, risks, expenses, logistics of treatment, and prognosis should be done before therapy. Counseling should be based on scientific and factual data. Duration of treatment should be discussed beforehand. They should be advised that the chance of conceiving in any one course is approximately 25%, and the average number of treatment courses needed to achieve a pregnancy is three. Overall, 60% of couples conceive within 6 months, with a smaller percentage between 6 and 9 months.[30] Cumulative pregnancy rates determined by life table analysis provide a more accurate assessment of treatment efficacy.

Patients who are clomiphene failures (both conception and ovulatory failures) may also be candidates for hMG therapy. Patients who ovulate on clomiphene alone or clomiphene plus hCG with normal prolactin concentration should be given at least a 6-month trial before choosing hMG. Clomiphene therapy can continue as long as normal luteal phases are documented on the treatment protocol by endometrial biopsy and no other adverse antiestrogenic effects of clomiphene citrate exist. Euprolactinemic women failing to ovulate on clomiphene plus hCG with normal semen analysis, HSG, and laparoscopy can be offered a trial of hMG–hCG therapy for induction of ovulation.

The successful use of hMG plus hCG in women with cervical-factor infertility after failed conventional therapy has been reported.[11-13] Despite the fact that hMG–hCG can also be associated with induction of a luteal-phase defect, hMG–hCG stimulation protocols have also been used to correct a preexisting luteal-phase defect (LPD).[57] In using hMG plus hCG for luteal-phase defect, Zimmerman reports a pregnancy rate of only 14.8% with a miscarriage rate of approximately 36%. Hyperstimulation syndrome occurred in 35% of cycles receiving hMG plus hCG for luteal-phase defect.[58]

Unexplained (idiopathic) infertility[15] is another indication for hMG plus hCG. Recently, a trial of controlled superovulation with hMG plus hCG in combination with intrauterine insemination (IUI) has been advocated in couples with unexplained infertility. Pregnancy rates comparable to gamete intrafollicular transfer have been reported (GIFT procedure).[59] We have used a similar protocol for couples who have completed evaluation and have the diagnosis of unexplained infertility. We attempt controlled superovulation combined with IUI therapy prior to in vitro fertilization (IVF) in couples previously demonstrating successful fertilization during IVF therapies who did not become pregnant.

Pregnancy rates that approach the fecundity of normal women and that equal or exceeds pregnancy rates reported for IVF and GIFT have been reported.[59] If the rationale for GIFT is the delivery of increased numbers of gametes at the site of fertilization in normal fallopian tubes, then the combination of hMG–hCG superovulation and IUI will accomplish that goal without the expense and risk of operative intervention. Cycle fecundities of 0.17 for endometriosis, 0.29 for cervical factor, and 0.19 for idiopathic infertility have been reported and seem to justify the expense and risks of controlled superovulation and IUI.[59] The major criticism of that study was its uncontrolled and retrospective analysis of cases. Prospective, controlled comparisons of IVF, GIFT, and superovulation with IUI are still lacking. Nonetheless, the data suggest that the provision of multiple gametes and/or the correction of subtle ovulatory dysfunction may be the mechanism(s) of improved fertilization and pregnancy rates seen.

Clinical Monitoring

Proper monitoring is mandatory to optimize benefits and minimize risks. Without proper monitoring, hMG may cause severe adverse reactions including superovulation, multiple pregnancy, and the ovarian hyperstimulation syndrome (OHSS). Early experiences with induction of ovulation with human gonadotropins demonstrated the dual risk of OHSS and the occurrence of multiple gestations.

Clinical Examination

The clinical assessment of early investigators utilized careful assessment of cervical mucus production and the monitoring of preovulatory ovarian sizes by pelvic examination. However, it became apparent that significant variations in responsive cervical mucus production among the individuals existed. A major source of this difficulty also lay in the fact that the cervical mucus response was insensitive to subtle estrogen changes and maximum at the estrogen concentrations that optimized the pregnancy rate. There was no room for increased response to signal ovarian hyperstimulation.

The detection of preovulatory ovarian enlargement by pelvic examination was the only other parameter available to signal hyperstimulation. The imprecision of the bimanual examination limited its ability to predict accurately the development of OHSS. Also, a lack of ovarian enlargement did not exclude the hyperstimulation syndrome. Because of the limitations of the clinical parameters experienced by earlier investigations, their use alone today for the purpose of monitoring ovarian response is inappropriate. Nonetheless, cervical mucus scoring continues to provide important adjunctive information relative to the patient's response and sperm survivability.

Serum Estradiol

Data indicating successful use of 24-hour serial urinary estrogen determinations for monitoring ovulation induction were published by Taymor.[60] Urinary determinations of estradiol, estrone, estriol, and pregnanediol have all been used to monitor the ovarian response in the past. The determination of a specific estrogen was not found to be superior to the determination of the total urinary estrogen secretion. An optimal excretion rate of total urinary estrogen was determined to be 50 to 60 μg per day, with the upper safe limits of total urinary estrogens being variably established as being between 100 and 150 μg per day.[61] The above estrogen ranges are consistent with maximum conception rates, and the incidence of hyperstimulation and multiple births is reduced. There is no significant effect of injection time on the urinary estrogen result as along as the injections are given once daily.

Difficulties in patients collecting complete 24-hour samples and determining 24-hour urinary total estrogens led many investigators to try radioimmunoassay of plasma estradiol when this method first became available. Because plasma estradiol was determined on a single sample of blood, the timing of the sampling in relation to the previous injection of gonadotropin became a critical variable. A study of the plasma estradiol concentrations over the 24-hour period following injection of the gonadotropins demonstrated that although the 24-hour plasma estradiol value correlated with the level of ovarian stimulation, plasma estradiol concentrations were maximum in the 8- to 10-hour postinjection interval.[62] At midcycle, in normal ovulatory women, the serum estradiol concentration is between 200 and 400 pg/mL.[63] It was recognized that higher levels of estradiol were necessary to increase the probability of conception, and Tredway concluded that the rate of ovulation could be increased by raising the range of estradiol from 500 to 1,000 pg/mL.[64] Associated with these higher plasma estradiol levels were increased rates of ovulation, and pregnancy rates but also ovarian hyperstimulation syndrome. Despite later experiments, no uniformity of range has been established, and there has been a tendency to allow higher levels of estrogen prior to hCG. This can be accomplished when ultrasound is also used to follow follicular development.

Consequently, the estrogen level above which hCG is withheld to minimize the development of ovarian hyperstimulation syndrome (OHSS) has also varied greatly (from greater than 500 to greater that 2,000 pg/mL.).[64–66] An excellent review of estradiol monitoring was recently published by Diamond.[35]

Ovarian Ultrasound for Follicular Sizes

The addition of follicular ultrasound scanning to the clinical monitoring protocol has allowed the use of hMG in a safer environment. Difficult patients can be pushed harder, and extremely brittle patients with rapid estradiol rises can be monitored more accurately with ultrasound. Improvements in ultrasound equipment and the development of vaginal probes with superior imaging qualities have yielded exquisite details of follicular development.

Ultrasound has been used to observe follicular growth during normal menstrual cycles[67] and also during gonadotropin treatments.[68,69] Follicular growth was noted to be linear during the ultrasonic examination, and there appeared to be strong correlations between follicular growth and estradiol measurements.[68-75] Furthermore, it became possible to observe development of multiple follicles and to assess the risk of multiple gestations or the occurrence of OHSS. Sonographic visualization may also be used to discriminate between single and multiple follicular growth and may therefore aid in clarifying the source of estradiol. Since prevailing evidence suggests that follicles with diameters between 17 and 22 mm will ovulate, then sonography may be a more precise predictor of the subsequent development of OHSS and become a more precise indicator for determining the time of hCG administration to cause ovum release.[69,72] Ultrasonic monitoring of follicular growth during ovulation induction is discussed in greater detail in Chapter 4.

Ultrasound has also been used to document and observe morphological changes in the cervix,[76] the endometrial cavity, and the endocervical canal during ovulation induction.[77] It should be emphasized that ultrasonography should not replace serum estradiol determinations. Ultrasound scanning of follicular growth is complementary to estradiol data. Serum estradiol levels coupled with cervical mucus evaluations and ultra-sonic findings will provide the most information on each individual's ovarian response and subsequent risks for OHSS.

Typical Treatment Cycle

Each patient responds uniquely and individually to hMG. Although multiple hMG dosages and treatment schedules have been advocated in the past and recently described in an excellent review article by Diamond,[35] only the individualized regimen can be considered the most commonly used dosage schedule (Table 6-3). The amount of medication and the duration of therapy vary not only in different patients but also from one treatment cycle to another within the same patient. Therefore, it is imperative to monitor the patient carefully each cycle to determine when a mature follicle is present, give hCG, and assess risks of OHSS.

The timing of hMG and hCG injections and the subsequent timing of blood drawing are important and critical to the success of ovulation induction. If urinary estrogens are to be monitored, then the timing of injections is less critical. If morning plasma sampling and morning injections are to be done, then a plasma estradiol window of 500 to 1000 pg/mL in the serum should be used. Ideally, a window of 600 to 800 pg/mL is optimum. If morning plasma sampling and injections between 5 and 9 p.m. are utilized, then a window of 1000 to 2000 pg/mL of plasma estradiol is recommended.[35] As noted above, the timing of plasma sampling is critical to the timing of injections of hMG.

The patient is usually begun on two am-

TABLE 6-3. Dosage schedules for hMG

1. Level
2. Gradual increase
3. Intermittent therapy
4. Initial step-up, then step-down
5. Sequential estrogen–hMG–hCG
6. Individualized based on response
7. Sequential clomiphene–hMG–hCG
8. Sequential GnRH agonist–hMG–hCG

pules of hMG (75 IU of both FSH and LH per ampule) daily very early in the follicular phase or after a progestin-induced menstrual period. A systematic flow sheet or a plot of the logarithm of the plasma estradiol versus linear days is very useful in following the ovulatory response to hMG as well as predicting the day of hCG injection. Extremely slow rises or no rise of serum estradiol indicate that the dose of hMG should be increased in increments and that these incremental rises should be maintained a minimum of 72 hours prior to further increases. Ideally, one should aim for a follicular length of approximately 9–12 days. Pregnancy rates are extremely low in patients given hCG before day 6.[35]

Follicular development should be monitored with frequent ultrasound studies. Ultrasound plays a critical role in assessing response to hMG and timing hCG administration. A baseline ultrasound scan is suggested in early follicular phase to determine the presence or absence of persistent follicles. When a significant increase in the estradiol level occurs, ultrasound imaging should be repeated every 2 to 3 days. Scanning should become more frequent when the follicle reaches 14 mm or greater. When a follicle 18 mm or greater is identified, hMG is discontinued, and hCG is given 24 hours later to cause ovum release. Usually 10,000 units of hCG is given to trigger ovulation. To maintain corpus luteum function, a supplemental dose of 5,000 units of hCG is given approximately 5 days after the initial ovumrelease injection. Some prefer multiple small injections of hCG (1,500 IU every 3 days) or progesterone suppositories for luteotropic support. If there are signs of ovarian enlargement or tenderness, the supplemental dosage of hCG (5,000 IU) is withheld.

In addition to the monitoring of estradiol levels and follicular ultrasound, patients are examined during each visit and before receiving hCG. Only mucus assessment is done. Ovarian size and growth are monitored more accurately and less traumatically by serial ultrasound and not bimanual examinations.

Bimanual examinations to determine ovarian size are imprecise and potentially damaging to enlarged ovaries. Lubricating gels should be avoided during examinations because they are spermicidal, and they can become a physical barrier to the cervix. A water-based gel can be utilized for vaginal ultrasonography, and patients are instructed on douching to remove the gel when ultrasounds are performed near the day of hCG administration.

The cervical score is determined during each visit, and a postcoital test can be done when appropriate. If the cervical mucus is scanty or the sperm survival is inadequate, then artificial inseminations are usually performed with the husband's semen and carefully timed for approximately 36 hours after the trigger hCG dosage is given. This can be accomplished either with cervical cup or by intrauterine insemination techniques.

The patient with a normal cervical factor is then instructed to have intercourse on the night of hCG injection and on the following two nights minimally. After hCG, she is instructed to record her weight every other day, and any total weight gain of 10 lbs or more or 5 lb in 24 hours is to be reported.

A serum pregnancy test is obtained approximately 16 to 20 days following the initial hCG injection if no menstrual bleeding has occurred. If the patient's hCG is positive, then ultrasound should be obtained 4 weeks (6 weeks of amenorrhea) following hCG injection to determine the number and location of fetuses present. This timely ultrasound allows for the early recognition of the multiple fetuses and gives time to plan for special care necessary for these high-risk pregnancies.

Ectopic pregnancies can also be diagnosed early by ultrasound, before tubal rupture and damage. Early recognition of ectopic gestations will allow for outpatient laparoscopic management and enhance opportunities for conservative surgical procedures to preserve the functional capacity of the fallopian tube. A typical treatment course is presented in Table 6-4.

TABLE 6-4. A typical hMG–hCG treatment protocol[a]

Baseline E_2[b] and ultrasound
Initiate therapy by cycle day 3
Individualized /graduated dosage
E_2 and scan every 2 to 3 days
Daily E_2 and scan when follicle > 14 mm
Cervical score
Postcoital test when appropriate
Continue scans until leading follicle > 18 mm
10,000 units hCG 24 hours after last hMG
Supplemental 5,000 hCG 5 days later
IUI[c] 36 hours after hCG (if necessary)
Serum hCG in 14 days
Scan 4 weeks after ovulation if pregnant

[a] Modified from March.[103]
[b] E_2, estradiol.
[c] IUI, intrauterine insemination.

Clinical Results

The results of a survey of several large series of patients receiving gonadotropin therapy from several institutions indicate that gonadotropin therapy is successful, and it has become widely accepted.[2–5,30,35] One survey included approximately 12,619 treatment cycles given to approximately 5,000 patients and resulting in more than 2,100 pregnancies.[30] The precise interpretation of the overall pregnancy rate for this series was difficult because of uncontrolled confounding variables. Consequently, a precise prognosis could not be given based on data obtained in that series. Blankstein reported the results of their series of patients undergoing gonadotropin therapy.[30]

Based on a simple classification of Insler,[78] patients were divided into two groups. Patients were either hypothalamic pituitary failure (group I) or patients with hypothalamic pituitary dysfunction (group II). Group I patients were hypoestrogenic and characterized by low or absent endogenous GnRH pulsatility. Group II patients had some endogenous GnRH pulsatility, albeit aberrant or dysfunctional. They were also estrogenized

and progestin responsive. Patients with clomiphene failure were more likely to be placed in group II.

The results of these series summarized by Blankstein showed a higher ovulatory and pregnancy rate in group I subjects. Of the 279 patients in group I, an 82% conception rate occurred in those patients receiving hMG–hCG treatments. The cumulative pregnancy rate for patients of group I was stated to be 91.2% after six cycles of treatment, and this is approximately 30% higher than the cumulative pregnancy rate in the normal nulliparous population. In contrast, of the 117 patients with hypothalamic pituitary dysfunction who failed to conceive following clomiphene citrate (group II), the pregnancy rate following hMG plus hCG was only 21.4%, and the ovulation rate was significantly less at 42%. Consequently, in their hands the success rates were 60.6% in group I versus 11.5% in group II in terms of the percentage of people who took home at least one living child. The mean number of ampules of hMG likewise differed between groups, being 40.0 for group I and 18.2 in group II patients.[30] In the patients who conceived, 94% did so within five cycles of treatment.

These findings all suggest that in patients with endogenous gonadotropin pulsatility, there exists greater patient variability, and they tend to be more difficult in management. This group also had a higher risk of ovarian hyperstimulation and treatment cancellation.

The poorer performance of patients in group II who have hypothalamic pituitary dysfunction led investigators to consider the use of GnRH agonists to create a temporary functional hypophysectomy to reduce circulating LH and to mimic the group I pituitary-failure patient. By abolishing the endogenous source of gonadotropin pulsatility, the investigator hoped to achieve a more uniform patient response and reduce individual variability and consequently reduce the risk of ovarian hyperstimulation. This subject is addressed in the section under ovulation for PCO.

Endocrine Consequences of hMG–hCG Therapy

Abnormal FSH/LH Ratio

Healy described the gonadotropic milieu presiding over the recruitment and selection of follicles during gonadotropin-induced ovulation in patients receiving human pituitary gonadotropin therapy (hPG).[79] These patients were clinically responsive with apparently normal ovulation and were without evidence of ovarian hyperstimulation. Gonadotropin therapy resulted in abnormally high circulating FSH levels during the follicular phase and an abnormal FSH/LH ratio. A marked increase in serum prolactin was seen before ovulation in patients receiving gonadotropins. This increase in serum prolactin was felt to be secondary to a synergy between circulating estrogens and progesterone. He concluded that excessive FSH levels and the elevated FSH/LH ratio orchestrated aberrant folliculogenesis, resulting in most of the clinical problems associated with gonadotropin therapies such as multiple ovulation and hyperstimulation.

Short Luteal Phases

Short luteal phases with luteal-phase lengths of 11 days or less have been reported to occur in approximately 18% of patients receiving hMG therapy.[80] Although luteal-phase defects have been well described in both spontaneous and clomiphene-induced cycles, it is less well described in patients receiving gonadotropin therapy. These short-luteal-phase cycles were associated with low hCG concentrations after exogenous hCG administration or peak preovulatory estradiol levels of 2,000 μg/mL or less than 200 μg/mL. This study suggests that both serum levels of hCG and estradiol values determine the normality of luteal phase length and function.

Blockade of Spontaneous LH Surge

It is now acceptable practice to administer exogenous hMG plus hCG to endocrinologic-

TABLE 6-5. Endocrine consequences of ovarian hyperstimulation

Abnormal FSH/LH ratio
Blockade of LH surge
Hyperprolactinemia
Premature luteinization
Short luteal phases
Follicular atresia/dyssynchrony
Heterogeneity of estradiol responses

ally normal women undergoing in vitro fertilization therapies. The primate served as an excellent model to study the endocrine consequences of a fixed-dose hMG administration protocol.[81] The endocrine consequences of prolonged ovarian hyperstimulation include (1) hyperprolactinemia in the luteal phase, (2) follicular atresia of growing follicles when timely hCG administration was withheld, (3) premature progesterone secretion and subsequent luteinization, (4) a heterogeneity of ovarian responses, and (5) the infrequent occurrence of a spontaneous LH surge (Table 6-5).

Blockade of the expected estrogen-induced spontaneous LH surge during hMG therapy is commonplace, and a surrogate LH surge, by way of hCG, is necessary to induce ovum release. This blockade is secondary to a yet unidentified factor that is highly immunogenic and presumably secreted from the ovaries.[82-84]

Follicular Atresia

Timely administration of hCG may be necessary to sustain viable follicles and the secretory potential of subsequent corporal lutea as well as to obtain oocytes competent for fertilization. Premature administration of hCG is deleterious to the developing follicle, yet delayed administration will result in postmature follicles receiving hCG. These postmature follicles will luteinize and fail to fertilize.

In the primate, it was demonstrated that estrogens promptly declined when hCG was not administered in a timely fashion.[81] This is critically important. Clinically, the pregnancy rate is noted to decline during fixed-dose administration regimens when hCG is given prior to 9 days or after 12 days of hMG administration. Pregnancy rates also decline during IVF therapy when hCG is delayed.[85]

Premature Luteinization

Premature luteinization occurred in a significant number of primates and is commonly seen in women. Although it was felt originally to be secondary to the LH content of the hMG, premature luteinization has been seen in patients receiving pure FSH therapies. Luteinization may be secondary to an attenuated endogenous LH surge. These subtle LH elevations may induce significant progesterone secretion by luteinizing the most advanced follicle that is latent with LH receptors on its granulosa cells. Luteinization precludes successful fertilization. Cervical mucus, endometrium, and tubal epithelium may also be adversely affected by premature luteinization. When documented clinically, patients usually respond to a combination regimen of GnRH agonist initially to completely remove endogenous LH secretion, followed by hMG therapy.

Hyperprolactinemia

Hyperprolactinemia has been observed in the primate and in women receiving gonadotropin therapy.[79,81] It has also been associated with ovarian hyperstimulation. It is secondary to a prolonged estrogen–progesterone synergy effect on the pituitary lactotrope. Despite increasing evidence that exogenous gonadotropin therapy enhances prolactin secretion in the human,[79] few data exist on the possible adverse effects or the potential diagnostic value of this transient condition. Further studies are warranted to clarify whether fertility is compromised by transient hyperprolactinemia or whether this may be the leading cause of early first-trimester losses experienced following hMG- plus hCG-induced ovulation.

Complications

A major complication of the use of hMG is the occurrence of ovarian hyperstimulation syndrome (OHSS). All complications of gonadotropin therapy are essentially related to the degree of ovarian stimulation during the induction of ovulation. Fortunately, with careful clinical, ultrasonographic, and biochemical monitoring, the severity and frequency of occurrence of complications can be reduced significantly. By controlling the degree of ovarian stimulation, the other complications of multiple pregnancy and pregnancy wastage can likewise be theoretically reduced. There are no published ovulation induction stimulation protocols that reduce the risk of ovarian hyperstimulation to zero.

Ovarian Hyperstimulation

Ovarian hyperstimulation syndrome is a major complication of hMG–hCG therapy.[86-93] The clinical presentation is quite variable. The syndrome is characterized by ovarian enlargement, ascites, hydrothorax, electrolyte imbalance, hypovolemia, and oliguria. In the severe forms, hemoconcentration, increased viscosity of blood, thromboembolic phenomena, and hypovolemic shock may occur, and death may ensue.

The incidence of ovarian hyperstimulation syndrome ranges from 3% to 23% for the mild form and from 0.4% to 4% for the severe and potentially lethal form.[35,86,87]

Three degrees of ovarian hyperstimulation have been suggested by Jewelewicz, and a modified version is reproduced here.[21]

Mild hyperstimulation. A feeling of bloating and lower abdominal discomfort. The ovaries are slightly enlarged but are no more than 5 × 5 cm. There is no marked weight gain.

Moderate hyperstimulation. More of a feeling of bloating and lower abdominal discomfort. The ovaries are enlarged up to 10 × 10 cm. There is some ascites, and weight gain is up to 10 lbs.

Severe hyperstimulation. The ovaries are extremely enlarged and easily palpated abdominally. Ascites, plural effusion, oliguria, hemoconcentration, hypertension, azotemia, and electrolyte imbalance occur. Increased blood coagulability and weight gain of more than 10 lbs are found.

According to that classification, Schenker and Weinstein reported mild hyperstimulation occurring in 8.4% to 23% of treatment cycles, moderate hyperstimulation in 6% to 7%, and severe in 0.8% to 2% of cycles.[87] The OHSS can usually be avoided when hCG is withheld, even in the presence of extremely high estrogen levels (Table 6-6).

The pathogenesis of OHSS is not entirely clear, but it is felt to be secondary to the acute hyperestrogenism and rapid fluid shifts. Ovarian hyperstimulation syndrome is associated with massive luteinization of the follicles and rarely occurs if hCG is withheld. However, hCG alone does not cause hyperstimulation. Both hMG and hCG must be administered. The increased capillary permeability associated with OHSS leads to hypovolemia, hemoconcentration, and decreased renal profusion, which together lead to a hypercoagulable state. Salt retention is also exacerbated by aldosterone secretion. Management involves careful monitoring of fluid and electrolytes. It is important to follow the hematocrit, since a fall in hematocrit may signal intraabdominal hemorrhage, and an increase in hematocrit seen in the early phase

is a good parameter for following the process of hemoconcentration. Optimal care lies in the prevention of the syndrome.

For mild to moderate OHSS, no specific therapy is necessary. Patients should be monitored for rapid increases in weight gain over 24 hours. There is a strong correlation among the total estrogen level, rate of estrogen rise,[88] degree of follicular development (total number and size of follicles),[90] and the subsequent development OHSS.

Navot et al.[88] investigated risk factors and prognostic variables in the development of OHSS. Significantly higher levels of estradiol and prolactin were seen in the follicular phase in the treatment group when compared to controls. Also, there was a tendency for greater follicular recruitment with significantly more smaller follicles (12 to 14 mm) present on day zero in all grades of OHSS. Out of 22 variables identified, an increased risk is seen in the young, lean patient. Using a mathematical model for the prediction of ovarian hyperstimulation, the authors in the above study suggested that three parameters (age, estradiol level on day zero, and basal prolactin levels) had a combined predicted value that could not be improved with additional parameters. A proposed clinical profile of the patient at the greatest risk for development of the syndrome is young, lean, receiving few ampules of hMG, with rapidly increasing estradiol levels, who subsequently develops multiple small follicles.[88]

Therapy for moderate to severe hyperstimulation requires hospitalizion and active management. Patients should be on bed rest with avoidance of pelvic examinations until the size of the ovaries decreases. Baseline and serial blood chemistry profiles and coagulation studies should be performed. Treatment is directed at maintaining vital signs, correction of electrolyte imbalances, and maintenance of adequate hydration. Patients who become severely oliguric or anuric require renal hemodialysis. Careful intake and output balance should be kept to prevent over hydration. Only fluid lost should be replaced.

In situations where the fluid status cannot

TABLE 6-6. The incidence of OHSS after hMG–hCG therapy[a]

Authors	Number of treatment cycles	Mild OHSS (%)	Severe OHSS (%)
Brown	222	3.2	?
Caspi	343	6.0	1.2
Ellis	322	5.0	0.6
Spadoni	225	4.4	1.8
Thompson	2,798	—	1.3
Lunenfeld	3,646	3.1	0.25
Total	11343	3.4	0.84

[a] Modified from Blankstein J et al.[30]

be adequately assessed, it may be appropriate to institute more invasive monitoring techniques such as a central venous pressure line or Swan–Ganz catheter. Diuretics should be avoided, since artificial diuresis may further diminish the depleted intravascular space during the acute situation. During resolution, diuretics may play a role. It seems logical to employ volume expanders that will increase the intravascular colloid osmotic pressure.

In the past 4 years, we have had occasion to treat two patients with severe ovarian hyperstimulation with a combination of human albumin and a potent diuretic, furosemide. During the acute resolution phase, albumin was administered, followed by furosemide 1 hour later. This was repeated once per 8 hours for 24 hours. There was a rapid diuresis with improvement in the patient's symptomatology.

Paracentesis has been suggested to control ascites. The risk of such a procedure is trauma to the massively enlarged and edematous ovaries. Trauma to the ovaries must be avoided. Because of the fragility of the ovaries, pelvic exams should be avoided. The possibility of ovarian rupture and torsion must be considered in every case of OHSS. A fall in hematocrit without an improvement in the patient's general status or considerable diuresis would suggest intraabdominal bleeding. Laparotomy is indicated in cases of ovarian rupture of torsion. One must be cautious in proceeding with laparotomy in that oophorectomy may then be unavoidable in order to achieve adequate hemostasis because of the massive enlargement and edema of the ovaries.

This OHSS syndrome is usually short-lived if the patient is not pregnant. Within 3 to 7 days after menses, diuresis begins, and the ascites disappears. In the presence of pregnancy, ovarian hyperstimulation persists, and slow improvement is expected over 6 to 8 weeks. The patient can be discharged when her condition stabilizes and urinary output is adequate.

In earlier clinical trials, investigators reported the occurrence of OHSS following the induction of ovulation with clomiphene citrate and pregnant urine gonadotropins. Rarely, it may eventually lead to death. Conservative management directed at maintaining vascular volume is sufficient to maintain renal profusion. Antihistamines and indomethacin have been used. Although the efficacy of these medications has been demonstrated in animal studies, there are insufficient data at present to establish efficacy in the human. During resolution, a fall in hematocrit is expected secondary to the return of third-space fluid to the intravascular compartment.

Pregnancy Wastage

Other complications of gonadotropin-induced ovulation include an increased spontaneous abortion rate, which has been reported in the literature to range between 12% and 31%. In the series of patients reported by Blankstein,[30] the overall abortion rate for their patients was 25.2%, with no significant differences existing between patients belonging to either group I or group II. However, a significant difference in abortion rate was observed in consecutive pregnancies (Table 6-7). In the initial pregnancy cycle following hMG–hCG treatment, the abortion rate was 28%. In contrast, in a subsequent pregnancy the abortion rate was only 12%, and this rate was comparable to the abortion rate in the normal population. The factors operative in the increased abortion rate observed in those patients were not identified, but ovarian hyperstimulation was suspected since approximately 50% of those patients with hyperstimulation ultimately aborted.

In contrast to pregnancies achieved with pulsatile GnRH for ovulation induction, the

TABLE 6-7. Pregnancy wastage after hMG plus hCG[a]

First conception	28%
Second conception	12%
No treatment after hMG	13%
Hyperstimulation	50%

[a] Modified from Blankstein et al.[30]

spontaneous abortion rate among pregnancies achieved by gonadotropin-induced ovulation is much higher.[94] In another study,[95] the authors examined several factors that may contribute to the high pregnancy wastage. They included age, history of previous miscarriages, duration of infertility, diagnostic category, weight, body surface area, duration and dose of gonadotropins, estradiol pattern, and whether the luteal phase was supported with additional hCG. They found a higher miscarriage rate in the treatment group versus control. All of the characteristics monitored were not different except for weight and age. A weight greater than 81.8 kg was a significant risk factor. The miscarriage rate was significantly higher, and patients older than age 35 had a miscarriage rate approximating 60%. Therefore, increased age and weight in that study were identified as risk factors for the occurrence of spontaneous first-trimester miscarriages in a population of women receiving combination gonadotropin therapy for ovulation induction.

Other factors leading to increased miscarriages include the degree of ovarian hyperstimulation, the presence of multiple pregnancies, and first pregnancies. Nonetheless, it can be shown that the high incidence of abortion in women receiving hMG plus hCG is not exclusively related to the abovementioned factors but may be linked to some other, as yet unknown, etiologic factor that remains to be investigated.

Multiple Births

The incidence of multiple births is also increased after gonadotropin therapy. In an early report by Gemzell and Roos[96] prior to the prospective use of estrogen data, the rate of multiple gestation was equal to the rate of single gestation. Recent advances have emphasized the control of hyperstimulation and the incidence of multiple gestation. Controlling the degree of ovarian stimulation by using either plasma or urinary estrogen determinations coupled with frequent monitoring by ultrasound has reduced the incidence

TABLE 6-8. Multiple gestation[a]

Pregnancies	Number (%)
Singleton	113 (69.8%)
Twins	41 (25.3%)
Triplets	5 (3.1%)
Quadruplets	3 (1.8%)
Total	162 (100%)

[a] Bettendorf et al.[97]

of multiple gestations. The reported incidences of multiple birth range from 11% to 44%, with the majority of the multiple gestations being twins.[97] Multiple gestations are to be avoided because of obstetrical complications. Apart from the increased incidence of spontaneous abortions and the increased obstetrical risks associated with multiple gestations, the outcome of pregnancies following ovulation induction with gonadotropins appears to be normal. In summary, the incidence of hyperstimulation has been reduced by careful monitoring; however, the incidence of twins and triplets has not been significantly reduced because those occur spontaneously in the population. Nonetheless, the frequency of fetuses greater than triplets appears to be reduced but not totally eliminated by careful monitoring of the patient's ovulatory response to exogenous gonadotropins (Table 6-8).

Sex Ratios

The incidence of male children in single pregnancies following hMG therapy was 51.8%.[97] The incidence for twins was 53.8%, and for triplets it was 66.7%. The expected ratio is 1.06.[98] The increased incidence of males in the Bettendorf series probably reflects the small numbers involved in the study. In the literature, the expected sex ratio is approximated when several series are combined. There is no increased tendency in either direction. In a large series of patients reported by Ben-Rafael, 256 children were born in 195 births among 176 women, and the secondary sex ratio was 50% male to 50% female. The same trend was observed for singletons and twin gestations.[99]

Spontaneous Conception after hMG–hCG Therapy

Few studies have reported on spontaneous pregnancy rates after gonadotropin-induced pregnancies. It is generally accepted that hMG–hCG treatment does not cure the patient permanently of her underlying ovulatory disorder. Spadoni[100] reported on spontaneous conceptions following hMG. A larger series reported by Ben-Rafael[101] showed that in 141 women who had previously conceived using hMG therapy, the cumulative spontaneous pregnancy rate was 30.4% after 5 years. The miscarriage rate was 29% in the hMG-induced pregnancy, whereas the subsequent pregnancy enjoyed a miscarriage rate of 8.8%. The cumulative pregnancy rate of 30.4% was much lower than that in a group of normal parous women. Another study by Lam[102] indicated a much lower spontaneous conception rate of 66.4% at 115 months when compared to 88.6% at 23 months during the first course of gonadotropin therapy. They conclude that the women receiving gonadotropin therapy have an 11-fold better chance of conceiving in a given cycle. Their fertility potential was not affected by the baseline estrogen and FSH hormone levels, diagnosis, previous result of gonadotropin therapy, age, or menstrual pattern. This contrasted with Ben-Rafael's study, which found a lower cumulative spontaneous pregnancy rate in patients with low baseline gonadotropin and estrogen levels.

Congenital Anomalies

The clinical data available in the literature do not indicate that babies born as a result of hMG- plus hCG-induced ovulation induction are at any greater risk of malformations than the general population (Table 6-9)[30,103]

TABLE 6-9. Congenital anomalies after hMG- plus hCG-induced conceptions[a]

Authors	Infants	Anomalies
Thompson et al.	358	5 (1.4%)
Schwartz et al.	211	2 (0.9%)
Hack et al.	115	4 (3.1%)
Spadoni et al.	36	2 (5.5%)
March	63	1 (1.6%)
Total	783	14 (1.8%)

[a] Modified from March.[103]

Ovulation Induction in Polycystic Ovarian Syndrome

Pure FSH

Polycystic ovarian syndrome is characterized as a chronic anovulatory condition with elevated circulating LH and ovarian hyperandrogenism. A hallmark for the disorder is relative FSH deficiency. Provision of pure FSH to patients with PCO appears to be a logical choice. Prior to the availability of pure FSH, ovulation induction was achieved in clomiphene-resistant patients using hMG plus hCG. Although successful, the therapeutic window utilizing hMG is quite narrow, and attempts to provide FSH in the form of hMG are often associated with multiple follicles and an increased incidence of ovarian hyperstimulation.[104] Gemzell[105] initially reported success in inducing ovulation in a single patient with PCO utilizing a FSH preparation. More recently, Seibel[46] and Schoemaker[106] utilized a pure FSH preparation to achieve successful ovulation in PCO patients. Both pituitary and urinary FSH have been used safely to correct the biochemical imbalances seen in PCO patients. Despite the successes, the PCO patient continues to be very sensitive to gonadotropin therapy, and ovarian hyperstimulation continues to be a real concern. The need for intensive clinical monitoring is not markedly reduced, if at all.[46,47,106]

Gonadotropin-Releasing Hormone Agonists and hMG–hCG Therapy

Individual variability during ovulation induction in the primate model is thought to be secondary to supraovarian factors.[44] The creation of a temporary medical hypophysectomy with either a GnRH agonist or an antagonist led to a more predictable ovulatory response in females receiving exogenous gonadotropins.

Clinically, the induction of ovulation in women with chronic anovulation secondary to polycystic ovarian disease (PCO) has led to discouraging results. In contrast, patients with hypothalamic amenorrhea receiving exogenous gonadotropins have a more predictable ovulatory response. The response in PCO has been quite variable, and fecundity has been low for these women who previously failed clomiphene citrate therapy. The continued endogenous gonadotropin secretion is felt to be responsible for the brittle response of these patients that frequently led to ovarian hyperstimulation without successful ovulation being induced. Earlier studies suggested that the employment of a GnRH analog to suppress endogenous LH secretion and perhaps premature LH surges may lead to a more predictable ovulatory response and hence improve the subsequent pregnancy rates. The rationale was to make group II patients (hypothalamic dysfunction, PCO, etc.) mimic group I patients in terms of estrogen status and absence of endogenous LH secretion. By removing circulating gonadotropins with the agonists, analogous to a selective hypophysectomy, supraovarian factors are eliminated, and a more predictable ovulatory response is expected.

We designed a study to investigate whether women with PCO would respond to exogenous gonadotropins to induce ovulation in a manner similar to women with hypothalamic failure. A GnRH agonist was employed to create a temporary medical hypophysectomy.[107] The study was designed to assess the effects of leuprolide acetate (Lupron, TAP Pharmaceuticals, Chicago, Illinois), a long-acting GnRH agonist, on the ovulatory response of the PCO patient and subsequent effects on pregnancy rates. Comparisons were made of hormonal profiles before and after leuprolide therapy, with each patient serving as her own control.

Ten women who were previously unresponsive or very brittle during previous hMG administration were selected to receive the GnRH agonist leuprolide. These women (mean age 30.8) underwent a standard infertility evaluation and had previously received from 3 to 16 months of hMG–hCG therapy. Leuprolide was then administered up to 14 days prior to hMG plus hCG to lower E_2 and LH; then concurrent hMG–hCG therapy began. Fifty percent of the women conceived within 3 months of concurrent leuprolide and hMG–hCG therapy. The mean duration of drug therapy and drug dose administered during a representative hMG–hCG cycle versus leuprolide plus hMG did not differ (Table 6-10). Maximum E_2 levels achieved did not differ (657.4 ± 589 versus 833.9 ± 276.9 pg/mL). However, significantly more follicles were 15 mm or greater in the leuprolide group on the day of hCG administration ($P < 0.05$).

We concluded that (1) the GnRH agonist leuprolide can be administered to safely induce a temporary medical hypophysectomy, which appears to be reversible; (2) concurrent administration of leuprolide with gonadotropins in PCO patients led to a more predictable ovulatory response and higher success rate in achieving pregnancy; and (3) in this study, the mean duration of therapy and the mean dose of gonadotropin required to achieve ovulation did not differ between

TABLE 6-10. Comparisons of hMG versus hMG–leuprolide in PCO subjects[a]

Measure	hMG–hCG plus leuprolide	hMG–hCG
Ampules of hMG	26.6 ± 13	27.6 ± 17
Days hMG given	10.8 ± 3	10.9 ± 4
Follicles > 15 mm	2.8 ± 1.3^b	1.7 ± 1.4
Estradiol on day of hCG (pg/mL)	833.8 ± 276	657.4 ± 589

[a] Values are mean $\pm$ SD ($N = 10$).
[b] $P < 0.05$.

groups. Our findings are in agreement with those of other authors.[108–111] This is in contrast to previous studies, where hypothalamic amenorrheic women or poorly responding patients in IVF treatments required significantly more gonadotropins and longer treatment.

Since the addition of leuprolide led to a more predictable ovulatory response in these very brittle patients, this study provides further evidence that individual variability during ovulation induction is secondary to supraovarian factors.

Adjuncts to hMG–hCG Treatment

Clomiphene Citrate

Clomiphene citrate is one of the adjuncts utilized to improve the follicular response to hMG (Table 6-11). In 1976, March et al. reported their experience utilizing clomiphene citrate pretreatment prior to hMG.[112] It was hoped that patients receiving clomiphene pretreatment would require less gonadotropin therapy to achieve ovulation. They found that only patients who had experienced withdrawal bleeding following intramuscular injection of progesterone and had normal FSH values would benefit from clomiphene citrate pretreatment. Patients who were hypoestrogenic with low FSH values and who failed to bleed after progesterone had no difference in the amount of hMG necessary to induce ovulation with or without clomiphene citrate pretreatment. Theoretically, a reduction in the incidence of ovarian hyperstimulation

TABLE 6-11. Adjuncts to hMG therapy

1. Clomiphene pretreatment
2. Estrogen pretreatment
3. Dexamethasone and hMG plus hCG
4. Pulsatile hMG
5. Pulsatile GnRH and hMG plus hCG
6. GnRH agonist down-regulation followed by hMG plus hCG

and multiple births could be achieved with combination therapy.[113] The concerns are the antiestrogenic effects of clomiphene citrate on cervical mucous and the milieu of the fallopian tube as well as the introduction of another factor contributing to the multiplicity of therapeutic responses.

Estrogen Pretreatment

Estrogen pretreatment may be necessary to induce adequate cervical mucus production in women with severe estrogen deficiency. Although ovulation is possible utilizing hMG, there have been discrepancies noted in cervical mucus production. To prime the endometrium in the cervix, estrogens are utilized for 2 months prior to hMG therapy. According to March, this protocol has resulted in a significantly higher pregnancy rate in the initial treatment cycle in the severely estrogen-deficient patient when compared to others who received no estrogen pretreatment.[103]

Dexamethasone

In a group of patients with PCO who were clomiphene citrate resistant and who also failed to conceive after hMG–hCG therapy alone, combination dexamethasone and hMG treatment was tried. Dexamethasone was given to suppress endogenous adrenal androgen production, which is ACTH dependent. The authors investigated whether suppression of androgen levels by low levels of dexamethasone could improve patient responsiveness to hMG therapy and consequently reduce complications. In this study,[114] 81% of patients ovulated, and 74% conceived, within four treatment cycles. Seventy-four percent were full-term deliveries with only one set of twins, and 25% experienced a first-trimester loss. Only one cycle was complicated by moderate OHSS. Androgen suppression by dexamethasone in androgenized patients unresponsive to clomiphene and/or hMG resistant resulted in successful ovulation and pregnancy.

Pulsatile hMG Therapy

To mimic the normal pulsatile delivery of pituitary gonadotropins to the gonad, several investigators have reported success utilizing computerized pumps for continuous pulsatile hMG administration. In an earlier report, the authors treated five women with prolonged anovulatory infertility for approximately 14 cycles. These women had previously failed to ovulate with daily administration of hMG or had repeatedly developed ovarian hyperstimulation syndrome. It was felt that pulsatile administration of exogenous gonadotropins would mimic the physiological circumstances during a normal menstrual cycle and therefore be more likely to control the development and maturation of mature follicles and reduce the risk of OHSS and multiple births. Ovulation was achieved in 12 of 14 cycles in that initial treatment cycle, and pregnancy occurred in 40% of the patients who had previously been hMG failures.[115] The authors concluded that the pulsatile administration of hMG was an alternative method when conventional routes of therapy failed to achieve successful ovulation or pregnancy. Others have reported similar experiences in ovulation-resistant patients by utilizing pulsatile hMG treatment.[116-118] More experience is required in order to determine the optimal route of administration, pulse frequency, daily dosage of hMG, and methods of monitoring this mode of treatment.

References

1. Gemzell CA, Diczfalusy E, Tillinger KG. Clinical effect of human pituitary follicle stimulating hormone (FSH). J Clin Endocrinol Metab. 1958;18:1333–48.
2. Jones KP, Ravnikar VA, Schiff I. Results of human menopausal gonadotropin therapy at the Boston Hospital for Women (1979–1981). Int J Fertil. 1987;32:131–34.
3. Kennedy JL, Adashi EY. Ovulation induction. Obstet Gynecol Clin North Am. 1987;14:831–64.
4. March CM, Davajan V, Mishell DR Jr. Ovulation induction in amenorrheic women. Obstet Gynecol. 1979;53:8–11.
5. March CM. Therapeutic regimens and monitoring techniques for human menopausal gonadotropin administration. J Reprod Med. 1978;21:198–204.
6. Raj SG, Berger MJ, Grimes EM, et al. The use of gonadotropins for the induction of ovulation in women with polycystic ovarian disease. Fertil Steril. 1977;28:1280–84.
7. Seibel MM, McArdle C, Smith D, et al. Ovulation induction in polycystic ovary syndrome with urinary follicle-stimulating hormone or human menopausal gonadotropin. Fertil Steril. 1985;43:703–08.
8. Venturoli S, Paradisi R, Fabbri R, et al. Comparison between human urinary follicle-stimulating hormone and human menopausal gonadotropin treatment in polycystic ovary. Obstet Gynecol. 1984;63:6–11.
9. Kurachi K, Aono T, Suzuki M. Results of hMG–hCG therapy in 1096 treatment cycles of 2166 Japanese women with anovulatory infertility. Eur J Obstet Gynecol Reprod Biol. 1985;19:43–52.
10. Kremmann E, Tavakoli F, Shelden RM, et al. Induction of ovulation with menotropins in women with polycystic ovary syndrome. Am J Obstet Gynecol. 1981;141:58–64.
11. Check JH. Treatment of cervical factor with combined high-dose estrogen and human menopausal gonadotropins. Fertil Steril. 1980;33:562–63.
12. Check JH, Adelson HG. Improvement of cervical factor by high-dose estrogen and human menopausal gonadotropin therapy with ultrasound monitoring. Obstet Gynecol. 1984;63:179–81.
13. Check JH, Wu CH, Dietterich C, et al. The treatment of cervical factor with ethinyl estradiol and human menopausal gonadotropins. Int J Fertil. 1986;31:148–52.
14. Lunenfeld B, Insler V. Gonadotropins. In: Diagnosis and treatment of functional infertility. Berlin: Grosse Verlag, 1978:76–89.
15. Welner S, DeCherney AH, Polan ML. Human menopausal gonadotropins: a justifiable therapy in ovulatory women with long-standing idiopathic infertility. Am J Obstet Gynecol. 1988;158:111–17.
16. Halme J, Hammond MG, Bailey L, et al. Lower doses of human menopausal gonadotropin are associated with improved success with in vitro fertilization in women with low body weight. Am J Obstet Gynecol. 1988;158:64–65.

17. Ben-Rafael Z, Benadiva CA, Ausmanas M, et al. Dose of human menopausal gonadotropin influences the outcome of an in vitro fertilization program. Fertil Steril. 1987;48:964–68.
18. Bernardus RE, Jones GS, Acosta M, et al. The significance of the ratio in follicle-stimulating hormone and luteinizing hormone in induction of multiple follicular growth. Fertil Steril. 1985;43:373–78.
19. Cohen JJ, Debache C, Pigeau F, et al. Sequential use of clomiphene citrate, human menopausal gonadotropin, and human chorionic gonadotropin in human in vitro fertilization. II. Study of luteal phase adequacy following aspiration of the preovulatory follicles. Fertil Steril. 1984;42:360–65.
20. Zondek B, Aschheim S. Des Hormon des hypophysenvorderlappens. Klin Wochenschr. 1928; 6:831–35.
21. Schwartz J, Jewelewicz R. The use of gonadotropins for induction of ovulation. Fertil Steril. 1981;35:3–12.
22. Smith PE, Engle ET. Experimental evidence regarding the role of anterior pituitary in the development and regulation of the genital system. Am J Anat. 1927;40:159–217.
23. Cole HH, Hart GH. The potency of blood serum of mares in progressive stages of pregnancy in effecting the sexual maturity of immature rats. Am J Physiol 1930;93:57–68.
24. Hamblen EC, Davis CD. Treatment of hypoovarianism by the sequential and cyclic administration of equine and chorionic gonadotropins. Am J Obstet Gynecol. 1945;50:137–46.
25. Borth R, Lunenfeld B, de Watteville H. Activite gonadotrope d'un extrait d'urines de femmes en menopause. Experientia. 1954;10: 264–68.
26. Borth R, Lunenfeld B, Riotton G, et al. Activite gonadotrope d'un extrait des femmes en menopause (2e communication). Experientia. 1957;13:115–17.
27. Lunenfeld B, Menzi A, Volet B. Clinical effects of a human postmenopausal gonadotropin. Rass Clin Ter Sci Affini. 1960;59:213–16.
28. Donini P, Puzuli D, Montezeniola R. Purification of gonadotropins from human menopause urine. Acta Endocrinol. 1964;45:329–34.
29. Borth R, Lunenfeld B, Menzi A. Pharmacologic and clinical effects of a gonadotropin preparation from human postmenopausal urine. In: Albert A, Thomas MC, eds. Human pituitary gonadotropins. Springfield: Charles C. Thomas, 1961:255.
30. Blankstein J, Mashiach, Lunenfeld B. Induction of ovulation with gonadotropins. In: Ovulation induction and in vitro fertilization. Chicago: Year Book, 1986:131–54.
31. Rosemberg E, Cortes-Prieto J. First demonstration of induction of ovulation with a hybrid human chorionic gonadotropin compound (AB1ER-CR-2XY). Fertil Steril. 1983; 40:790–97.
32. Richards JA, Hedin L. Molecular aspects of hormone action in ovarian follicular development, ovulation and luteinization. Annu Rev Physiol. 1988;50:441–64.
33. Dlugi AM, Laufer N, DeCherney AH, et al. The day of initiation of human menopausal gonadotropin stimulation affects follicular growth in in vitro fertilization cycles. J In Vitro Fertil Embryo Transfer. 1985;2:33–40.
34. Vermesh M, Kletzky OA. Follicle-stimulating hormone is the main determinant of follicular recruitment and development in ovulation induction with human menopausal gonadotropin. Am J Obstet Gynecol. 1987;157:1397–1402.
35. Diamond MP, Wentz AC. Ovulation induction with human menopausal gonadotropins. Obstet Gynecol Surv. 1986;41:480–90.
36. Filicori M, Santoro N, Merriam GR, et al. Characterization of the physiological pattern of episodic gonadotropin secretion throughout the human menstrual cycle. J Clin Endocrinol Metab. 1986;62:1136–44.
37. Collins RL, Sopelak V, Williams RF, et al. Prevention of GnRH antagonist-induced luteal regression by concurrent exogenous pulsatile gonadotrophin administration in monkeys. Fertil Steril. 1986;46:945–53.
38. Groff T, Raj HGM, Talbert LM, et al. Effects of neutralization of luteinizing hormone on corpus luteum function and cyclicity in *Macaca fascicularis*. J Clin Endocrinol Metab. 1984;59:1054–57.
39. Coelingh Bennink HJT. Pulsatile administration of LHRH for ovulation induction. In: Shaw RW, Marshall JC, eds. LHRH and its analogues. Their use in gynaecological practice. London: Wright Press, 1989:92–112.
40. Mais V, Kazer RR, Cetel NS, et al. The dependency of folliculogenesis and corpus luteum function on pulsatile gonadotropin secretion in cycling women using a gonadotropin-releasing hormone antagonist as a probe. J Clin Endocrinol Metab. 1986;62:1250–55.
41. Weinstein FG, Seibel MM, Taymor ML. Ovu-

lation induction with subcutaneous pulsatile gonadotropin-releasing hormone: the role of supplemental human chorionic gonadotropin in the luteal phase. Fertil Steril. 1984;41: 546–50.

42. Zeleznik AJ, Hutchison JS. The use of pulsatile GnRH treatment to investigate the regulation of the primate corpus luteum. In: Coelingh Bennink HJT, Dogterom AA, Lappohn RE, et al., eds. Pulsatile GnRH 1985. Naarlem, The Netherlands: Ferring, 1986:71–79.

43. Berger NG, Zacur HA. Exogenous progesterone for luteal support following gonodatropin-releasing hormone ovulation induction: case report. Fertil Steril. 1985;44:133–35.

44. Kenigsberg D, Littman BA, Williams RF, et al. Medical hypophysectomy. II: variability of ovarian response to exogenous gonadotropins. Fertil Steril. 1984;42:116–26.

45. Cook AS, Webster BW, Terranova PF, et al. Variation in the biologic and biochemical characteristics of human menopausal gonadotropin. Fertil Steril. 1988;49:704–12.

46. Seibel M. Toward understanding the pathophysiology and treatment of polycystic ovarian disease. Semin Reprod Endocrinol. 1984; 2:297–304.

47. Traub Al, McFaul PB, Sheridan B, et al. Pure FSH induces ovulation in polycystic ovary syndrome despite rising androgen levels. Clin Reprod Fertil. 1987;5:167–71.

48. Hoffman DI, Lobo RA, Campeau J, et al. Ovulation induction in clomiphene-resistant anovulatory women: differential follicular response to purified urinary follicle-stimulating hormone (FSH) versus purified urinary FSH and luteinizing hormone. J Clin Endocrinol Metab. 1985;60:922–27.

49. Couzinet B, Lestrat N, Brailly S, et al. Stimulation of ovarian follicular maturation with pure follicle-stimulating hormone in women with gonadotropin deficiency. J Clin Endocrinol Metab. 1988;66:552–56.

50. Reid RL, Fretts R, Van Vugt DA. The theory and practice of ovulation induction with gonadotropin-releasing hormone. Am J Obstet Gynecol. 1988;158:173–85.

51. Sueldo CE, Swanson JA. The economics of inducing ovulation with human menopausal gonadotropins versus pulsatile subcutaneous gonadotropin-releasing hormone. Fertil Steril. 1986;45:128–29.

52. Dawood MY, Jarrett JC 2d, Choe JK. Partial

hypopituitarism and hyperprolactinemia: successful induction of ovulation with bromocriptine and human menopausal gonadotropins. Fertil Steril. 1982;38:415–18.

53. Farine D, Mashiach S, Ben-Rafael Z, et al. Retrospective evaluation of human menopausal gonadotropin and human chorionic gonadotropin induction of ovulation in galactorrheic and hyperprolactinemic women. Fertil Steril. 1982;38:187–89.

54. Tang GW, Tang LC, Ho PC. Transient hyperprolactinaemia in human menopausal gonadotropin induction of ovulation. Int J Fertil. 1984;29:136–40.

55. Check JH, Chase JS. Ovulation induction in hypergonadotropic amenorrhea with estrogen and human menopausal gonadotropin therapy. Fertil Steril. 1984;42:919–22.

56. Fleming R, Hamilton MP, Barlow DH, et al. Pregnancy after ovulation induction in a patient with menopausal gonadotropin levels after chemotherapy [letter]. Lancet. 1984; 1399.

57. Jones GS, Aziz A, Urbina G. Clinical use of gonadotropins in conditions of ovarian insufficiency of various etiologies. Fertil Steril. 1961;12:217–35.

58. Zimmerman R, Soor B, Braendle W, et al. Gonadotropin therapy of female infertility: analysis of results in 416 cases. Gynecol Obstet Invest. 1982;14:1–6.

59. Dodson WC, Whitesides DB, Hughes CL, et al. Superovulation with intrauterine insemination in the treatment of infertility: a possible alternative to gamete intrafallopian transfer and in vitro fertilization. Fertil Steril. 1987; 48:441–45.

60. Taymor ML, Yussman MA, Gmisnki D. Estrogen monitoring in ovulation induction. Fertil Steril. 1970;21:759–62.

61. Webb-Wilson GJ, Arronet GH. Ovulation induction with human menopausal gonadotropins: an evaluation of a variable daily dosage regimen. Int J Fertil. 1977;22:225–29.

62. Klopper A, Aiman J, Besser M. Ovarian steroidogenesis resulting from treatment with menopausal gonadotropin. Eur J Obstet Gynecol Reprod Biol. 1974;4:25–28.

63. Shaaban MM, Klopper A. Plasma oestradiol and progesterone concentration in the normal menstrual cycle. J Obstet Gynaecol Br Commonw. 1973;80:776–80.

64. Tredway DR, Goebelsmann U, Thorneycroft IH, et al. Monitoring induction of ovulation

with human menopausal gonadotropin by a rapid estrogen radioimmunoassay. Am J Obstet Gynecol 1974;120:1035–39.

65. Schenker JG, Weinstein D. Ovarian hyperstimulation syndrome: a current survey. Fertil Steril. 1978;30:255–68.

66. Haning RV, Levin RM, Behrman HR, et al. Plasma estradiol window and urinary estriol glucuronide determinations for monitoring menotropin induction of ovulation. Obstet Gynecol. 1979;54:442–47.

67. Duff GB. Ultrasound and ovulation. NZ Med J. 1987;100:657–59.

68. Robinson RD, Packer RH, Wilson PC, et al. Assessment of ovulation by ultrasound and plasma estradiol determination. Obstet Gynecol. 1979;54:686–91.

69. O'Herlihy C, deCrespigny LJC, Robinson HP. Monitoring ovarian follicular development with real-time ultrasound. Br J Obstet Gynaecol 1980;87:613–17.

70. Cabau A, Bessis R. Monitoring of ovulation induction with human menopausal gonadotropin and human chorionic gonadotropin by ultrasound. Fertil Steril. 1981;36:178–82.

71. Dornbluth NC, Potter JL, Shepard MK, et al. Assessment of follicular development by ultrasonography and total serum estrogen in human menopausal gonadotropin-stimulated cycles. J Ultrasound Med. 1983;2:407–12.

72. Hull ME, Moghissi KS, Magyar DM, et al. Correlation of serum estradiol levels and ultrasound monitoring to assess follicular maturation. Fertil Steril. 1986;46:42–45.

73. Marrs RP, Vargyas JM, March CM. Correlation of ultrasonic and endocrinologic measurements in human menopausal gonadotropin therapy. Am J Obstet Gynecol. 1983;145:417–21.

74. Seibel MM, McArdle CR, Thompson IE, et al. The role of ultrasound in ovulation induction: a critical appraisal. Fertil Steril. 1981;36:573–77.

75. Tulandi T, Hamilton EF, Arronet GH, et al. Ovulation induction by human menopausal gonadotropin with ultrasonic monitoring of the ovarian follicles. Int J Fertil. 1987;32:312–15.

76. Hill LM, Coulam CB, Kislak SL, et al. Sonographic evaluation of the cervix during ovulation induction. Am J Obstet Gynecol. 1987;157:1170–74.

77. Fleischer AC, Pittaway DE, Beard LA, et al. Sonographic depiction of endometrial changes occurring with ovulation induction. J Ultrasound Med. 1984;3:341–46.

78. Insler V, Melmed H, Mashiach S, et al. A Functional classification of patients selected for gonadotropic therapy. Obstet Gynecol. 1968;32:620–26.

79. Healy DL, Burger HG. Serum follicle-stimulating hormone, luteinizing hormone, and prolactin during the induction of ovulation with exogenous gonadotropin. J Clin Endocrinol Metab. 1983;56:474–78.

80. Olson JL, Rebar RW, Schreiber JR, et al. Shortened luteal phase after ovulation induction with human menopausal gonadotropin and human chorionic gonadotropin. Fertil Steril. 1983;39:284–91.

81. Collins RL, Williams RF, Hodgen GD. Endocrine consequences of prolonged ovarian hyperstimulation: Hyperprolactinemia, follicular atresia and premature luteinization. Fertil Steril. 1984;42:436–45.

82. Hodgen GD. The dominant ovarian follicle. Fertil Steril. 1982;38:281–300.

83. Stillman RJ, Williams RF, Lynch A, et al. Selective inhibition of follicle-stimulating hormone by porcine follicular fluid extracts in the monkey: effects on midcycle surges and pulsatile secretion. Fertil Steril. 1983;40:823–28.

84. Schenken RS, Hodgen GD. Follicle-stimulating hormone induced ovarian hyperstimulation in monkeys: blockade of the luteinizing hormone surge. J Clin Endocrinol Metab. 1983;57:50–55.

85. Laufer N, DeCherney AH, Tarlatzis BC, et al. Delaying human chorionic gonadotropin administration in human menopausal gonadotropin-induced cycles decreases successful in vitro fertilization of human oocytes. Fertil Steril. 1984;42:198–203.

86. Tulandi T, McInnes RA, Arronet GH. Ovarian hyperstimulation syndrome following ovulation induction with human menopausal gonadotropin. Int J Fertil. 1984;29:113–17.

87. Schenker JG, Weinstein D. Ovarian hyperstimulation syndrome: a current survey. Fertil Steril. 1978;30:255–68.

88. Navot D, Relou A, Birkenfeld A, et al. Risk factors and prognostic variables in the ovarian hyperstimulation syndrome. Am J Obstet Gynecol. 1988;159:210–15.

89. Kirshon B, Doody MC, Cotton DB, et al. Management of ovarian hyperstimulation syndrome with chlorpheniramine maleate, man-

nitol, and invasive hemodynamic monitoring. Obstet Gynecol. 1988;71:485–87.

90. Blankstein J, Shalev J, Saadon T, et al. Ovarian hyperstimulation syndrome: prediction by number and size of preovulatory ovarian follicles. Fertil Steril. 1987;47:597–602.

91. McArdle C, Seibel M, Hann LE, et al. The diagnosis of ovarian hyperstimulation (OHS): the impact of ultrasound. Fertil Steril. 1983; 39:464–67.

92. Narita O, Shimosuka Y, Suzuki M, et al. Induction of ovulation with human menopausal gonadotropin, with special reference to ovarian hyperstimulation syndrome and hormone excretion. Nagoya J Med Sci. 1980;43:7–13.

93. Thaler I, Yoffe N, Kaftory JK, et al. Treatment of ovarian hyperstimulation syndrome: the physiologic basis for a modified approach. Fertil Steril. 1981;36:110–13.

94. Ben-Rafael Z, Dor J, Mashiach S, et al. Abortion rate in pregnancies following ovulation induced by human menopausal gonadotropin/ human chorionic gonadotropin. Fertil Steril. 1983;39:157–61.

95. Kemmann E, Bohrer M. Risk factors for spontaneous abortion in menotropintreated women. Fertil Steril. 1987;48:571–75.

96. Gemzell C, Roos P. Pregnancies following treatment with human gonadotropins. Am J Obstet Gynecol. 1966;94:490–94.

97. Bettendorf G, Braendle W, Sprotte C, et al. Overall results of gonadotropin therapy. In: Insler V, Bettendorf G, eds. Advances and diagnosis in treatment of infertility. New York: Elsevier North-Holland, 1981:21–34.

98. Tricomi V, Ferrd M, Solish G. The ratio of male and female embryo as determined by the sex chromosome. Am J Obstet Gynecol. 1960; 75:504–09.

99. Ben-Rafael Z, Matalon A, Blankstein J, et al. Male to female ratio after gonadotropin-induced ovulation. Fertil Steril. 1986;45:36–40.

100. Spadoni LR, Cox DW, Smith DC. Use of human menopausal gonadotropin for the induction of ovulation. Am J Obstet Gynecol. 1974; 120:988–93.

101. Ben-Rafael Z, Mashiach S, Oelsner G, et al. Spontaneous pregnancy and its outcome after human menopausal gonadotropin/human chorionic gonadotropin-induced pregnancy. Fertil Steril. 1981;36:560–64.

102. Lam SY, Baker G, Pepperell R, et al. Treatment-independent pregnancies after cessation of gonadotropin ovulation induction in women with oligomenorrhea and anovulatory menses. Fertil Steril. 1988;50:26–30.

103. March CM. The use of Pergonal for the induction of ovulation. Clin Obstet Gynecol. 1984; 27:966–74.

104. Wang CF, Gemzell C. The use of human gonadotropins for induction of ovulation in women with polycystic ovary disease. Fertil Steril. 1980;33:479–86.

105. Gemzell C. Induction of ovulation with human gonadotropins. Recent Prog Horm Res. 1965;21:179–97.

106. Schoemaker J, Wentz AC, Jones GS, et al. Stimulation of follicular growth with "pure" FSH in patients with anovulation and elevated LH levels. Obstet Gynecol. 1978;51: 270–77.

107. Collins RL, Gidwani GP, Seiler JC. Improved ovulation in women with PCO receiving exogenous gonadotropins and a GnRH agonist concurrently. 70th Meeting of the Endocrine Society. New Orleans, LA, 1988;840.

108. Lewinthal D, Taylor PJ, Pattison HA, et al. Induction of ovulation with leuprolide acetate and human menopausal gonadotropin. Fertil Steril. 1988;49:585–88.

109. Dodson WC, Hughes CL, Whitesides DB, et al. The effect of leuprolide acetate on ovulation induction with human menopausal gonadotropins in polycystic ovary syndrome. J Clin Endocrinol Metab. 1987;65:95–100.

110. Charbonnel B, Krempf M, Blanchard P, et al. Induction of ovulation in polycystic ovary syndrome with a combination of a luteinizing hormone-releasing hormone analog and exogenous gonadotropins. Fertil Steril. 1987; 47:920–24.

111. Lanzone A, Fulghesu AM, Spina MA, et al. Successful induction of ovulation and conception with combined gonadotropin-releasing hormone agonist plus highly follicle-stimulating hormone in patients with polycystic ovarian disease. J Clin Endocrinol Metab. 1987;65:1253–58.

112. March CM, Tredway DR, Michelle DR Jr. Affect of clomiphene citrate upon amount and duration of human menopausal gonadotropin therapy. Am J Obstet Gynecol. 1976;125: 699–704.

113. Jarrell J, McInnes R, Cooke R, et al. Observations on the combination of clomiphene citrate-human menopausal gonadotropin-human chorionic gonadotropin in the man-

agement of anovulation. Fertil Steril. 1981;
35:634–37.

114. Evron S, Navot D, Laufer N, et al. Induction
of ovulation with combined human gonadotropins and dexamethasone in women with
polycystic ovarian disease. Fertil Steril. 1983;
40:183–86.

115. Diamant YZ, Friedler S. Ovulation induction
with pulsatile human menopausal gonadotropins (HMG) administration. Eur J Obstet Gynecol Reprod Biol. 1987;25:303–13.

116. Friedler S, Diamant YZ. Ovulation induction
with pulsatile human menopausal gonadotropin (HMG) administration. Eur J Obstet Gynecol Reprod Biol. 1987;25:303–13.

117. Yuen BH, Pride SM, Sime MO. Successful
induction of ovulation and conception with
pulsatile intravenous administration of human menopausal gonadotropins in anovulatory infertile women resistant to clomiphene
and pulsatile gonadotropin-releasing hormone therapy. Am J Obstet Gynecol. 1984;
148:508–12.

118. Kemmann E, Brandeis VT, Shelden RM, et
al. The initial experience with the use of a
portable infusion pump in the delivery of human menopausal gonadotropins. Fertil Steril.
1983;40:448–53.

7
"Pulsatile" Gonadotropin-Releasing Hormone for Ovulation Induction

DANIEL KENIGSBERG AND ROBERT L. COLLINS

There are many names that describe anovulatory disorders, but for purposes of this chapter, all nonmenopausal anovulatory states in the reproductive age group can grouped lumped according to estrogen status. As described elsewhere in this volume, when endogenous estrogen is adequate to produce progestin challenge withdrawal bleeding, antiestrogen therapy such as clomiphene citrate is usually successful. Failing that, human menopausal gonadotropin therapy serves as a last resort. Clearly, the treatment can sometimes be modified to target the specific etiology for anovulation such as the use of bromocriptine for hyperprolactinemia or corticosteroids for adrenal enzyme deficiency-associated anovulation. This chapter focuses on to the anovulatory states associated with low estrogen levels also known as hypothalamic amenorrhea or eugonadotropic euprolactinemic amenorrhea. This term is apt because these are the disorders most amenable to treatment with the hypothalamic hormonal peptide gonadotropin-releasing hormone (GnRH), also known as luteinizing hormone-releasing hormone (LHRH).

Background

The search for hypothalamic hormones began in the mid-1950s, when it was shown conclusively by Geoffrey Harris that the mechanism of communication between the hypothalamus and pituitary was hormonal.[1] Although the releaser of ACTH was the initial quest, the first hypothalamic hormone isolated and fully characterized was the tripeptide thyrotropin-releasing hormone (TRH) in 1969.[2]

The isolation of GnRH was a major accomplishment for two independent investigators.[3-5] The relative simplicity of its 10-amino-acid structure and its short half-life in peripheral circulation made direct physiological studies of this releaser of LH and FSH difficult to perform or interpret. What did become clear in a matter of a few years was that this substance was not analogous to its pituitary counterparts, LH and FSH, where ever-increasing dosages would produce corresponding ever-increasing stimulation of gonadal function.

In 1978, using subhuman primate models, Knobil[6] conclusively demonstrated that the frequency and amplitude of administration were the key to the stimulatory potential of GnRH. The critical concept was that pulsatile as opposed to continuous administration was necessary to promote prolonged pituitary and ensuing gonadal function. Indeed, when applied via a pulsatile infusion pump, GnRH could provide ongoing, chronic gonadal function in both males and females devoid of endogenous GnRH secretion.

Physiology of GnRH

Gonadotropin-releasing hormone is a decapeptide that is common to all mammals tested. The gene for the precursor peptide for GnRH has been isolated and fully characterized.[7] The second and third amino acids, histidine and tryptophan, are critical for the activation of the second messenger system. Gonadotropin-releasing hormone is a membrane-bound peptide, and subsequent gonadotropin release is dependent on calcium mobilization. The short half-life of GnRH in the serum is a result of enzymatic cleavage, which occurs principally at position six. Appropriate substitutions in the native molecule will result in superactive analogs that resist enzymatic degradation, thereby prolonging their half-life.

Gonadotropin-releasing hormone is produced in the hypothalamus, and the pulsatile center is the arcuate nucleus. Novel research studies by Ernest Knobil[6] characterized the nature of gonadotropin pulsatility and subsequently GnRH itself. Knobil[6] demonstrated in monkeys that destruction of the arcuate nucleus in the hypothalamus resulted in a loss of peripheral LH pulsatility. The LH pulsatility could be restored by exogenous pulsatile administration of GnRH but not by continuous or extremely infrequent GnRH pulse administration. Therefore, the destruction of the arcuate nucleus in the monkey, the so-called "hypothalamic clamp" model, resulted in peripheral abolition of LH pulsatility. When exogenous GnRH results in normal gonadotropin secretion patterns in the primate, this unequivocally demonstrates the requisite pulsatile nature of GnRH presentation to the pituitary gland. These remarkable neurophysiological experiments were soon followed by confirmation in several clinical models with endogenous GnRH deficiency states such as Kallmann's syndrome.

The activation of cyclic gonadotropin–ovarian function in patients with hypogonadotropic amenorrhea represented a major challenge in the clinical management of infertility. Initial attempts to achieve ovulation with GnRH were unsuccessful. Early investigators administered GnRH once daily or one to three times per day in large dosages. The resulting initial failure to induce ovulation is now understandable in the view of the physiological background just reviewed. It

is necessary to deliver GnRH in a pulsatile manner in order to achieve successful activation of the pituitary gland and subsequent folliculogenesis.

Follicular Maturation

The experience in elucidating the physiological activity of GnRH and the pulsatile nature of its secretion has shed light on the understanding of normal hypothalamic pituitary–ovarian interactions. In humans, the control of timely ovarian follicular development resulting in a regular single ovulation is now understood to occur in the ovary itself, since it has been shown that any unvarying hypothalamic activity as represented by pulsatile infusion with a mechanical pump can produce average cycle lengths with repetitive ovulations. In the face of this unvarying message, the pituitary modulates its output of FSH and LH according to ovarian hormonal feedback. It follows then that ovarian follicular feedback is the timekeeper of the menstrual cycle.

In the normal sequence of follicular development in the ovary, simple primary follicles are recruited and begin to grow and accumulate supporting gonadal stromal cells, granulosa and theca, and a fluid-filled cavity adjacent to the oocyte, the antrum. Of the antral follicles, only one is selected to attain a dominant status and continue development to the point of ovulation and subsequent corpus luteum formation. The other recruited and unselected follicles undergo atresia.[8]

Human menopausal gonadotropins (hMG) override this normal physiology and cause multiple follicles to reach a preovulatory state. This is the underlying mechanism behind both multiple pregnancy and the ovarian hyperstimulation syndrome with its attendant fluid shifts from the edematous and distended ovaries. The mechanism of follicular development with the GnRH mimics the natural cycle, with only one dominant follicle emerging, thereby obviating the risks of multiple pregnancy and hyperstimulation. The only possible exception to this might be in the first month of treatment, when a readjustment of pituitary synthesis, storage, and secretion of FSH and LH could result in multiple follicular development.[9] However, the wide clinical experience with GnRH has proven this to be uncommon, and certainly once the first cycle has occurred, all continuous subsequent cycles should have but one dominant follicle and ovulation.

Before the advent and the availability of GnRH, exogenous gonadotropins (hMG) were available for use to achieve ovulation. Attendant with the use of such medication were the risks of multiple births, risk of ovarian hyperstimulation syndrome, and the added expense associated with extensive clinical monitoring of the patient's follicular response. Theoretically, the employment of GnRH could avoid some of the risks of hMG therapy. The GnRH would utilize intact feedback mechanisms because the site of action is at the level of the pituitary gland. Patients who are suitable candidates for GnRH therapy must possess an intact pituitary gland and functional ovaries. In contrast, exogenous gonadotropins stimulate the ovaries directly. Pulsatile GnRH allows appropriate secretion of physiological ratios of FSH and LH in the serum to achieve ovulation, and usually one dominant follicle emerges, resulting in ovulation. Theoretically, the risk of ovarian hyperstimulation is reduced by the employment of GnRH therapy. The cost of monitoring the patient response is reduced as well, thereby making the treatment cycle less expensive when compared to gonadotropin therapy.[10]

Clinical Application

The essential component in GnRH therapy for ovulation induction is a pulsatile infusion pump.[11] The peptide is only active parenterally, and the necessity of 12 to 24 pulses per day makes automation almost mandatory.

Route of administration can be either subcutaneous or intravenous.[12] The authors prefer the former, as it can be as efficacious without the potential complications of directly contaminating or invading the circulatory system. Also, access to subcutaneous areas such as the abdomen and thigh provide greater patient comfort than venous access in the arms.

Dosages of GnRH are effective over at least a fourfold range of 5 to 20 μg, and effective frequencies have at least a twofold range of one pulse every 60 to 120 minutes. The variables of dosages, route of administration, and pulse frequency are addressed later.

Patient Selection

Ovulation induction with GnRH appears to be most successful for anovulatory women with diminished or absent endogenous LH pulses, as depicted in Table 7-1. Patients with Kallmann's syndrome[13,14] or hypothalamic amenorrhea[15-22] (e.g. caused by weight loss or exercise) fall into this category. Other anovulatory conditions such as partial adrenal enzyme deficiencies and polycystic ovarian syndrome may be treated with pulsatile GnRH, but the results are less than satisfactory.[23-27] Therefore, before one considers GnRH therapy for ovulation induction, one should make a concerted effort to diagnose the specific cause of anovulation. Pubertal disorders[28-30] and other conditions of anovulatory infertility[31-36] also respond. Although anovulatory patients with hyperprolactinemia[37] and lactational amenorrhea[38] also respond because of their decreased endogenous GnRH secretion, other agents may prove more efficacious. Except for Kallmann's syndrome and hypothalamic amenorrhea, more specific therapies may be appropriate for other categories of anovulation.

Patients with constitutional delayed puberty have responded to pulsatile GnRH; however, long-term treatment is necessary to allow for normal pubertal progression to occur once the hypothalamic-pituitary-ovarian axis is activated. Certain patients with anovulatory infertility have been treated successfully. Pulsatile GnRH is also appropriate for men with decreased GnRH pulsatility, e.g., Kallmann's syndrome, hypogonadotropic hypogonadism, and cryptorchidism.[39]

Patient Monitoring

Standardized guidelines do not exist for monitoring patients receiving GnRH to induce ovulation. In general, plasma estradiol levels are obtained at periodic intervals, as are pelvic ultrasounds to assess the ovarian response during folliculogenesis. Duration of therapy prior to ovulation is extremely variable and in some cases may take up to 30 days for an initial treatment cycle. Usually, after the first ovulatory menstrual cycle, the subsequent cycles are more predictable, between 28 and 30 days. Since patients retain normal feedback mechanisms, they will usually experience a normal endogenous LH surge. Consequently, periodic methods to detect ovulation may be necessary to allow for precise timing of coital activity. In the past, urinary LH detection kits have been employed to assist patients in the timing of coitus. This is in contrast to exogenous human menopausal gonadotropin therapy, where the endogenous LH surge is usually suppressed, and a surrogate LH surge, such as hCG, is usually necessary to induce the release of the egg from the maturing follicle.[35]

Clinical Results

It is now appreciated that the best effectiveness of GnRH in promoting ovulation induction is in those states where there is a likely deficiency of endogenous GnRH, e.g., hypoestrogenism (Table 7-1). In Table 7-2, 14 series of intravenous pulsatile GnRH use for ovulation induction in hypothalamic amenorrhea (low estrogen level) are summarized. Pulsatile GnRH is highly efficacious in low-estrogen conditions resulting in (1) a high efficiency rate of 89% ovulation rate per patient, (2) 93% ovulation rate per cycle, and (3) a 30% pregnancy rate per cycle. Pulsatile GnRH is effective over a wide range of dosages (pulse amplitude) and pulse frequencies. Because of low or absent GnRH in the circulation, luteal-phase supplementation is required.

Subcutaneous administration is as effective as intravenous treatment. Ten series of subcutaneous pulsatile GnRH for ovulation induction in hypothalamic (low estrogen level) amenorrhea are summarized in Table 7-3. Like intravenous therapy, subcutaneous treatment results in a high efficiency rate of 91% ovulation per patient, 89% ovulatory rate per cycle, and a 32% pregnancy rate per cycle. A wide range of dosages (pulse amplitude) and pulse frequencies were effective. Again, luteal-phase supplementation is required.

Administration of GnRH via portable pulsatile infusion pumps is not nearly as effective when there is underlying, albeit disordered, pituitary and gonadal function such as in the nonhypoestrogenic states or patients demonstrating pituitary dysfunction (Table 7-4). Nine series of intravenous pulsatile GnRH for ovulation induction in hyperestrogenic amenorrhea (polycystic ovarian disease) are summarized in Table 7-4. A reduced rate of efficiency is noted in these patients despite the intravenous route of administration. The data show a 74% ovulation rate per patient, a 64% ovulation rate per cycle, and a low 19% pregnancy rate per cycle. Although a wide range of dosages (pulse amplitude) and pulse frequencies are effective, an optimal dose and frequency have yet to be established. A larger dosage is required for subcutaneous treatment compared to intravenous. Unlike patients with low estrogen status, luteal-phase supplementation is usually not required.

Subcutaneous therapy for hyperestrogenic patients (pituitary dysfunction) is less effective that intravenous. Five series of subcu-

TABLE 7-1. Current indications for pulsatile GnRH therapy

  I. Female: Hypothalamic amenorrhea
    1. Kallmann's syndrome
    2. Lactational amenorrhea
    3. Hyperprolactinemia
    4. Polycystic ovarian disease
    5. Delayed puberty
    6. In vitro fertilization
  II. Male
    1. Cryptorchidism
    2. Male hypogonadotropic hypogonadism
    3. Kallmann's syndrome

TABLE 7-2. Intravenous pulsatile GnRH therapy for hypothalamic amenorrhea

Investigator	Patients/ ovulation	Cycles/ ovulation	Preg/ mult/ ABs[a]	Dosages (μg)	Pulse interval (min)	Luteal phase
Leyendecker[15]	33/33	143/143	38/5/9	2.5–2.0	90	hCG/GnRH
Miller[17]	8/8	23/20	7/0/3	1–5	96–120	hCG/GnRH
Berg[18]	12/9	14/10	4/0/2	20	90	hCG
Crowley[13]	8	11/9	3	25 ng/kg	60	GnRH
	9	13/13	10	100 ng/kg	60	GnRH
Jansen[54]	12/12	22/22	9/2	2.5–5	90	hCG
Loucopoulos[19]	8/5	16/9	2	2–20	90–180	GnRH/hCG
Goerzen[55]	6/6	10/10	4	10	120	hCG
Bringer[20]	15	31/26	4	8	69–128	GnRH
Lorign[32]	18		9/1/4	5	90	GnRH
Schriock[31]	14/13	24/23	7/0/2	1.2–10	90	hCG
Reid[33]	3/3	8/7	1	2.5–5	90–120	hCG
Jacobs[24]	3/3	6/6	3	10–25	90	hCG/GnRH
Molloy[23]	9/4	20/20	1/0/0	25–200 ng/kg	60–90	hCG/GnRH
Total	108/96 (89%)	341/318 (93%)	102/8/20			

[a] Preg, pregnancies; multi, multiple births; ABs, spontaneous abortions.

TABLE 7-3. Subcutaneous pulsatile GnRH therapy for hypothalamic amenorrhea

Investigator	Patients/ ovulation	Cycles/ ovulation	Preg/ mult/ ABs[a]	Dosages (μg)	Pulse interval (min)	Luteal phase
Loucopoulos[19]	2/0	5/0	0	2–20	90–180	GnRH/hCG
Reid[33]	2/0	3/0		5–10	120–180	hCG
	3/2	8/2		2–20	60–240	GnRH
Jacobs[24]	25/25	83/80	25/1/8	10–25	90	hCG/GnRH
Hurley[16]	14/14	36/30	13/0/2			
Skarin[34]	19/17		12/1/3	20	90	GnRH
Keogh[56]	14/10		6	50–200	60–120	GnRH
Woodhouse[21]	4/4	9/9	4	2.5–15	90	GnRH
Seibel[22]		10/10	2	20	120	hCG
Saffan[26]	10/10	15/15	4/1	12.5–20	120	hCG
Molloy[23]	14/15	44/44	2/1	25–200 ng/kg	60–90	hCG/GnRH
Total	107/97 (91%)	213/190 (89%)	68/2/11			

[a] Preg, pregnancies; multi, multiple births; ABs, spontaneous abortions.

taneous pulsatile GnRH for ovulation induction in hyperestrogenic amenorrhea (polycystic ovarian disease) are summarized in Table 7-5. Note the following: (1) a very low efficiency rate of 27% ovulatory rate per patient, and (2) a 4% ovulation rate per cycle and a 20% pregnancy rate per ovulation.

The same general prognostic factors hold true for gonadotropin therapy; that is, hypoestrogenic patients with gonadotropin deficiency are more predictable in their response. However, the difference between GnRH and gonadotropin therapy in the nonhypoestrogenic patient is that the latter can override the endogenous system, whereas pulsatile GnRH may not.

TABLE 7-4. Intravenous pulsatile GnRH in hyperestrogenic amenorrhea (PCO)[a]

Investigator	Patients/ ovulation	Cycles/ ovulation	Preg/ mult/ ABs[a]	Dosages (μg)	Pulse interval (min)	Luteal phase
Bringer[20]	7	15/6	3	8	69–128	GnRH
Lorign[32]	4		0	5	90	GnRH
Schriock[31]	10/6	17/10	1	10–20	90	GnRH
Bennink[25]	15/10	42/29	8	10–20	90	GnRH
Berg[18]	15/13	26/26	7/1/1	20	90	hCG
Loucopoulos[19]	2/1	9/1	0	2–20	90–180	GnRH/hCG
Tucker[50]	6	17/11	2/0/2	10–25	90	GnRH/hCG
Tucker[50]	4	7/7	6/0/2	10–25	90	hCG/GnRH
Ory[27]	4/4	6/5	0	0.025 ng/kg	90	GnRH
Total	46/34 (74%)	139/95 (68%)	27/1/5			

[a] PCO, polycystic ovarian disease.
[b] Preg, pregnancies; multi, multiple births; ABs, spontaneous abortions.

TABLE 7-5. Subcutaneous pulsatile GnRH for polycystic ovarian disease

Investigator	Patients/ ovulation	Cycles/ ovulation	Preg/ mult/ ABs[a]	Dosages (μg)	Pulse interval (min)	Luteal phase
Tucker[50]	13	33	11/0/3	10–25	90	hCG/GnRH
Tucker[50]	16	23	3/0/0	10–25	90	hCG/GnRH
Loucopoulos[19]	3	9	0	2–20	90–180	GnRH/hCG
Saffan[26]	3	5	0	5–20	120	GnRH
Hull[57]	5		0	7.5–15	90	GnRH
Total	11/3 (27%)	70/32 (46%)	14/0/3			

[a] Preg, pregnancies; multi, multiple births; ABs, spontaneous abortions.

With proper patient case selection of hypothalamic (hypoestrogenic) cases, pulsatile GnRH has been repeatedly shown to be highly effective at ovulation induction. The first reported series by Leyendecker[15] was closely modeled after the animal studies of Knobil.[6]

Controversies

Controversies surrounding GnRH therapy center around the best route of administration, dosage, pulse frequency, pulse interval variations, and luteal-phase support.

Gonadotropin-releasing hormone can be administered successfully intravenously, subcutaneously, intranasally, or intramuscularly. Comparisons of the pharmacology of gonadotropin-releasing hormone when administered either subcutaneously or intravenously have been reported.[12] After intravenous administration, GnRH plasma levels peak rapidly compared to the subcutaneous route. Intravenous therapy appears to be more physiological and more effective. The subcutaneous route requires higher dosages per pulse and has lower efficacy with a longer time to ovulation. Ovulatory rates are somewhat less when compared to intravenous.[31,40] Nonetheless, successes have been reported with the subcutaneous route of administration (Table 7-3). The advantages of subcutaneous over intravenous is that it is easier to perform and manage as an outpatient, and there is a lower risk of systemic infection.

A wide range of pulse dosages have been successfully used in the treatment of anovulatory states. They range from 1.0 to 40 μg per pulse. Some investigators have attempted to correlate the severity of hypothalamic amenorrhea with subsequent pulse dosages.[41] Crowley attempted to chose a dosage of GnRH that may mimic the physiological situation. The dose range appears to be between 25 ng/kg and 100 ng/kg. The lower dosage is threshold for folliculogenesis. At the upper limits of 100 ng/kg, essentially 100% of women ovulated, but that dosage carried a slightly increased risk of multiple follicular development and multiple pregnancy. In Crowley's study, 75 ng/kg (4 μg per pulse) elicited gonadotropin patterns in women with hypothalamic amenorrhea consistent with normal controls. These data were obtained with intravenous administration. It has been shown that subcutaneous routes require higher pulses of approximately 15 to 20 μg per pulse. The threshold dosage for subcutaneous administration is much higher than for the intravenous route.

The ideal goal during GnRH therapy is to mimic the physiological pulse frequency during an ovulatory menstrual cycle. The LH pulse frequency varies throughout the menstrual cycle with fairly frequent pulses every 60 to 90 minutes during the follicular phase and gradual slowing during the luteal phase secondary to progesterone inhibition.[41,42] No investigator has reported varying pulse frequency during GnRH administration, yet successful ovulation has been achieved with unvarying dosages and pulse frequency. This suggests a permissive role of GnRH therapy during ovulation induction. Data from women of various anovulatory states receiving varying pulse frequencies were reviewed recently. The results are shown in Table 7-6. The best ovulatory rates and resulting pregnancies were achieved when the pulse interval was between 90 and 120 minutes. Ovula-

TABLE 7-6. Results of various GnRH pulse frequencies

Pulse intervals (min)	Ovulation/cycle	Pregnancy
60	2/12*	0/2
90	12/19	4/4
120	7/8	2/4
180	5/9	0/2

*$p < .05$.

tion rates and percentages of pregnancies fell when the pulse intervals were as short as 60 or as long as 180 minutes.

The primate corpus luteum is dependent on continuous pituitary LH support. Several studies have demonstrated the dependence of the corpus luteum on LH support.[42-45] Neutralization of LH by antibodies[44] or suppression of LH with the use of GnRH agonist or antagonist treatment in the luteal phase resulted in the early demise of the corpus luteum, a decline in serum progesterone, and premature menstruation.[43,46] Kallmann's patients receiving pulsatile GnRH for ovulation induction, when not supported in the luteal phase, demonstrated short menstrual cycles.[47]

Studies by Zeleznik[48] in GnRH-deficient monkeys have shown that premature menses and truncation of corpus luteum function occur within a few days of discontinuation of exogenous GnRH therapy. Corpus luteum function is recoverable if pulsatile GnRH therapy is reinstituted. Therefore, in women with hypothalamic amenorrhea supplemental luteal phase support is required, either by continuous pulsatile GnRH or by supplemental human chorionic gonadotropin (hCG) injections. Continued pulsatile GnRH may prove to be more physiological.

Most investigators have chosen to continue the same pulse frequency utilized in the follicular phase without decreasing the frequency as normally expected during the luteal phase. Continued luteal-phase support in women with polycystic ovarian disease may not be as critical as in women with hypothalamic amenorrhea. Progesterone suppositories may be sufficient in the former situation,[49] whereas either pulsatile GnRH or hCG support is required throughout the luteal phase for patients devoid of endogenous LH secretion.

Complications

Complications of GnRH therapy include mild ovarian hyperstimulation, and multiple pregnancies have been reported.[50,51] An accurate estimate of the true incidence of multiple pregnancy remains to be elicited. It appears to be a phenomenon of the first cycle of GnRH administration.

A second complication is possible antibody formation.[52,53] This reaction to a naturally occurring peptide may occur more frequently in patients with a congenital absence of GnRH such as a patient with Kallmann's syndrome or severe hypothalamic amenorrhea. The development of such antibodies has been documented by Clayman[52] in the setting of long-term treatment during puberty induction. The most extensive published experience reported five of 163 patients with the development of antibodies Meakin.[53] Some of these antibodies may be capable of obliterating the biological response to GnRH in addition to their associations with allergic reactions.

Since GnRH is an exact replica of the endogenous hormone, the true incidence of antibody formation is very small. It has also been reported in long-term use in men receiving pulsatile subcutaneous GnRH to achieve pubertal progression and maturation. It is not seen during intravenous administration.[53]

Spontaneous abortion risk is less than in patients receiving pulsatile GnRH when compared to human menopausal gonadotropins. Malformation risk remains to be determined, but several small series have detected no increased risk for birth defects.

Localized concerns include infection at the injection site and hematoma formation at the site of new placement, the latter being secondary to the low-dose heparin that is required to maintain intravenous lines. Local treatment has been sufficient for care, and infection has been localized and self-limited. Heparin should be avoided in patients receiving subcutaneous therapy.

Summary

In conclusion, pulsatile GnRH administered via computerized pumps is currently being used successfully to induce ovulation in many clinical situations. Remaining controversy centers around the precise dosage required, the timing of GnRH pulse frequency in the luteal phase, and route of administration. Subcutaneous therapy is quite efficacious and should be the first choice, with intravenous therapy reserved for more resistant patients such as polycystic ovarian disease. Clinical experience with the medication remains limited, and exact risks of hyperstimulation, multiple pregnancy rate, and spontaneous abortion need to be precisely determined. Nevertheless, GnRH represents a physiological approach to ovulation induction and an attractive alternative to consider when recommending therapy for certain types of anovulatory patients.

References

1. Harris GW. Humours and hormones. J Endocrinol. 1972;53:2–23.
2. Guillemin R, Sakiz E, Ward DN. Further purification of TSH releasing factor from sheep hypothalamic tissues with observations on the amino acid composition. Proc Soc Exp Biol Med. 1965;118:132–37.
3. Matsuo H, Baba Y, Nair RM, et al. Structure of the porcine LH- and FSH-releasing hormone, I. the proposed amino acid sequence. Biochem Biophys Res Commun. 1971;43:1334–40.
4. Schally AV, Arimura A, Bowers CY, et al. Purification of hypothalamic releasing hormones of human origin. J Clin Endocrinol Metab 1970;31:291–300.
5. Burgus R, Butcher M, Amoss N, et al. Primary structure of the hypothalamic luteinizing hormone-releasing factor (LRF) of ovine origin. Proc Natl Acad Sci USA. 1972;69:278–82.
6. Knobil E. The neuroendocrine control of the menstrual cycle. Recent Prog Horm Res. 1980;36:53–88.

7. Seeburg PH, Adelman JP. Characterization of CDNA for precursor of human luteinizing hormone releasing hormone. Nature. 1984;311: 666–68.

8. Hodgen GD. The dominant ovarian follicle. Fertil Steril. 1982;38:281–300.

9. Adams J, Franks S, Polson DW, et al. Multifollicular ovaries: clinical and endocrine features and response to pulsatile gonadotropin releasing hormone. Lancet. 1985;2:1375–79.

10. Sueldo CE, Swanson JA. The economics of inducing ovulation with human menopausal gonadotropins versus pulsatile subcutaneous gonadotropin-releasing hormone. Fertil Steril. 1986;45:128–29.

11. Chambers GR, Sutherland IA, White S, et al. A new generation of pulsatile infusion devices. Ups J Med Sci. 1984;89:91–95.

12. Handelsman DJ, Jansen RP, Boylan LM, et al. Pharmacokinetics of gonadotropin-releasing hormone: comparison of subcutaneous and intravenous routes. J Clin Endocrinol Metab. 1984;59:739–46.

13. Crowley WF Jr, MacArthur JW. Simulation of the normal menstrual cycle in Kallmann's syndrome by pulsatile administration of luteinizing hormone-releasing hormone (LHRH). J Clin Endocrinol Metab. 1980;51:173–75.

14. Seibel MM, Claman P, Oskowitz SP, et al. Events surrounding the initiation of puberty with long term subcutaneous pulsatile gonadotropin-releasing hormone in female patient with Kallmann's syndrome. J Clin Endocrinol Metab. 1985;61:575–79.

15. Leyendecker A, Wildt L. Induction of ovulation with chronic intermittent (pulsatile) administration of GnRH in women with hypothalamic amenorrhea. J Reprod Fertil. 1983;69: 397–404.

16. Hurley DM, Brian RJ, Dutch K, et al. Induction of ovulation and fertility in amenorrheic women by pulsatile low-dose gonadotropin-releasing hormone. N Engl J Med 1984;310: 1069–74.

17. Miller DS, Reid RL, Cetel NS, et al. "Pulsatile administration of low-dose gonadotropin-releasing hormone. JAMA 1983;250: 2937–41.

18. Berg D, Mickan H, Michael S, et al. Ovulation and pregnancy after pulsatile administration of gonadotropin releasing hormone. Arch Gynecol 1983;233:205–10.

19. Loucopoulos A, Ferin M, Van de Wiele RL.

Pulsatile administration of gonadotropin-releasing hormone for induction of ovulation. Am J Obstet Gynecol 1984;148:895–900.

20. Bringer J, Hedon B, Jaffrol C. Influence of the frequency of gonadotropin-releasing hormone (GnRH) administration on ovulatory responses in women with hypothalamic anovulation (HA) and polycystic ovarian syndrome (PCO). Excerpta Medica Cong Ser. 1984;652:470.

21. Woodhouse NJY, Niles N, Othnan HO. Hypothalamic hypogonadism—induction of ovulation and pregnancy by subcutaneous pulsatile injections of gonadotropin-releasing hormone. Horm Res. 1984;20:172–77.

22. Seibel MM, Kamrava M, McArdle C, et al. Ovulation induction and conception using subcutaneous pulsatile luteinizing hormone-releasing hormone. Obstet Gynecol. 1983;61: 292–98.

23. Molloy BG, Hancock KW, Glass MR. Ovulation induction in clomiphene nonresponsive patients: the place of pulsatile gonadotropin-releasing hormone in clinical practice. Fertil Steril. 1985;43:26–33.

24. Jacobs HS, Adams J, Franks S. Induction of ovulation with LHRH—problems, indications and contraindications. J Steroid Biochem 1984;20:A36.

25. Coelingh-Bennink HJT, Weber HW, Alsbach GPJ, et al. Induction of ovulation by pulsatile intravenous administration of GnRH in polycystic ovarian disease. Excerpta Medica Cong Ser. 1984;652:432.

26. Saffan D, Seibel MM. Ovulation induction with subcutaneous pulsatile gonadotropin-releasing hormone in various ovulatory disorders. Fertil Steril. 1986;45:475–82.

27. Ory SJ, London SN, Tyrey L, et al. Ovulation induction with pulsatile gonadotropin-releasing hormone administration in patients with polycystic ovarian syndrome. Fertil Steril. 1985;43:20–25.

28. Wagner TO, Brabant G, Warsch F, et al. Pulsatile gonadotropin-releasing hormone treatment in idiopathic delayed puberty. J Clin Endocrinol Metab. 1986;62:95–101.

29. Stanhope R, Adams J, Brook CG. Disturbances of puberty. Clin Obstet Gynaecol. 1985;12: 557–77.

30. Stanhope R, Abdulwahid NA, Adams J, et al. Problems in the use of pulsatile gonadotrophin-releasing hormone for the induction of puberty. Horm Res. 1985;22:74–77.

31. Schriock ED, Jaffe RB. Induction of ovulation

with gonadotropin-releasing hormone. Obstet Gynecol Surv. 1986;41:414–23.

32. Lorijn RH, Rolland R. Induction of ovulation with pulsatile LH-RH in infertile women. Ups J Med Sci. 1984;89:47–51.

33. Reid RL, Sauerbrei E. Evaluation of techniques for induction of ovulation in patients employing pulsatile gonadotropin releasing hormone. Am J Obstet Gynecol. 1984;148:648–56.

34. Skarin G, Nillus SJ, Wide L. Pulsatile subcutaneous low-dose gonadotropin-releasing hormone treatment of anovulatory infertility. Fertil Steril. 1983;40:454–60.

35. Eckstein N, Vagman 1, Eshel A, et al. Induction of ovulation in amenorrheic patients with gonadotropin-releasing hormone and human menopausal gonadotropin. Fertil Steril. 1985;44:744–50.

36. O'Herlihy C, Stanley J, Powell D. Successful pregnancy following ovulation induction with pulsatile GnRH. Ir Med J. 1985;78:133–34.

37. Bergh T, Skarin G, Nillius SJ, et al. Pulsatile GnRH therapy—an alternative successful therapy for induction of ovulation in infertile normo and hyperprolactinaemic amenorrhoeic women with pituitary tumours. Acta Endocrinol. 1985;110:440–44.

38. Glasier A, McNeilly AS, Baird DT. Induction of ovarian activity by pulsatile infusion of LHRH in women with lactational amenorrhoea. Clin Endocrinol. 1986;24:243–52.

39. Santoro N, Filicori M, Crowley WF Jr. Hypogonadotropic disorders in men and women: diagnosis and therapy with pulsatile gonadotropin-releasing hormone. Endocr Rev. 1986;7:11–23.

40. Zacur HA. Ovulation induction with gonadotropin-releasing hormone. Fertil Steril. 1985;44:435–48.

41. Crowley WF Jr, Filicori M, Spratt D, et al. The physiology of a gonadotropin-releasing hormone (GnRH) secretion in men and women. Rec Prog Horm Res. 1985;41:473–531.

42. Filicori M, Santoro N, Merriam GR, et al. Characterization of the physiological pattern of episodic gonadotropin secretion throughout the human menstrual cycle. J Clin Endocrinol Metab. 1986;62:1136–44.

43. Collins RL, Sopelak V, Williams RF, et al. Prevention of GnRH antagonist-induced luteal regression by concurrent exogenous pulsatile gonadotrophin administration in monkeys. Fertil Steril. 1986;46:945–53.

44. Groff T, Raj HGM, Talbert LM, et al. Effects of neutralization of luteinizing hormone on corpus luteum function and cyclicity in *Macaca fascicularis*. J Clin Endocrinol Metab. 1984;59:1054–57.

45. Coelingh Bennink HJT. Pulsatile administration of LHRH for ovulation induction. In: Shaw RW, Marshall JC, eds. LHRH and its analogues. Their use in gynaecological practice. London: Wright Press, 1989:92–112.

46. Mais V, Kazer RR, Cetel NS, et al. The dependency of folliculogenesis and corpus luteum function on pulsatile gonadotropin secretion in cycling women using a gonadotropin-releasing hormone antagonist as a probe. J Clin Endocrinol Metab. 1986;62:1250–55.

47. Weinstein FG, Seibel MM, Taymor ML. Ovulation induction with subcutaneous pulsatile gonadotropin-releasing hormone: the role of supplemental human chorionic gonadotropin in the luteal phase. Fertil Steril. 1984;41:546–50.

48. Zeleznik AJ, Hutchison JS. The use of pulsatile GnRH treatment to investigate the regulation of the primate corpus luteum. In: Coelingh Bennink HJT, Dogterom AA, Lappohn RE, et al., eds. Pulsatile GnRH 1985. Haarlenu, The Netherlands: Ferring, 1986:71–79.

49. Berger NG, Zacur HA. Exogenous progesterone for luteal support following gonodatropin-releasing hormone ovulation induction: case report. Fertil Steril. 1985;44:133–35.

50. Tucker M, Adams J, Mason WP, et al. Multiple cystic ovarian disease—a new classification. Excerpta Medica Cong Ser. 1984;652:1588.

51. Schweditsch MO, Keller PJ, Floersheim Y, et al. Ovarian hyperstimulation during chronic pulsatile GnRH therapy. Gynecol Obstet Invest. 1984;17:276–77.

52. Claman P, Elkind-Hirsch K, Oskowitz SP, et al. Urticaria associated with antigonadotropin-releasing hormone antibody in a female Kallmann's syndrome patient being treated with long-term pulsatile gonadotropin-releasing hormone. Obstet Gynecol 1987;69:503–05.

53. Meakin JL, Keogh EJ, Martin CE. Human anti-luteinizing hormone releasing hormone antibodies in patients treated with synthetic luteinizing hormone releasing hormone. Fertil Steril. 1985;43:811–13.

54. Jansen RPS, Hendelsman DJ, Boylan LM. Induction of ovulation with pulsatile intravenous injections of gonadotropin-releasing hor-

mone (GnRH). Excerpta Medica Cong Ser.
1984;652:709.

55. Goerzen J, Corenblum B, Wiseman D, et al.
Ovulation induction and pregnancy in hypothalamic amenorrhea using self-administered
intravenous gonadotropin-releasing hormone.
Fertil Steril. 1984;41:319–21.

56. Keogh EJ, Mallal SA, Giles PFH, et al. Ovulation induction with intermittent subcutaneous
LHRH. Lancet 1981;1:147.

57. Hull ME, Kenigsberg DJ. Gonadotropin releasing hormone: function and clinical use.
Lab Management. 1987;25:51–55.

8
Luteal Function after Ovulation Induction

Marc A. Fritz

Luteal-phase inadequacy is a diagnosis that should be considered in any woman presenting with reproductive failure, whether manifested by repetitive pregnancy wastage or infertility. Although, in general, a deficient luteal phase will be found in fewer than 10% of women who seek evaluation for infertility, the diagnosis is made significantly more often in certain subsets of the infertile population. The extremes of reproductive age, hyperprolactinemia, regular strenuous exercise, elevated circulating androgens, oligoovulation, and treatment with ovulation-inducing agents all are associated with a higher incidence of the disorder, as is the interval immediately after termination of pregnancy. The focus of this discussion is deficiencies of luteal function that may follow ovulation induction.

Although there is some controversy over the importance of ruling out luteal-phase defects in the routine evaluation of the infertile couple, few would deny the importance of considering this diagnosis in women undergoing medical induction of ovulation. A relatively high incidence of luteal-phase deficiency has been observed in anovulatory women treated with clomiphene citrate (CC),[1-3] but inadequate luteal function may also complicate ovulation induction with bromocriptine, human menopausal gonadotropins (hMG), and gonadotropin-releasing hormone (GnRH).

The mechanisms responsible for the deficient luteal function that may follow induced ovulation are varied. A luteal-phase defect may result from as yet incomplete correction of the underlying ovulatory disturbance and merely indicate that corrective therapy is still inadequate. In this sense, ovulatory dysfunction might be viewed as a spectrum, with luteal-phase deficiency falling somewhere between normal ovulatory function and frank anovulation (Fig. 8-1). In other words, in attempting to induce normal ovulatory cycles in the anovulatory woman, an ovulatory but relatively poor quality cycle may result, one manifestation of which is luteal-phase inadequacy. Alternatively, the drug(s) used to induce ovulation may more directly interfere with processes that influence the nature of the subsequent luteal phase. The factors that may affect the quality of luteal function and the mechanisms underlying the luteal inadequacy that may follow ovulation induction with CC, bromocriptine, hMG, and GnRH are unique to each agent, and each is considered separately.

Luteal Function after Clomiphene Citrate Therapy

Clomiphene citrate is the most commonly used drug for the induction of ovulation in the anovulatory infertile patient. It competitively binds to the estrogen receptor (ER) in numerous tissues throughout the reproductive system, including the hypothalamus, pituitary, ovary, endocervix, and endome-

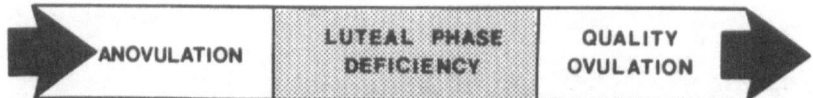

FIGURE 8-1. Spectrum of ovulatory dysfunction, with luteal-phase deficiency falling between frank anovulation and normal ovulatory function.

trium. Under normal circumstances, estrogen binds to its specific intracellular receptor and, in so doing, induces a conformational change in the hormone–receptor complex that allows binding of the complex to nuclear chromatin, where it may then direct the production of specific messenger RNAs and ultimately the production of specific cellular proteins. Among the proteins produced is the ER itself in a process known as ER replenishment. Specific intracellular progesterone receptors (PR) are another of the important proteins produced through the action of estrogen (Fig. 8-2).

In induction of ovulation, CC is believed to act by inhibiting ER replenishment at the level of the hypothalamus and thereby interfering with the normal negative feedback

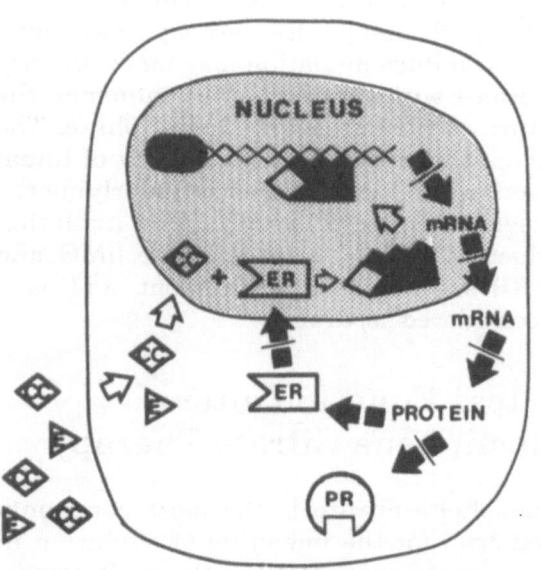

FIGURE 8-2. Mechanism of action of clomiphene citrate (CC). E, estrogen; ER, estrogen receptor; PR, progesterone receptor. Broken arrows denote processes inhibited by clomiphene.

effect of endogenous estrogens on gonadotropin secretion, probably by altering the pattern of hypothalamic GnRH release.[4] The result is an appropriate response to a perceived hypoestrogenic state at the hypothalamic–pituitary level: an increase in the release of gonadotropins. Consequently, during CC administration, peripheral serum levels of follicle-stimulating hormone (FSH) rise as in the early follicular phase of the normal cycle. This relative increase in circulating FSH levels is crucial because the effectiveness of CC in ovulation induction stems from its ability to promote the many FSH-dependent processes that are involved in effective follicular development. Emergence and maturation of the dominant ovarian follicle, proliferation of the granulosa cell layer, induction of the luteinizing hormone (LH) receptors that will mediate ovulation and luteinization, renewed endometrial proliferation and PR induction, and stimulation of the LH surge itself are all directly dependent on follicular-phase FSH, the estrogen produced by FSH-induced aromatase activity, or both. Each of these follicular-phase events is also an important prerequisite for subsequent normal luteal function.

Together, FSH and the high local concentrations of estradiol that result from FSH-induced aromatization of thecal androgens in the granulosa cell layer promote rapid proliferation of the granulosa cell mass as the follicle grows and matures.[5] It is these same granulosa cells that hypertrophy and accumulate lipid during luteinization and ultimately become the granulosa-luteal cells of the corpus luteum. Obviously, the ultimate size of the functional cell mass of the corpus luteum, to some degree, predetermines its steroidogenic capacity. The relative quality of FSH-dependent folliculogenesis influences not only the size of the granulosa cell contribution to the corpus luteum but the process of luteinization as well.

In order to induce an effective LH surge, one capable of initiating both the ovulatory sequence and luteinization, estrogen produced by the proliferating granulosa must be sufficient to achieve and maintain a critical threshold concentration of estradiol. Levels below the threshold are unsuccessful in inducing a normal LH surge, as are those above the threshold but abnormally brief in duration.[6] Effective luteinization, however, even in response to an LH surge of normal amplitude and duration, also requires that the granulosa first acquire the LH receptors necessary to mediate a response. This too is an FSH-dependent process. Selective binding of FSH induces the appearance of LH receptor on granulosa cells of larger antral follicles in a time- and dose-dependent manner, an action that is further enhanced by estradiol.[7,8] A deficiency in FSH may thus result in a reduced number of LH receptors, which are required to mediate not only luteinization at midcycle but the trophic action of LH on the corpus luteum during the luteal phase as well. This mechanism may explain why treatment with human chorionic gonadotropin (hCG) frequently fails to improve luteal function in women with a short luteal phase and the observation that monkey luteal cells obtained in FSH-deficient cycles induced by treatment with porcine follicular fluid exhibit suppressed basal as well as hCG-stimulated progesterone synthesis *in vitro*.[9]

Clearly, the functional capacity of the corpus luteum is in many ways dependent on normal growth and maturation of the preovulatory follicle that is its progenitor. Anything less than optimal follicular development may result in inadequate luteal function despite the apparently successful induction of ovulation. Several lines of evidence have linked a short or otherwise inadequate luteal phase to a relatively subtle follicular-phase FSH deficiency.[10-11] In both monkeys and humans, luteal-phase deficiency is frequently preceded by subnormal serum concentrations of FSH and low FSH:LH ratios

during the early and midfollicular phase.[10,11] Experimentally, the selective suppression of FSH during the follicular phase is associated with lower preovulatory estradiol levels, depressed midluteal progesterone production, and a decrease in luteal cell mass.[12] Similarly, in women, reduced follicular-phase FSH levels induced by treatment with a potent, long-acting GnRH agonist result in a shortened luteal phase and reduced concentrations of both estradiol and progesterone.[13]

It should be clear that as induction of ovulation is attempted with CC in the usual empirical incremental manner, a given dose of the drug may be adequate to induce an increase in FSH sufficient to promote meaningful follicular development and even achieve ovulation but still be inadequate to ensure normal luteal function. Although whether a given dose of CC has succeeded in inducing ovulation is usually relatively easily determined, the quality of that ovulatory cycle and, specifically, of the subsequent luteal phase cannot in any case be assumed. A grossly short luteal phase as judged by the basal body temperature (BBT) pattern certainly does suggest that one has not yet achieved optimal follicular development and truly successful induction of ovulation. Recall that a short luteal phase is highly correlated with follicular-phase FSH deficiency. In addition, the histological maturation delays that are observed in endometrial biopsy specimens obtained in short-luteal-phase cycles are typically more severe than defects that occur in cycles having a luteal phase of normal duration.[14,15] Unfortunately, a BBT pattern that exhibits a short luteal phase is not reliable in identifying those individuals who may be receiving an inadequate dose of CC because the majority of luteal-phase defects are accompanied by a luteal phase of normal duration[14] (Fig. 8-3). Therefore, specific evaluation of the quality of luteal function must be undertaken if one is to ensure that each and every treatment cycle is potentially fertile. The failure to do so may easily lead to continued use of an ineffective dose of CC, the erroneous conclusion that additional factors are responsible for the

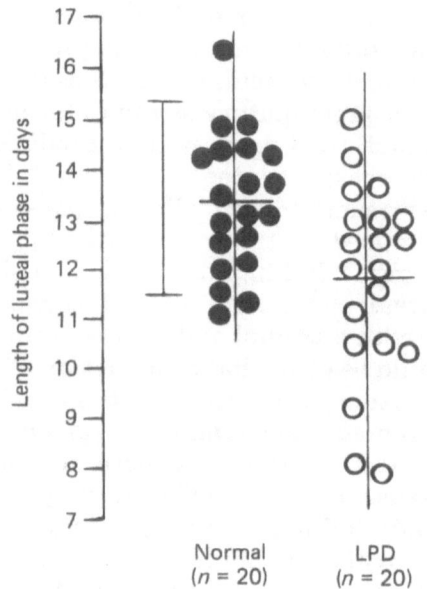

FIGURE 8-3. Mean luteal-phase length averaged for three cycles as derived from basal body temperature charts for subjects with biopsy-proven normal luteal phases (●) and subjects with biopsy-confirmed luteal-phase defects (o). Horizontal bars indicate the mean ± 2 standard deviations ($P < 0.05$). (From Downs KA, Gibson M. Basal body temperature graph and the luteal phase defect. Fertil Steril 1983, 40:466. Reproduced with permission of the publisher, The American Fertility Society.)

couple's infertility, and, further, often more invasive and ultimately unnecessary methods of evaluation.

Whereas luteal-phase deficiency may be only the consequence of inadequate CC therapy, the drug itself may also be more directly responsible for many of the luteal-phase defects that have been observed in association with its use. Luteal-phase inadequacy may complicate induction of ovulation with CC even when the dose employed is appropriate and effective in promoting the development of an optimally mature preovulatory follicle. Clomiphene citrate binds to the ER in all estrogen-dependent tissues and not only to those at the hypothalamic–pituitary level. In addition to the desirable central actions of CC that are the basis for its effectiveness in ovulation induction, the drug may also exert its antiestrogenic influence at the level of the

ovary, endocervix, and endometrium, some of which may not be at all desirable (Fig. 8-4). Interference with the action of estrogen within the ovary may attenuate the response of the follicle to the increase in FSH that CC induces centrally.[16] Remember that estrogen is important in enhancing FSH-induced granulosa proliferation and LH receptor induction within the follicle. Recent evidence that CC may even compromise the developmental capacity of the maturing ovum is also of concern.[17,18] The drug's ability to affect adversely the quantity and quality of mucus produced by the endocervical glands is widely recognized.

But perhaps most importantly, at the endometrial level, CC may interfere with the actions of estrogen produced by the maturing follicle that the CC earlier helped to emerge. Rising levels of estradiol serve to stimulate renewed endometrial proliferation after the functionalis is shed in the preceding menses. As in all estrogen-dependent tissues, this action of estrogen is mediated by specific ER and, in addition to stimulating further production of its own endometrial receptor, estrogen induces the appearance of endometrial PR. Consequently, endometrial PR levels rise throughout the follicular phase and become maximal coincident with the preovulatory surge in estradiol concentrations[19] (Fig. 8-5). Progesterone is widely accepted as the principal mediator of the orderly sequence of secretory endometrial development that characterizes the luteal phase of the menstrual cycle in women. Presumably, progesterone exerts its action on the endometrium by first combining with these specific, estrogen-induced PR. Normal secretory development of the preimplantation endometrium must then depend on estrogen induction of an effective PR population. If receptor concentrations are inadequate or receptor function is otherwise impaired, optimal secretory endometrial development may not occur.[20] Interference with ER-mediated endometrial ER and PR induction has been considered the mechanism most likely to be responsible for the increased incidence of luteal phase deficiency associated with CC treatment.

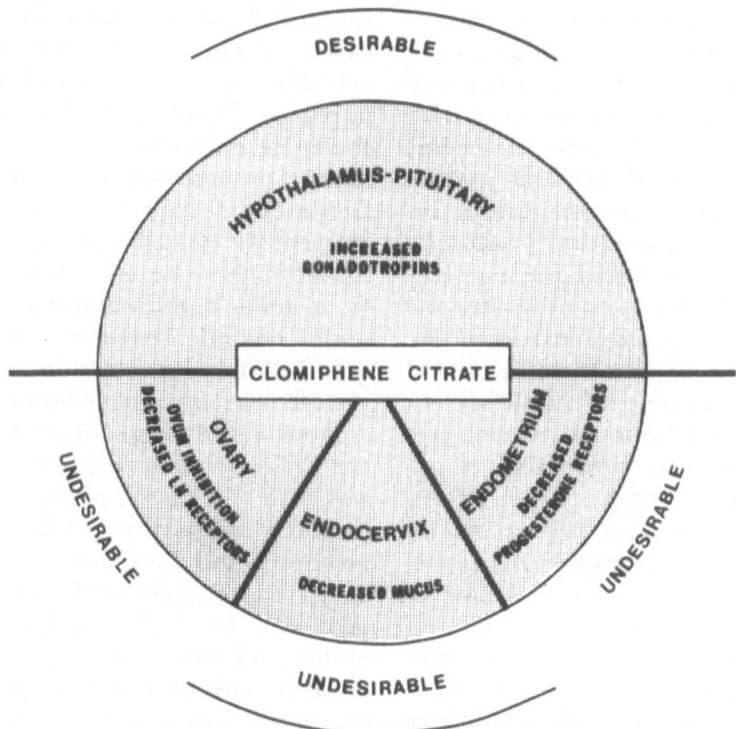

FIGURE 8-4. Actions of clomiphene citrate at various sites throughout the reproductive system.

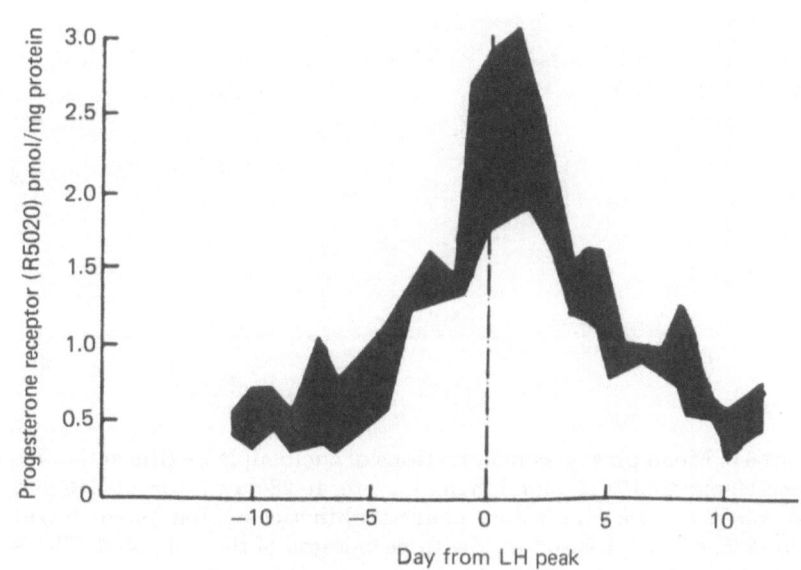

FIGURE 8-5. Endometrial progesterone receptor concentrations during the menstrual cycle. (Reprinted by permission from Edman, CD. *Seminars in Reproductive Endocrinology*, Vol. 1, No. 3. New York: Thieme Medical Publishers, 1983.)

During CC treatment estrogen levels are typically higher in the late follicular phase, a fact suggesting that, if anything, the population of endometrial PR induced should be greater than that normally seen. However, CC administration is also frequently associated with a premature peri-ovulatory increase in progesterone production[21] that may limit or prevent any such enhancement of steroid receptor induction, as progesterone inhibits ER production and, indirectly, the induction of its own receptor. In addition, CC has been reported capable of reducing endometrial ER and PR concentrations, presumably by antagonizing the action of endogenous estrogens.[22] Which of these effects will predominate when the drug is administered—that of higher estrogen or progesterone levels or the antiestrogenic action of the drug itself—and whether there is dose–response relationship has been uncertain. Interestingly, recent data now demonstrates that CC treatment in normal, ovulatory women neither enhances nor inhibits overall endometrial steroid receptor induction.[23,24]

Regardless of the dose of CC administered or time of sampling, the concentration and subcellular distribution of both ER and PR were unchanged from spontaneous cycle values in the same individuals, despite a dramatic increase in preovulatory estradiol after CC treatment.[24] Nevertheless, the link drawn between CC treatment and increased risk of luteal-phase deficiency derives from observations made in anovulatory infertile patients under chronic therapy. The entended half-life of CC and its corresponding potential for significant systemic accumulation have been demonstrated (Fig. 8-6).[25] Impressive residual CC concentrations almost certainly persist into the luteal phase and beyond, particularly in patients who fail to conceive promptly and therefore continue treatment for extended periods of time, and high circulating CC levels during the luteal phase are associated with consistently delayed endometrial maturation.[26] A dose-and/or time-dependent adverse effect of CC on endometrial steroid receptor populations therefore cannot be excluded.

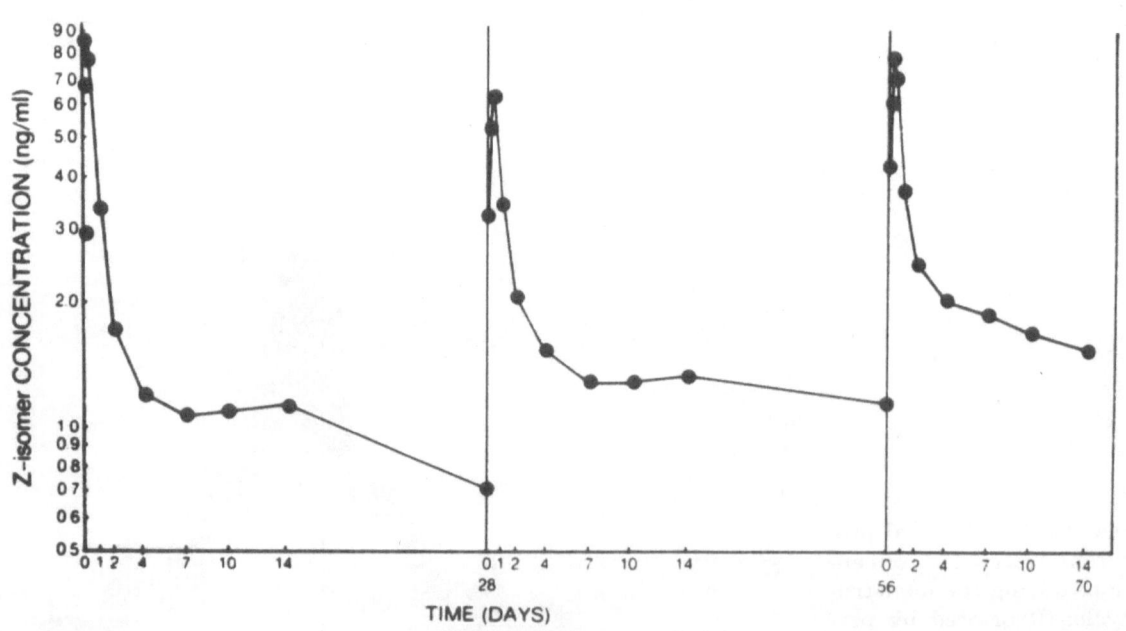

FIGURE 8-6. Mean plasma concentrations of zuclomiphene (the active isomer) after oral administration of one 50-mg tablet of clomiphene citrate at 28-day intervals. (From Mikkelson TJ, Kroboth PD, Cameron WJ, et al. Single-dose pharmacokinetics of clomiphene citrate in normal volunteers. Fertil Steril 1986, 46:392. Reproduced with permission of the publisher, The American Fertility Society.)

It would appear likely that other mechanisms unrelated to endometrial steroid receptor concentration and/or function are involved in CC-associated luteal-phase deficiency. First of all, direct adverse effects of CC that operate through postreceptor mechanisms remain a possibility. The marked elevation of luteal-phase estradiol that occasionally follows CC-induced ovulation and that consistently accompanies elevated luteal-phase CC concentrations[26,27] may directly interfere with the process of endometrial decidualization.[28] Moreover, residual levels of CC may be capable of directly inhibiting steroidogenesis in the corpus luteum.[29,30] Progesterone production by luteinized human granulosa cells in vitro can be inhibited by CC at concentrations known to exist in both serum and follicular fluid on the day of ovulation[30,31] and to persist in the circulation at the time of expected nidation of the blastocyst.[32] Subtle CC-induced disruption of the pattern of pulsatile gonadotropin secretion is another possibility. An abnormally increased follicular-phase LH pulse frequency has been implicated in the pathogenesis of luteal-phase defects.[33] Interestingly, the mechanism of action of CC in ovulation induction appears to involve just such an increase in LH pulse frequency, presumably a reflection of an induced increase in pulsatile hypothalamic GnRH secretion.[4] It may be that excess CC, whether it results from frank overdosage and/or accumulation due to chronic administration, will provoke an abnormally rapid and thus ineffective pattern of gonadotropin secretion that predisposes to inadequate corpus luteum function.

Clearly, there are many plausible explanations for the relatively high incidence of luteal-phase deficiency observed in association with the use of CC for ovulation induction. Luteal-phase inadequacy may result from inadequate therapy and subsequent marginal gonadotropin stimulation and incomplete folliculogenesis. On the other hand, there is ample reason to contend that CC treatment may itself directly cause luteal-phase deficiency by antagonizing essential actions of estrogen at the ovarian or endometrial level in either the follicular or luteal phase. The dilemma then is how to interpret the luteal-phase defect that is diagnosed in a patient receiving CC for ovulation induction. Clinically, if the luteal-phase inadequacy is the result of not yet having achieved optimal preovulatory follicular development, an increase in dose may be effective in providing the added stimulation necessary to ensure development of a fully mature preovulatory follicle and a subsequent normally functional corpus luteum. Consistent with this approach is the fact that CC has been demonstrated effective in treating luteal-phase defects diagnosed in spontaneous ovulatory cycles.[34,35]

Alternatively, luteal-phase deficiency may be directly related to the estrogen-antagonistic actions of the drug itself. In the latter case, there is a further question as to how the abnormality can be best be corrected if the patient will not ovulate at all without the use of CC. Furthermore, if treatment is continued, it is uncertain whether increasing the circulating concentration of progesterone with supplemental therapy or even adjunctive hCG will have any effect on an endometrium possibly deficient in the PR required for response. Regardless of the mechanism involved, the potential for luteal-phase deficiency to accompany either too much or too little drug suggests that the effective therapeutic range for CC may be narrower than previously appreciated, at least in some individuals.

When a luteal-phase defect is diagnosed in association with CC therapy, a one-step increment in dose might seem the most logical initial approach to its correction. This is particularly true when the luteal phase is abnormally brief in duration, because follicular-phase FSH deficiency is characteristic of cycles having a short luteal phase.[10] If, in fact, ovulation has been induced but luteal function is inadequate because of marginal follicular development, the measure should help to compete folliculogenesis, provide an LH surge of normal amplitude, and ensure effective luteinization. Should an increase in the dose of CC fail to correct the abnormality, the estrogen-antagonistic actions of the drug itself are clearly implicated. Supplementing the probably deficient steroid production of the corpus luteum with progesterone vaginal suppositories or stimulating greater endogenous production with exogenous hCG is likely to be successful. However, increasing the circulating concentration of progesterone may also fail if the defect is related to CC interference with the development of an effective endometrial PR population.

An alternative to the empirical approach to correction of luteal-phase defects that accompany the use of CC is first to undertake a careful evaluation of the quality of folliculogenesis that precedes the inadequate luteal phase using ultrasound and serum estradiol determinations.[36,37] Documented normal preovulatory estradiol concentrations together with serial sonograms that provide objective evidence for the development of a follicle of mature size should eliminate concerns about the quality of CC-induced follicular development. Guided by these findings, progesterone supplementation is the treatment of choice[38] since an increase in the dose of CC could only be counterproductive. Conversely, hormone and sonographic evidence of inadequate folliculogenesis suggests a need for additional gonadotropin stimulation.

Even when management is specifically guided by the apparent quality of preovulatory follicular development, an occasional CC-associated luteal-phase defect will prove refractory to treatment. Consideration should then be given to determining whether the patient may have elevated androgen levels, particularly dehyroepiandrosterone sulfate (DHEAS). When present in excess, androgens may interfere with normal estrogen-induced endometrial PR development.[39,40] A DHEAS level above 200 μg/dL identifies those patients in whom an ovulatory response might be maintained with a reduced dose of CC when they are also treated with dexamethasone.[41] The combination should succeed in overcoming the inhibitory influences of both excess androgen and the higher dose of CC. In the event that a reduced dose of CC is met with a return to anovulation or fails to correct the luteal-phase defect, discontinuation of CC altogether and taking a more direct approach to ovulation induction with exogenous gonadotropins (e.g., purified FSH or hMG) is the logical alternative.

Luteal-phase deficiency may be responsible for the much-quoted discrepancy between ovulation and pregnancy rates that is associated with the use of CC. Effective use of CC requires careful titration in an attempt to establish that dose of the drug that will produce the desired effect on gonadotropin secretion centrally but not interfere with important estrogen-mediated processes in the periphery. The goal is to identify the lowest dose of CC that is compatible with both successful ovulation induction and normal luteal function. To achieve it, specific evaluation of the quality of luteal function that follows CC-induced ovulation is essential.

Luteal Function after Bromocriptine Therapy

Hyperprolactinemia is not infrequently found in association with anovulation in the infertile woman. The mechanisms whereby elevated prolactin levels may disrupt normal ovulatory function are several. Inhibition of effective folliculogenesis may occur as a result of interference with central dopaminergic mechanisms[42,43] as well as a number of more direct actions at the ovarian level.[44-54] Clearly, it is important to consider the diagnosis and obtain a prolactin determination in any woman suspected of having ovulatory dysfunction. The identification of a prolactin disorder offers the unusual opportunity to use therapy specific for the apparent underlying cause of the ovulatory disturbance. In addition, when hyperprolactinemia is unrecognized, other possible treatment options are also unlikely to succeed.

Bromocriptine is clearly the treatment of choice for ovulatory dysfunction associated with hyperprolactinemia. However, as was the case with the use of CC, the quality of ovulatory cycle induced with bromocriptine should not be assumed. Normalization of prolactin levels with any given dose of the drug must be confirmed because the inhibitory influence of even modestly elevated prolactin levels is impressive if it is also often subtle. A growing body of literature supports the notion of a pathological association between chronic and even transient hyperprolactinemia and luteal-phase deficiency.[55-59] Although many hyperprolactinemic women are frankly anovulatory if not amenorrheic, an elevated prolactin level may also cause only a short or otherwise inadequate luteal phase. Following the discontinuation of bromocriptine treatment in hyperprolactinemic patients, a shortening of the luteal phase is often the first clinical indication of a return to elevated levels, followed in turn by recurrent galactorrhea, frank anovulation, and, finally, amenorrhea[56] (Fig. 8-7). Thus, luteal-phase deficiency may be one of the earliest manifestations of an emerging prolactin disorder. Conversely, it may accompany the ovulatory cycle induced with bromocriptine as prolactin levels are reduced. Failure to achieve euprolactinemia during treatment may easily result in apparently successful induction of ovulation but continued infertility because of an unrecognized and consistent luteal-phase defect.

Various mechanisms have been proposed to explain the association of luteal-phase deficiency with hyperprolactinemia. The weight of evidence suggests that the adverse effect of elevated prolactin levels on the quality of luteal function results from interference with normal preovulatory follicular development and the process of luteinization. Several lines of experimental evidence support the view that luteal-phase deficiency is the consequence of disturbed follicular-phase events and not the result of a direct action of prolactin on the corpus luteum itself. First of all, successful suppression of prolactin concentrations in hyperprolactinemic women with short-luteal-phase cycles is followed by an increase in follicular-phase FSH, increased amplitude of the midcycle gonadotropin surge, and a normal luteal-phase duration that is accompanied by increased serum concentrations of progesterone, 17α-hydroxyprogesterone, and estradiol.[42] Second, a number of in vitro studies have demonstrated direct prolactin inhibition of FSH-induced aromatization and granulosa cell estrogen production.[47-49] This effect has been observed in the presence of prolactin concentrations as low as 10 ng/mL in vitro,[54] but, since follicular fluid prolactin levels are generally lower than those present in serum,[60] significant inhibition is unlikely except in hyperprolactinemic states.

In addition to both direct and indirect interference with estrogen biosynthesis within the follicle, prolactin has recently been implicated as a luteinization inhibitor. At concentrations within the range that can be

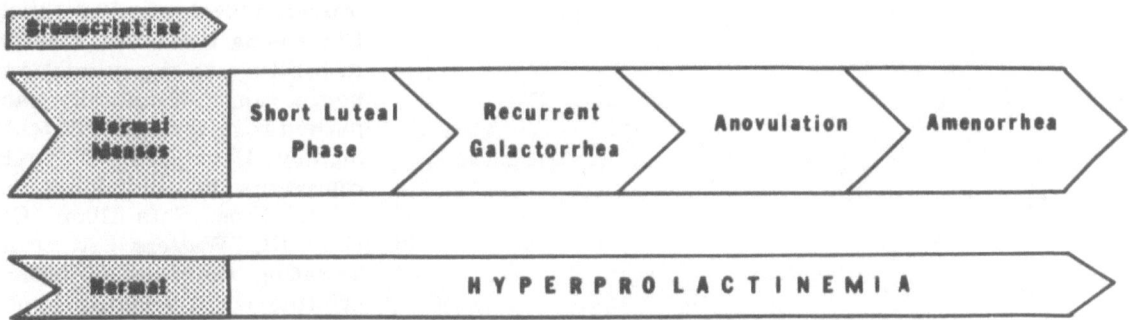

FIGURE 8-7. Sequence of clinical events following the discontinuation of bromocriptine in the hyperprolactinemic patient.

achieved in follicular fluid in vivo, prolactin inhibits FSH-induced LH binding to rat granulosa cells, an effect further associated with a significant reduction in hCG-stimulated progesterone production in vitro.[53] Observations of an inverse correlation between human follicular fluid prolactin levels and the extent of follicular maturity as judged by follicular size and steroid content[60] provide further evidence that luteal-phase inadequacy in hyperprolactinemic women results from similarly inadequate preovulatory follicular development. In a more clinical perspective, serial follicular sonograms in cycling women with metoclopramide-induced hyperprolactinemia have demonstrated a decrease in the size of the largest follicle in association with reduced steroid production.[61]

Also noteworthy is one study of 20 hyperprolactinemic anovulatory women in which bromocriptine treatment was limited to only the follicular phase; there were 15 successful pregnancies in the group despite consistent elevations of prolactin levels during the luteal phase of conception cycles.[62] For all of the reasons discussed earlier in reference to CC, any interference with the many essential estrogen-mediated processes during folliculogenesis may prevent the development of an optimally mature preovulatory follicle and risk creation of a functionally incompetent corpus luteum or an endometrium ill prepared to respond. Hyperprolactinemia appears to cause luteal-phase deficiency by altering the normal patterns of gonadotropin secretion and by direct interference with LH receptor acquisition and FSH-induced aromatase activity within the follicle.

Whereas a lowering of prolactin concentrations is clearly the objective of bromocriptine treatment, oversuppression is also best avoided. There is some evidence that prolactin, at physiological concentrations, may play an important permissive or mildly trophic role in support of normal luteal function. Progesterone produced by luteinized human granulosa cells maintained in culture is significantly reduced when prolactin present in the culture medium is neutralized with a specific antiserum.[51] In addition, when administered together, bromocriptine and estradiol induce luteolysis in the monkey

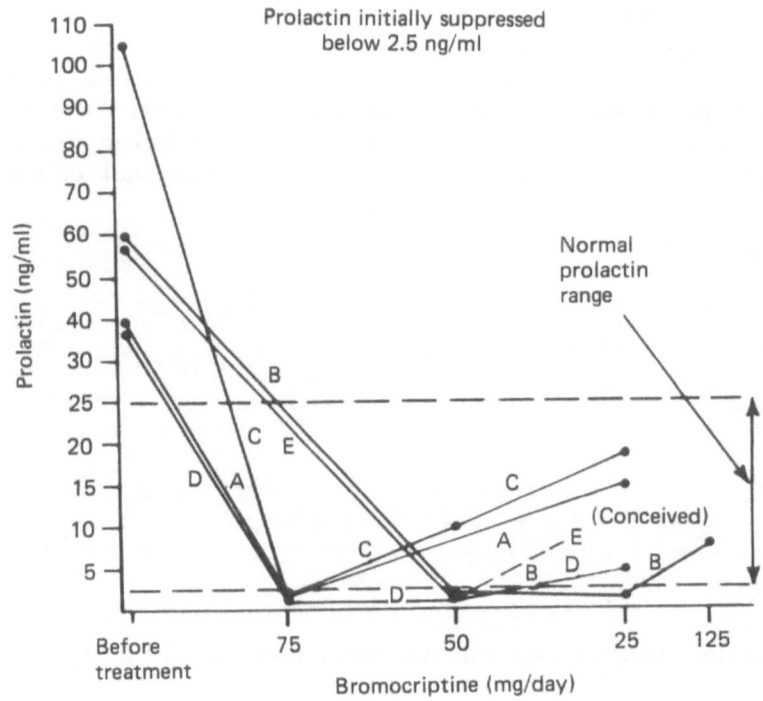

FIGURE 8-8. In these five patients treated "routinely" with 5.0 to 7.5 mg/day of bromocriptine, the prolactin level was <2.6 ng/mL. Decreasing their dose resulted in a return to the normal prolactin range. Eventually each patient required only 1.25 to 2.5 mg/day. Each letter (A to E) represents an individual patient. (From Soto-Albors CE, Daly DC, Walters CA, et al. Titrating the dose of bromocriptine when treating hyperprolactinemic infertile women. Fertil Steril 1985, 43:485. Reproduced with permission of the publisher, The American Fertility Society.)

when the same dose of either alone is ineffective.[63,64] Addition of bromocriptine to an already luteolytic dose of estradiol enhances the effect.[64] Moreover, continuous administration of bromocriptine throughout the cycle of normal individuals may reduce luteal-phase progesterone production.[65] The importance of prolactin to normal luteal function remains open to question, however. The report of a woman with an isolated prolactin deficiency who conceived without assistance, delivered but did not lactate, and had undetectable prolactin levels even with provocative testing is difficult to reconcile with an essential role for prolactin.[66] On the other hand, her menstrual cycles between pregnancies were short, and luteal-phase progesterone concentrations were lower than normal.

It seems that normal luteal function may require prolactin levels that are neither too high nor too low. The dose of bromocriptine that is required to normalize the prolactin concentration generally correlates with the extent of hyperprolactinemia, but many patients exhibit an exquisite sensitivity to the drug.[67] It is also important to note that the dose of bromocriptine necessary to maintain euprolactinemia may ultimately be less than that required to achieve it initially[67] (Fig. 8-8). Ovulation induction with bromocriptine must therefore be carefully monitored in order to ensure that euprolactinemia is both induced and maintained and that oversuppression is also avoided. Clearly, as was the case with CC-induced ovulation, a specific effort should be made to confirm that ovulation induced with bromocriptine is followed by a normal luteal phase.

Luteal Function after Human Menopausal Gonadotropin Therapy

Human menopausal gonadotropin (hMG, menotropins) is usually the choice for induction of ovulation in the euprolactinemic patient who fails to respond to CC and in women with functional hypogonadotropism. On the surface, it would seem that luteal-phase deficiency should be virtually unknown after induction of ovulation with hMG. After all, hMG therapy is usually associated with luteal-phase progesterone concentrations that are substantially higher than those observed in spontaneous ovulatory cycles[68,69] (Fig. 8-9). One suggested estimated is that normal values should be adjusted upward by a factor of 3.0 following the use of menotropins.[68] In all probability, the higher progesterone levels result from unavoidable stimulation of multiple follicular development and the subsequent formation of more than a single cor-

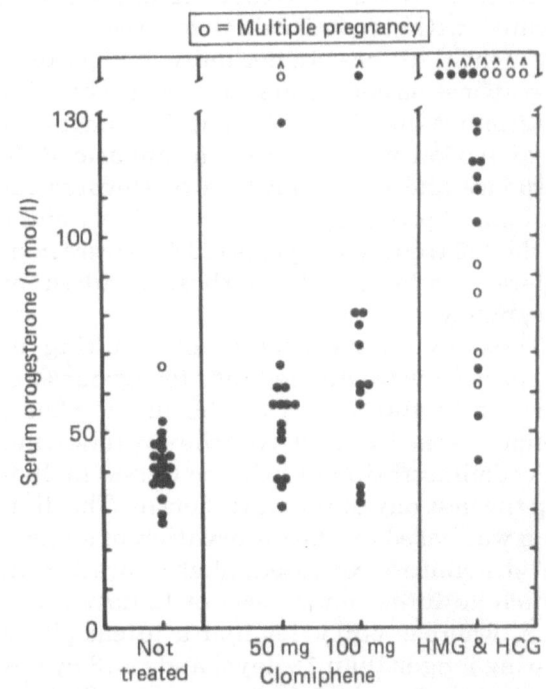

FIGURE 8-9. Midluteal serum progesterone concentration in conception cycles after treatment with clomiphene in two different daily doses or with gonadotropins, compared with untreated conception cycles. 1 ng/mL = 3.18 nmol/L. (From Hull MGR, Savage PE, Bromham DR, et al. The value of a single serum progesterone measurement in the midluteal phase as a criterion of a potentially fertile cycle ("ovulation") derived from treated and untreated conception cycles. Fertil Steril 1982, 37:355. Reproduced with permission of the publisher, The American Fertility Society.)

pus luteum. Surprisingly, despite these facts, inadequate luteal function may not be altogether rare following ovulation induction with hMG.

In actuality, very little data regarding the quality of luteal function that follows a course of hMG–hCG treatment are available. Outside of the context of in vitro fertilization and embryo transfer (IVF-ET) cycles in which endocrinologically normal women are usually involved, the only systematic analysis of the quality of luteal function in anovulatory patients treated with hMG–hCG is that undertaken by Olson and colleagues.[70] In that study, the hormonal profiles in 126 treatment cycles from 24 consecutive patients receiving hMG therapy were characterized. Each was treated with an individualized regimen of hMG–hCG tailored to her individual pattern of response as determined by serum estradiol determinations. The presumptive diagnosis of ovulation was based on a biphasic BBT response and demonstration of elevated luteal-phase progesterone levels. Ninety-eight of the 126 treatment cycles (76.5%) were considered ovulatory; 20 of these resulted in pregnancy.

Those ovulatory cycles not resulting in conception were divided into two groups according to the length of the luteal phase, defined as the interval from the day following the administration of hCG up to and including the first day of the next menses. The division was based on the observation of a bimodal distribution of luteal-phase duration in which no luteal phase was of 12 days duration, whereas 60 cycles had a luteal phase lasting longer than 12 days, and in 18 cycles the luteal phase was 11 days or less. Sixteen of the 18 (89%) cycles having a short luteal phase were characterized by one or more of the following features: (1) a serum hCG concentration of less then 75 mIU/mL 24 hours after hCG administration, (2) peak preovulatory estradiol levels either less than 200 pg/mL or greater than 2,000 pg/mL, or (3) a midluteal serum progesterone level less than 10 ng/mL. In only one instance was low midluteal serum progesterone unaccompanied by an abnormal midcycle estradiol or serum

hCG level. Furthermore, rarely was any of these same features present in a conception cycle, an observation that led the authors to conclude that serum estradiol and hCG levels (as defined above) will predict the quality of luteal function that follows hMG- and hCG-induced ovulation.[70]

The results of the study by Olson and associates[70] demonstrate that inadequate luteal function can and does occur in ovulatory cycles induced by hMG–hCG treatment. In the series overall, 14% of all treatment cycles were characterized by a shortened luteal phase. Although endometrial biopsies were not performed in the study, and multiple serial progesterone determinations were not always available, the data do suggest that the luteal phase was inadequate in these cycles because they were endocrinologically so distinct from those in which pregnancy was achieved. The results further suggest that the cause of luteal-phase deficiency that may follow ovulation induction with menotropins is either inadequate follicular development (as judged by low preovulatory estradiol levels), incomplete luteinization (because of inadequate hCG administration), or both. These same two mechanisms were also implicated in the luteal-phase deficiency that is associated with the use of CC or bromocriptine for ovulation induction.

Methods for ovulation induction with menotropins have since been significantly refined. Typically, the progress and quality of induced follicular development are under careful scrutiny and routinely monitored with both serial determinations of serum estradiol and ultrasound examinations. The quality of preovulatory folliculogenesis is therefore not often in question. As discussed as length elsewhere in this volume, (R. L. Collins, Chapter 6), in contemporary practice hCG is not normally administered until estradiol levels are at least 500 pg/mL and ultrasound demonstrates the existence of one or more follicles of mature size (generally ≥ 16.0 mm). Consequently, if luteal-phase inadequacy occurs, it is not likely to be related to inadequate development of the preovulatory follicle(s).

The influence of the amount and timing of hCG administration also seems to be important, however. In the study by Olson and colleagues,[70] the usual single dose of 10,000 IU hCG was not always adequate to achieve a serum hCG level above 75 mIU/mL 24 hours later, a level that correlated well with a subsequent luteal phase of normal duration. Inadequate hCG administration would be analogous to a spontaneous LH surge of low amplitude in normal ovulatory cycles, and both apparently increase the risk of incomplete luteinization and luteal-phase deficiency. A recent study comparing the luteal-phase duration and serum steroid concentrations observed in hMG-treated cycles in which 10,000 IU exogenous hCG was administered, either as a single midcycle bolus or divided doses of 5,000 IU each 1 week apart, demonstrated improved luteal function with the split-dose regimen.[71] The levels of serum hCG achieved with the two regimens was not reported, however. The question of what is an optimal regimen of hCG administration in hMG-treated cycles is an important one and deserves further study because it appears that inadequate hCG treatment may be one cause of luteal-phase deficiency following ovulation induction with hMG.

There are other, unique mechanisms that may be involved when luteal-phase deficiency complicates induction of ovulation with hMG plus hCG. The relative ovarian hyperstimulation that accompanies exogenous gonadotropin therapy enhances prolactin secretion in both human[72–74] and nonhuman primates.[75,76] The mechanism of this effect appears to involve an estrogen–progesterone synergy.[77] Not infrequently, prolactin levels may rise to clearly abnormal levels in the immediate periovulatory interval and remain elevated throughout the luteal phase. An increase in follicular fluid prolactin levels may result and ultimately adversely affect the outcome of such cycles.[78,79] Relatively little is known about the possible adverse effects of such transient hyperprolactinemia, but, as discussed earlier, follicular fluid hyperprolactinemia may compromise the extent of LH receptor induction and thereby prevent nor-

mal luteinization and/or limit the steroidogenic response of the corpus luteum to LH–hCG. In addition, there is the possibility that luteal-phase hyperprolactinemia may directly inhibit steroid production by the corpus luteum and further predispose to unrecognized luteal-phase deficiency following ovulation induction with hMG plus hCG.

The far from physiological pattern of gonadotropin stimulation that occurs during the course of menotropin therapy suggests another possible mechanism for the luteal-phase dysfunction that may be seen. In response to hMG, as contrasted with spontaneous ovulatory cycles, multiple follicular development is the rule rather than the exception. Consequently, follicular-phase estradiol levels and luteal-phase estradiol and progesterone concentrations are typically well above those generally observed in unstimulated cycles. The older but elegant studies of the effects of various doses of steroid hormones on the development of the secretory endometrium in macaques performed by Good and Moyer[80] provide evidence that such abnormal patterns of steroid hormone production during the luteal phase may have significant adverse influence on the development of the preimplantation endometrium (Fig. 8-10). Specifically, endometrial development was abnormally advanced when concentrations of both estradiol and progesterone were increased; there was extensive glandular involution and stromal hypermaturation. Abnormal patterns of development were also observed in association with normal progesterone levels but elevated or deficient concentrations of estradiol.[80]

Clinically, elevated levels of estradiol during the preimplantation period of gonadotropin-stimulated cycles are associated with a high incidence of implantation failure and pregnancy loss.[81,82] These findings may well be related to the abnormally advanced degree of early secretory development that has been observed in endometrial biopsy specimens obtained in the first 3 days of the luteal phase from patients treated with hMG–hCG for the purpose of IVF–ET.[83] Aberrant patterns of steroid production during the luteal

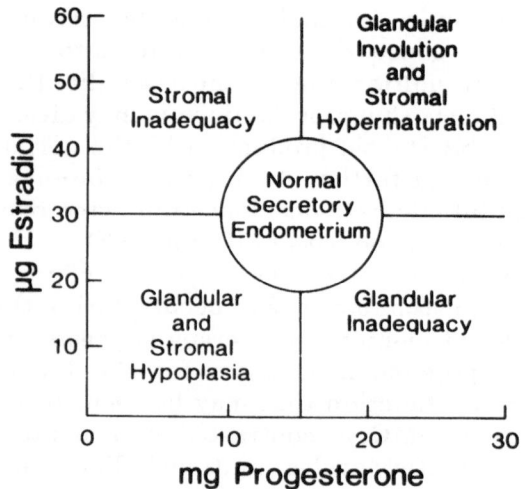

FIGURE 8-10. Relationship between the morphology of the endometrium and various doses of estrogen and progesterone replacement in ovariectomized rhesus macaques. (From Good RG, Moyer DL. Estrogen-progesterone relationships in the development of secretory endometrium. Fertil Steril 1968, 19:37. Reproduced with permission of the publisher, The American Fertility Society.)

phase may thus cause a temporal distortion of the endometrial "window of receptivity" and thereby predispose to the relatively high incidence of implantation failure and early abortion observed in pregnancies achieved with hMG- and hCG-induced ovulation and following IVF–ET.

Despite the fact that induction of ovulation with menotropins involves direct gonadotropin stimulation, often to a supraphysiological degree, and the frequent development of multiple corpora lutea, the quality of luteal function is not necessarily assured. Whereas the treatment regimens currently in use will most often guarantee an adequate stimulus to follicular development and the emergence of one or more mature follicles, endocrinological aberrations that occur only in association with ovarian hyperstimulation may adversely affect corpus luteum function or disrupt the normal sequence of maturation in the preimplantation endometrium. The results of recent studies designed to characterize better the nature of

luteal function that follows hMG- and hCG-induced ovulation suggest that disordered events in the luteal phase may in fact be responsible for the failure of many such treatment cycles that appear to have been otherwise conducted successfully.

Luteal Function after Gonadotropin-Releasing Hormone Therapy

Ovulation induction with synthetic GnRH, administered in a pulsatile fashion either intravenously or subcutaneously by means of small, portable, and programmable infusion pumps, has now become possible. This form of therapy has emerged as a viable alternative to hMG–hCG and appears best suited to the anovulatory patient with hypothalamic amenorrhea, although some success has been achieved in CC-resistant patients with polycystic ovarian disease as well. Particularly when used in patients with suppressed endogenous gonadotropin levels, the issue of how best to ensure that successful ovulation induction will be followed by a normal luteal phase remains unsettled.

A fixed dose of GnRH, when administered in a pulsatile fashion to monkeys bearing radiofrequency lesions of the arcuate nucleus (which destroys the endogenous source of GnRH), consistently results in ovulation and a normal luteal phase.[84] Whereas such an unvarying pattern of GnRH administration can reestablish normal cyclic ovarian function, studies in both humans and subhuman primates have demonstrated that LH pulse amplitude and frequency vary throughout the normal cycle, most strikingly during the luteal phase.[85] The obvious inference is that these changes in the pattern of pulsatile LH secretion reflect similar variations in the pattern of hypothalamic GnRH release, probably induced by the feedback effects of ovarian sex steroids.[85]

Ideally, if the normal luteal phase is characterized by a distinct pattern of hypothalamic GnRH secretion, the pattern of exogenous pulsatile administration used to induce ovulation should be similarly altered in efforts to provide a more physiological stimulus for pituitary gonadotropin secretion. Although there is still some controversy,[86,87] it is generally accepted that normal function of the corpus luteum requires a continued low-level exposure to LH.[88] The critical importance of GnRH to the maintenance of trophic LH support during the luteal phase is unquestioned. Abrupt discontinuation of an exogenous GnRH infusion after ovulation is induced in arcuate-lesioned monkeys consistently causes the premature onset of menses.[89] Similar results are obtained when potent GnRH agonists or antagonists are administered to normally cycling women in the early or midluteal phase.[90-94]

The influence that a specific pattern of GnRH administration may have on luteal function is suggested by a more recent study in which the pituitary and luteal responsiveness to a bolus of GnRH was examined at various stages of the luteal phase.[95] Whereas GnRH elicited an increase in plasma LH and FSH at all times, a significant steroidogenic response to the increase in gonadotropins occurred consistently only in the mid- and late luteal phases; increased steroid production was sometimes observed in the premenstrual phase and not at all in the early luteal phase.[95] The results indicate a variable dependence of the corpus luteum on the functional activity of the hypothalamic–pituitary axis. Thus, the pattern of exogenous GnRH administration that will consistently optimize luteal function after ovulation induction is uncertain and remains a source of continuing debate.

Discontinuation of pulsatile GnRH infusions soon after induced ovulation results in defective luteal function in humans, just as it does in experimental animals.[96] Nevertheless, an abnormally brief or otherwise deficient luteal phase has not infrequently been observed even when the GnRH infusion is continued in an unaltered fashion during the luteal phase.[97-99] Understandably, there is speculation that the same fixed-dose regimen of GnRH that successfully promotes progressive follicular development and induces ovu-

lation may not support normal or sustained luteal function. Despite these concerns, in the majority of clinical trials undertaken to date, an unvarying pattern of GnRH administration has been employed throughout the cycle, and the same course of treatment repeated until pregnancy is achieved.[100-102] Alternatively, the GnRH infusion has been discontinued after ovulation, and the luteal phase supported with progesterone vaginal suppositories.[103] Still others prefer to support luteal function with hCG injections,[100,102,104-106] and some advocate that GnRH therapy be continued but enhanced with exogenous hCG.[97] Which of these many approaches will provide the most physiological form of luteal support and prove most effective in achieving pregnancy is not yet clear. The use of exogenous hCG to support luteal function deserves special mention, however.

Exogenous hCG has been advocated as an easy and effective means to ensure that normal luteal function follows ovulation induction with either hMG or pulsatile GnRH therapy. It is also the logical choice in newer approaches to ovulation with hMG in which confounding endogenous gonadotropin secretion is first suppressed with a GnRH agonist, since essential LH secretion during the luteal phase may be eliminated as well.[107] The principle underlying the use of exogenous hCG is straightforward; hCG directly stimulates steroidogenesis in the corpus luteum. Its use appears to be a sound physiological approach in that it is the same hormone that normally serves to rescue the corpus luteum and prolong luteal support except in those instances where the steroidogenic capacity of the corpus luteum is limited by inadequate LH receptor induction and defective luteinization prior to ovulation. The corpus luteum might then be rendered relatively insensitive to hCG stimulation.

The timing, dose, and frequency of hCG administration are somewhat empirical, and clinical recommendations have varied.[108-110]

To date, there have been no studies specifically designed to determine which regimen will reliably optimize luteal function.

This question does appear important in light of evidence that premature hCG administration promotes atresia rather than luteinization[111] and that the character of the steroidogenic response varies with the age of the corpus luteum under treatment.[112,113] Unless the preovulatory follicle is fully mature, hCG disrupts the final stages of development and causes ovulation to fail altogether.[111] When administered to monkeys immediately after the LH surge in a pattern mimicking that observed in early pregnancy, hCG fails to elicit an increase in estradiol or progesterone concentrations over that seen in its absence.[112] If it is withheld until the midluteal phase, circulating levels of progesterone closely approximate the pattern normally observed in early macaque pregnancy: concentrations transiently increase but then decline despite continued treatment, whereas estradiol levels remain elevated.[112,113] Finally, when hCG treatment begins late in the luteal phase, the progesterone response is brief and attenuated, and levels thereafter fall steadily for the duration of treatment.[112,113] These results suggest that the qualitative and quantitative response of the primate corpus luteum to hCG is temporally related. If so, the question of what time and frequency of hCG administration will best support luteal function after ovulation induction is important and worthy of specific investigation. Clinically, the various hCG treatment regimens that have been recommended all involve intermittent bolus administration, which, depending on the time that each injection is given, may produce a continuously changing pattern of response. Importantly, these data further suggest that the corpus luteum response to one pattern of exogenous hCG administration in no way predicts what might be expected using any other treatment regimen.

Conclusions

If ovulation induction is ultimately to achieve its intended goal, careful attention must be paid to the quality of the ovulatory cycle that is induced. The many unique characteristics of the cycle stimulated with each of the ovulation-inducing agents must be kept in mind. Regardless of whether ovulation is achieved with CC, bromocriptine, hMG plus hCG, or even a pulsatile GnRH infusion, a normal luteal phase cannot be confidently assumed. Specific investigation of the quality of luteal function is an integral part of any ovulation-induction regimen. Without it, therapy is at best incomplete and, at worst, ineffectual.

References

1. Garcia J, Jones GS, Wentz AC. The use of clomiphene citrate. Fertil Steril. 1977;28:707–17.
2. Cook CL, Schroeder JA, Yussman MA, et al. Induction of luteal phase defect with clomiphene citrate. Am J Obstet Gynecol. 1984;149:613–16.
3. Jones GS, Maffezzoli RD, Strott CA, et al. Pathophysiology of reproductive failure after clomiphene-induced ovulation. Am J Obstet Gynecol. 1970;108:847–67.
4. Kerin JF, Liu JH, Phillipou G, et al. Evidence for a hypothalamic site of action of clomiphene citrate in women. J Clin Endocrinol Metab. 1985;61:265–68.
5. Richards JS. Hormonal control of ovarian follicular development: a 1978 perspective. Recent Prog Horm Res. 1979;35:343–73.
6. Knobil E. On the control of gonadotropin secretion in the rhesus monkey. Recent Prog Horm Res. 1974;30:1–46.
7. Zeleznik AJ, Midgley AR, Reichert LE. Granulosa cell maturation in the rat: increased binding of human chorionic gonadotropin following treatment with follicle-stimulating hormone in vivo. Endocrinology. 1974;95:818–25.
8. Richards JS, Midgley AR. Protein hormone action: a key to understanding ovarian follicular and luteal cell development. Biol Reprod. 1976;14:82–94.
9. Stouffer RL, Hodgen GD. Induction of luteal phase defects in rhesus monkeys by follicular fluid administration at the onset of the menstrual cycle. J Clin Endocrinol Metab. 1980;51:669–71.
10. Strott CA, Cargille CM, Ross GT, et al. The short luteal phase. J Clin Endocrinol Metab. 1970;30:246–51.

11. diZerega GS, Hodgen GD. Luteal phase dysfunction infertility: a sequel to aberrant folliculogenesis. Fertil Steril. 1981;335:489–99.
12. Stouffer RL, Coensgen JL, diZerega GS, et al. Induction of defective corpus luteum function by administration of follicular fluid to monkeys during the follicular phase of the menstrual cycle. In: Schwartz NB, Hunzicker-Dunn M, eds. Dynamics of ovarian function. New York: Raven Press, 1981:185–90.
13. Sheehan KL, Casper RF, Yen SSC. Luteal phase defects induced by an agonist of luteinizing hormone-releasing factor: a model for fertility control. Science. 1982;215:170–72.
14. Downs KA, Gibson M. Basal body temperature graph and the luteal phase defect. Fertil Steril. 1983;40:466–68.
15. Lenton EA, Landgren B, Sexton L. Normal variation in the length of the luteal phase of the menstrual cycle: identification of the short luteal phase. Br J Obstet Gynaecol. 1984;91:685–89.
16. Marut EL, Hodgen GD. Antiestrogenic action of high-dose clomiphene in primates: pituitary augmentation but with ovarian attenuation. Fertil Steril. 1982;38:100–04.
17. Yoshimura Y, Hosoi Y, Atlas SJ, et al. Effect of clomiphene citrate on in vitro ovulated ova. Fertil Steril. 1986;45:800–04.
18. Schmidt GE, Kim MH, Mansour R, et al. The effects of enclomiphene and zuclomiphene citrates on mouse embryos fertilized in vitro and in vivo. Am J Obstet Gynecol. 1986;154:727–36.
19. Edman CD. The effects of steroids on the endometrium. Semin Reprod Endocrinol. 1983;1:179–87.
20. Spirtos NJ, Yurewicz EC, Moghissi KS, et al. Pseudocorpus luteum insufficiency: a study of cytosol progesterone receptors in human endometrium. Obstet Gynecol. 1985;65:535–40.
21. Fedele L, Brioschi D, Marchini M, et al. Enhanced preovulatory progesterone levels in clomiphene citrate-induced cycles. J Clin Endocrinol Metab. 1989;69:681–83.
22. Kokko E, Janne O, Kauppila A, et al. Cyclic clomiphene citrate treatment lowers cytosol estrogen and progestin receptor concentrations in the endometrium of postmenopausal women on estrogen replacement therapy. J Clin Endocrinol Metab. 1981;52:345–49.
23. Hecht BR, Khan-Dawood FS, Dawood MY. Peri-implantation phase endometrial estrogen and progesterone receptors: effect of ovulation induction with clomiphene citrate. Am J Obstet Gynecol. 1989;161:1688–93.
24. Fritz MA, Holmes RT, Keenan EJ. Effect of clomiphene citrate treatment on endometrial estrogen and progesterone receptor induction in women. Presented at the 37th Annual Meeting of the Society for Gynecologic Investigation, March 21–24, 1990, St Louis, MO.
25. Mikkelson TJ, Kroboth PD, Cameron WJ, et al. Single-dose pharmacokinetics of clomiphene citrate in normal volunteers. Fertil Steril. 1986;46:392-96 .
26. Fritz MA, Westfahl PK, Graham RL. Effect of luteal phase estrogen antagonism on endometrial development and luteal function in women. J Clin Endocrinol Metab. 1987;1006–13.
27. Maruncic M, Casper RF. The effect of luteal phase estrogen antagonism on luteinizing hormone pulsatility and luteal function in women. J Clin Endocrinol Metab. 1987;64:148–52.
28. Daly DC, Maslar IA, Riddick DH. Prolactin production during in vitro decidualization of proliferative endometrium. Am J Obstet Gynecol. 1983;145:672–78.
29. Sgarlata CS, Mikhail G, Hertelendy R. Clomiphene and tamoxifen inhibit progesterone synthesis in granulosa cells: comparison with estradiol. Endocrinology. 1984;114:2032–38.
30. Yuen BH, Mari N, Duleba AJ, et al. Direct effects of clomiphene citrate on the steroidogenic capability of human granulosa cells. Fertil Steril. 1988;49:626–31.
31. Oelsner G, Barnea ER, Mullen MV, et al. Simultaneous measurements of clomiphene citrate in plasma and follicular fluid in women undergoing IVF and ET. Presented at the 42nd annual meeting of The American Fertility Society. Toronto, Ontario, Canada, September 27 to October 2, 1986.
32. Geier A, Lunenfeld B, Pariente C, et al. Estrogen receptor binding material in blood of patients after clomiphene citrate administration: determination by a radioreceptor assay. Fertil Steril . 1987;47:778–84 .
33. Soules MR, Clifton DK, Cohen NL, et al. Luteal phase deficiency: abnormal gonadotropin and progesterone secretion patterns. J Clin Endocrinol Metab. 1989;69:813–20.
34. Quagliarello J, Weiss G. Clomiphene citrate in the management of infertility associated with shortened luteal phase. Fertil Steril. 1979;31:373–77.

35. Hammond MG, Talbert LM. Clomiphene citrate therapy of infertile women with low luteal phase progesterone levels. Obstet Gynecol. 1982;59:275–79.

36. Check JH, Goldberg BB, Kurtz A, et al. Pelvic ultrasonography to help determine the appropriate therapy for luteal phase defect. Int J Fertil. 1984;29:156–58.

37. Daly DC. Luteal phase defects. In: Gondos B, Riddick DH, eds. Pathology of infertility. New York: Thieme Medical, 1987:169–84.

38. Check JH, Adelson PG. The efficacy of progesterone in achieving successful pregnancy: II. In women with pure luteal phase defects. Int J Fertil. 1987;32:139–41.

39. Kreitmann B, Bugat R, Bayard F. Estrogen and progestin regulation of the progesterone receptor concentration in human endometrium. J Clin Endocrinol Metab. 1979;49:926–29.

40. Bayard F, Damilano S, Robel P, et al. Cytoplasmic and nuclear estradiol and progesterone receptors in human endometrium. J Clin Endocrinol Metab. 1978;46:635–48.

41. Daly DC, Walters CA, Soto-Albors CE, et al. A randomized study of dexamethasone in ovulation induction with clomiphene citrate. Fertil Steril. 1984;41:844–48.

42. Knobil E. The neuroendocrine control of the menstrual cycle. Recent Prog Horm Res. 1980; 36:53–88.

43. Moult PJA, Rees LH, Besser GM. Pulsatile gonadotropin secretion in hyperprolactinemic amenorrhea and the response to bromocriptine therapy. Clin Endocrinol. 1982;16:153–62.

44. Lee MS, Ben-Rafael Z, Meloni F, et al. Effects of prolactin on steroidogenesis by human luteinized granulosa cells. Fertil Steril. 1986; 46:32–36.

45. Soto EA, Turek RW, Strauss JF III. Effects of prolactin on progestin secretion by human granulosa cells in culture. Biol Reprod. 1985; 32:541–45.

46. Wang C, Hsueh AJW, Erickson GF. Prolactin inhibition of estrogen production by cultured rat granulosa cells. Mol Cell Endocrinol. 1980;20:135–44.

47. Dorrington JH, Gore-Langton RE. Prolactin inhibits oestrogen synthesis in the ovary. Nature. 1981;290:600–02.

48. Tsai-Morris C-H, Gosh M, Hirshfield AN, et al. Inhibition of ovarian aromatase by prolactin in vivo. Biol Reprod. 1983;29:342–46.

49. Uilenbroek J, Van der Linden R. Effects of prolactin on follicle oestradiol production in the rat. J Endocrinol. 1984;102:245–50.

50. Munabi AK, Mericq V, Koppleman MCS, et al. The effects of prolactin on rat ovarian function. Steroids. 1984;43:631–37.

51. McNatty KP, Sawers RS, McNeilly AS. A possible role for prolactin in control of steroid secretion by the human graafian follicle. Nature. 1974;250:653–55.

52. Demura R, Ono N, Demura H, et al. Prolactin directly inhibits basal as well as gonadotropin-stimulated secretion of progesterone and 17β-estradiol in the human ovary. J Clin Endocrinol Metab. 1982;54:1246–50.

53. Adashi EY, Resnick CE. Prolactin as an inhibitor of granulosa cell luteinization: implications for hyperprolactinemia-associated luteal phase dysfunction. Fertil Steril. 1987;48:131–39.

54. Cutie RE, Andino NA. Prolactin inhibits the steroidogenesis in mid-follicular phase human granulosa cells cultured in a chemically defined medium. Fertil Steril. 1988;49:632–37.

55. Corenblum B, Pairaudeau N, Schewchuk AB. Prolactin hypersecretion and short luteal phase defects. Obstet Gynecol. 1976;47:486–88.

56. Seppala M, Hirvonen E, Ranta T. Hyperprolactinemia and luteal insufficiency. Lancet. 1976;1:229–30.

57. Del Pozo E, Wyss H, Tolis G, et al. Prolactin and deficient luteal function. Obstet Gynecol. 1979;53:282–86.

58. Fredricsson B, Bjork G, Carlstrom K. Short luteal phase and prolactin. Lancet. 1977;1:1210.

59. Muhlenstedt D, Wuttke W, Schneider HPG. Short luteal phase and prolactin. Int J Fertil. 1978;23:213–18.

60. McNatty KP. Relationship between plasma prolactin and the endocrine microenvironment of the developing human antral follicle. Fertil Steril. 1979;32:433–38.

61. Kauppila A, Leinonen P, Vihko R, et al. Metoclopramide-induced hyper-prolactinemia impairs ovarian follicle maturation and corpus luteum function in women. J Clin Endocrinol Metab. 1982;54:955–60.

62. Coelingh Bennink HJT. Intermittent bromocriptine treatment for the induction of ovulation in hyperprolactinemic patients. Fertil Steril. 1979;31:267–72.

63. Castracane VD, Shaikh AA. Synergism of estrogen and bromoergocryptine in the induction of luteolysis in cynomolgus monkeys. J Clin Endocrinol Metab. 1980;51:1311–15.

64. Blackwell RE, Boots LR, Potter HD. Evaluation of delestrogen and parlodel as a luteolytic agent in humans. Fertil Steril. 1982;37:213–17.

65. Castracane VD, Goldzieher JW. The luteolytic and abortifacient potential of an estrogen-bromoergocryptine regimen in the baboon. Fertil Steril. 1982;37:258–62.

66. Kauppila A, Chatelain P, Kirkinen P, et al. Isolated prolactin deficiency in a woman with puerperal lactogenesis. J Clin Endocrinol Metab. 1987;64:309–12.

67. Soto-Albors CE, Daly DC, Walters CA, et al. Titrating the dose of bromocriptine when treating hyperprolactinemic infertile women. Fertil Steril. 1985;43:485–87.

68. Hull MGR, Savage PE, Bromham DR, et al. The value of a single serum progesterone measurement in the midluteal phase as a criterion of a potentially fertile cycle ("ovulation") derived from treated and untreated conception cycles. Fertil Steril. 1982;37:355–60.

69. Bohnet PG, Dato K, Trapp M, et al. Different hormonal patterns in human menopausal gonadotropin-treated, clomiphene citrate-treated, and untreated conception cycles. Fertil Steril. 1986;45:469–74.

70. Olson JL, Rebar RW, Schreiber JR, et al. Shortened luteal phase after ovulation induction with human menopausal gonadotropin and human chorionic gonadotropin. Fertil Steril. 1983;39:284–91.

71. Graze RV, Taney FH, Gagliardi CL, et al. Progesterone levels, estradiol levels and luteal phase lengths in hMG/hCG-stimulated cycles: effects of two hCG regimens. Presented at the 43rd annual meeting of the American Fertility Society. Reno, Nevada, September 28 to 30, 1987.

72. Healy DL, Burger PG. Serum follicle-stimulating hormone, luteinizing hormone, and prolactin during the induction of ovulation with exogenous gonadotropin. J Clin Endocrinol Metab. 1983;56:474–78.

73. Kemmann E, Gemzell CA, Beinert WC, et al. Plasma prolactin changes during the administration of human menopausal gonadotropins in nonovulatory women. Am J Obstet Gynecol. 1977;129:145–49.

74. Yuen BH, Cannon W. Regulation of ovarian follicular and luteal function during treatment with exogenous gonadotropins in anovulatory infertility. Am J Obstet Gynecol. 1981;140:629–35.

75. Williams RF, Hodgen GD. Hyperprolactinemia: induction by an estrogen-progesterone synergy. Fertil Steril (Abstr suppl). 1983;39:430–31.

76. Collins RL, William RF, Hodgen GD. Endocrine consequences of prolonged ovarian hyperstimulation: hyperprolactinemia, follicular atresia, and premature luteinization. Fertil Steril. 1984;42:436–45.

77. Williams RF, Barber DL, Cowan BD, et al. Hyperprolactinemia in monkeys: induction by an estrogen-progesterone synergy. Steroids. 1981;38:321–31.

78. Laufer N, Botero-Ruiz HR, DeCherney AH, et al. Gonadotropin and prolactin levels in follicular fluid of human ova successfully fertilized in vitro. J Clin Endocrinol Metab. 1984;58:430–34.

79. Bohnet PG, Baukloh V. Prolactin concentrations in follicular fluid following ovarian hyperstimulation for in vitro fertilization. Hormone Res. 1985;22:189–95.

80. Good RG, Moyer DL. Estrogen-progesterone relationships in the development of secretory endometrium. Fertil Steril. 1968;19:37–49.

81. Lejeune B, Dehou MF, Leroy F. Tentative extrapolation of animal data to human implantation. Ann NY Acad Sci. 1986;476:63–74.

82. Gidley-Baird AA, O'Neill C, Sinosich MJ, et al. Failure of implantation in human in vitro fertilization and embryo transfer patients: the effects of altered progesterone/estrogen ratios in humans and mice. Fertil Steril. 1986;45:69–74.

83. Garcia JE, Acosta AA, Hsiu J-G, et al. Advanced endometrial maturation after ovulation induction with human menopausal gonadotropin/human chorionic gonadotropin for in vitro fertilization. Fertil Steril. 1984;41:31–35.

84. Knobil E, Plant TM, Wildt L, et al. Control of the rhesus monkey menstrual cycle: permissive role of hypothalamic gonadotropin-releasing hormone. Science. 1980;207:1371–73.

85. Soules MR, Steiner RA, Clifton DK, et al. Progesterone modulation of pulsatile luteinizing hormone secretion in normal women. J Clin Endocrinol Metab 1984;58:378–83.

86. Asch RH, Abou-Samra M, Braunstein GD, et al. Luteal function in hypophysectomized rhesus monkeys. J Clin Endocrinol Metab. 1982;55:154–61.

87. Balmaceda JP, Borghi MR, Coy DH, et al. Suppression of postovulatory gonadotropin levels does not affect corpus luteum function in rhesus monkeys. J Clin Endocrinol Metab. 1983;57:866–68.

88. Stouffer RL. Perspectives on the corpus luteum of the menstrual cycle and early pregnancy. Semin Reprod Endocrinol. 1988;6:103–13.

89. Hutchison JS, Zeleznik AJ. The rhesus monkey corpus luteum is dependent on pituitary gonadotropin secretion throughout the luteal phase of the menstrual cycle. Endocrinology. 1984;115:1780–86.

90. Sheehan KL, Casper RF, Yen SSC. Luteal phase defect induced by an agonist of luteinizing hormone-releasing factor; a model for fertility control. Science 1982;215:170–72.

91. Casper RF, Yen SSC. Induction of luteolysis in the human with a long acting analog of luteinizing hormone-releasing factor. Science. 1979;205:408–10.

92. Lemay A, Labrie F, Ferland L, et al. Possible luteolytic effects of luteinizing hormone-releasing hormone in normal women. Fertil Steril. 1979;31:29–34.

93. Caldwell BV, Rotchell YE, Pang CY, et al. Comparative study of high-dose chorionic gonadotropin on the human and rat corpus luteum and effect of gonadotropin-releasing hormone on human luteal function. Am J Obstet Gynecol. 1980;136:458–64.

94. Monroe SE, Henzl MR, Martin MC, et al. Ablation of folliculogenesis in women by a single dose of gonadotropin-releasing hormone agonist: significance of time in cycle. Fertil Steril. 1985;43:361–68.

95. Caruso A, Lanzone A, Fulghesu AM, et al. Luteal responses to gonadotropin-releasing hormone during the luteal phase: relation to the age of corpus luteum. J Clin Endocrinol Metab. 1987;64:244–78.

96. Weinstein FG, Seibel MM, Taymor ML. Ovulation induction with subcutaneous pulsatile gonadotropin-releasing hormone: the role of supplemental human chorionic gonadotropin in the luteal phase. Fertil Steril. 1984;41:546–50.

97. Nillius SJ, Wide L. Gonadotropin-releasing hormone treatment for induction of follicular maturation and ovulation in amenorrheic women with anorexia nervosa. Br Med J. 1975;3:405–08.

98. Nillius SJ, Fries H, Wide L. Successful induction of follicular maturation and ovulation by prolonged treatment with LH-releasing hormone in women with anorexia nervosa. Am J Obstet Gynecol. 1975;122:921–28.

99. Casas PR, Badano AR, Aparicio N, et al. Luteinizing hormone-releasing hormone in the treatment of anovulatory infertility. Fertil Steril. 1975;26:549–53.

100. Molloy BG, Hancock KW, Glass MR. Ovulation induction in clomiphene nonresponsive patients: the place of pulsatile gonadotropin-releasing hormone in clinical practice. Fertil Steril. 1985;43:26–33.

101. Schoemaker J, Simons AHM, van Osnabrugge GJC, et al. Pregnancy after prolonged pulsatile administration of luteinizing hormone-releasing hormone in a patient with clomiphene-resistant secondary amenorrhea. J Clin Endocrinol Metab. 1981;52:882–85.

102. Mason P, Adams J, Morris DV, et al. Induction of ovulation with pulsatile luteinizing hormone-releasing hormone. Br Med J. 1984;288:181–85.

103. Zacur HA. Ovulation induction with gonadotropin-releasing hormone. Fertil Steril. 1985;44:435–48.

104. Goerzen J, Corenblum B, Wiseman DA, et al. Ovulation induction and pregnancy in hypothalamic amenorrhea using self-administered intravenous gonadotropin-releasing hormone. Fertil Steril. 1984;41:319–21.

105. Hurley DM, Brian RJ, Burger PG. Ovulation induction with subcutaneous pulsatile gonadotropin-releasing hormone: singleton pregnancies in patients with previous multiple pregnancies after gonadotropin therapy. Fertil Steril. 1983;40:575–79.

106. Skarin G, Nillius SJ, Wide L. Pulsatile subcutaneous low-dose gonadotropin-releasing hormone treatment of anovulatory infertility. Fertil Steril. 1983;40:454–60.

107. Lewinthal D, Taylor PJ, Pattinson HA, et al. Induction of ovulation with luprolide acetate and human menopausal gonadotropin. Fertil Steril. 1988;49:585–88.

108. Jones GS. The luteal phase defect. Fertil Steril. 1976;27:351–56.

109. Wentz AC. Physiologic and clinical considerations in luteal phase defects. Clin Obstet Gynecol. 1979;22:169–85.

110. Jones GS. [Editorial]. Obstet Gynecol Surv. 1986;41:706–09.

111. Williams RF, Hodgen GD. Disparate effects of human chorionic gonadotropin during the late follicular phase in monkeys: normal ovulation, follicular atresia, ovarian acyclicity, and hypersecretion of follicle-stimulating hormone. Fertil Steril. 1980;33:64–68.

112. Ottobre JS, Stouffer RL. Persistent vs. transient stimulation of the macaque corpus luteum during prolonged exposure to hCG: a function of age of the menstrual cycle. Endocrinology. 1984;114:2175–82.

113. Wilks JW, Noble AS. Steroidogenic responsiveness of the monkey corpus luteum to exogenous chorionic gonadotropin. Endocrinology. 1983;112:1256–66.

9
Bromocriptine and Related Compounds for Ovulation Induction in Hyperprolactinemia

Vivian Lewis and Anna K. Parsons

Causes of Hyperprolactinemia

In order to understand the treatment of hyperprolactinemia, it is helpful to know the causes of hyperprolactinemia and its effects on fertility. To this end, the normal regulation of pituitary secretion of prolactin is reviewed, along with alterations of the normal physiology by disease or drugs.

The Physiological Role of Prolactin

Lactation

Prolactin is a polypeptide hormone secreted by the lactotrophs in the anterior pituitary. These cells are located in the lateral aspects of the gland and are identifiable by routine histochemistry, immunocytochemistry, and electron microscopy. During pregnancy and lactation the entire pituitary enlarges because of the increased number and size of these cells.

Prolactin is found in the circulation in several forms: glycosylated, "big," "big-big," and "little." [1-3] Although the significance of the various forms is unknown, there are reports of a predominance of one or another form. For example, one report cites a patient with increased levels of only "big-big" prolactin. [4] Another study shows that pregnant women have only very small amounts of nonglycosylated prolactin in contrast to normal men and nonpregnant women. [2] For most people, however, "little" prolactin make up 80% to 85% of total circulating prolactin.

The only established physiological role of human prolactin is initiation and maintenance of lactation. Despite this, prolactin receptors have been found in many tissues including the liver, ovaries, adrenals, kidneys, fetal lung, testes, and prostate. [3] The importance of these receptors is unknown. However, prolactin is practically ubiquitous in animal phyla and is responsible for many actions, such as osmoregulation, promotion of fetal lung maturation, and induction of maternal behavior. Other roles for prolactin in humans remain speculative. Since the known role of prolactin is to prepare for lactation, the changes that occur in pregnancy are easily understood.

Prolactin levels increase throughout pregnancy until parturition, primarily because of the very high estrogen levels. Estrogens can cause lactotroph hyperplasia and stimulation of transcription of the prolactin gene. [5] Furthermore, estrogens can also modify hypothalamic infuences on pituitary prolactin secretion levels as well as gonadotropin-releasing hormone (GnRH) and thyrotropin-releasing hormone (TRH) receptor levels. The latter two may not be so important in pregnancy, but estrogen regulation of prolactin levels probably occurs by similar mechanisms in both pregnant and the nonpregnant women.

Lactation during pregnancy is blocked by the elevated estradiol levels, which drop at parturition. Subsequent suckling causes sharp bursts of prolactin release, which gradually taper off by about 6 months postpartum, when basal and suckling-induced prolactin levels are normal. Sensory afferent neural fibers from the nipple carry impulses through the spinal cord to the midbrain and hypothalamus. It is not known what neurotransmitters and/or peptides mediate subsequent prolactin and oxytocin release; however, changes in dopamine levels, serotonin, and TRH have all been implicated.[6] Similar mechanisms are probably important in the hyperprolactinemia seen in the herpes zoster patients and patients with chest-wall trauma.

Physiological Regulators of Prolactin Secretion

In nonpregnant women, prolactin secretion is principally regulated by tonic inhibition through a number of factors. Locally, dopamine is the most potent inhibitor of prolactin secretion (Fig. 9-1).[6] The arcuate nucleus, the hypothalamic periventricular area, and the preoptic area are the principal sites of cell bodies where dopamine is synthesized. Axons from these areas project onto the median eminence, the infundibular stalk, and the pituitary.[7] Evidence that dopamine inhibits prolactin secretion comes from several clinical observations. Systemic administration of dopamine by intravenous infusion lowers the serum prolactin in normal women and women with tumors.[8] Blockade of dopamine receptors by administration of phenothiazines causes hyperprolactinemia.[9] In vitro studies of pituitary cells show that dopamine can directly inhibit prolactin synthesis and release.[10] In addition to dopamine, which is the well-established prolactin inhibitor, recent evidence suggests the existence of another physiological prolactin-inhibiting factor. The precursor to GnRH contains a peptide (GnRH-asociated peptide, GAP) that has been found to inhibit prolactin synthesis and release by rat pituitary cells in culture.[11] Further work is needed to determine GAP's importance in humans. At present dopamine remains the principal physiological regulator of prolactin through tonic inhibition.

A number of physiological influences can

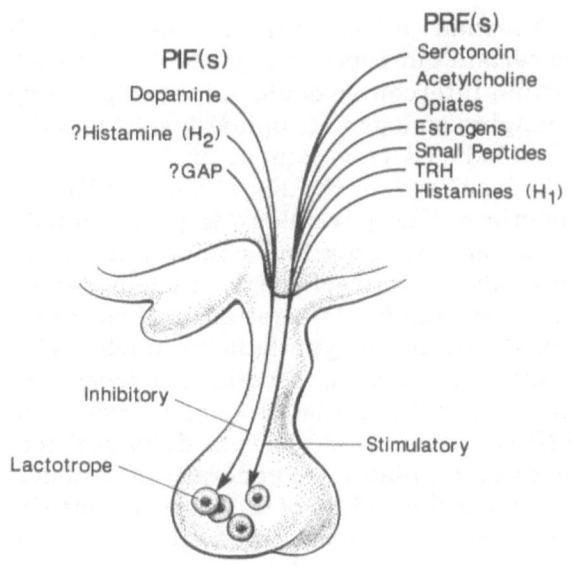

FIGURE 9-1. Prolactin regulatory substances. Prolactin inhibitory factors (PIFs), especially dopamine, maintain basal prolactin levels through tonic inhibition. Prolactin-releasing factors (PRFs) mediate increases in prolactin under a variety of circumstances (see text). Reprinted with permission from Krieger DT, Hughes JC (eds): *Neuroendocrinology.* Copyright © 1980 by HP Publishing Co., Inc., New York, N.Y. Illustration by Nancy Lou Makris.

overcome this tonic inhibition; some act directly, and others act indirectly. Thyrotropin-releasing hormone and vasoactive intestinal protein (VIP) act directly on the pituitary. Whereas endogenous opioids and possibly serotonin can stimulate prolactin indirectly through their effects on hypothalamic dopamine, many neuropeptides, such as angiotensin II, neurotensin, and oxytocin, as well as certain neurotransmitters (e.g., norepinephrine, histamine, and acetylcholine), can also stimulate prolactin release.[6]

These local regulators may mediate some of the systemic activators of prolactin release such as stress, food, exercise, intercourse, and sleep.[12] For example, some of these regulators are stress hormones (e.g., catecholamines, opioids, angiotensin II, TRH), and certain physiological stresses can stimulate prolactin release, such as exercise or hypoglycemia. Food intake will cause the release of prolactin, perhaps by increasing levels of tryptophan (a serotonin substrate) as well as certain gut peptides (e.g., VIP and CCK). Sexual intercourse could raise prolactin by changing endogenous opioid levels, and the sleep-induced elevation in prolactin parallels the circadian rhythm of most endocrine functions. The physiology is poorly understood, but such rhythms could be mediated through the suprachiasmic nucleus, which receives input from the retina and has projections onto many hypothalamic nuclei. This nucleus is rich in several neuropeptides known to affect prolactin (e.g., neurotensin, VIP, somatostatin).[13] The physiology of most of these regulators is generally not understood, but the finding of increased insensitivity in women suggests that estrogens are important natural modulators.

However, the fluctuations in estrogens seen during a normal menstrual cycle do not consistently affect prolactin levels. The midcycle estradiol peak may cause transient hyperprolactinemia, although this has not been observed by all investigators. In fact, controversy remains whether prolactin levels vary from the follicular to the luteal phase of the cycle. Clinical evidence suggests that prolactin is not required for ovulation, since some women ovulate in the presence of disturbed prolactin secretory dynamics.[14]

Pathological Causes of Hyperprolactinemia

Prolactin-secreting pituitary adenomas are the most common cause of hyperprolactinemia. They are slow-growing tumors that are usually found in the lateral aspects of the pituitary, where normal lactotrophs are present. Normal lactotroph regulation of prolactin secretion is somewhat paralleled by these tumors. These tumors possess functionally normal dopamine receptors in concentrations similar to normal pituitaries.[15] Patients with pituitary adenomas can show partial suppression of prolactin secretion in response to dopamine infusion.[8] However, administration of the dopamine antagonists metoclopramide and sulpiride may not affect prolactin levels in adenoma patients.[16,17]

This suggests a possible role for dopamine deficiency in the pathogenesis of pituitary adenomas. Perhaps these tumors develop as a result of a local deficiency of dopamine or vascular abnormalities that affect local dopamine concentrations.

Hyperprolactinemia is also seen with other causes of lactotroph compressions, including other pituitary tumors. About 15% to 25% of acromegalic patients also have hyperprolactinemia.[18,19] In addition, hypothalamic tumors, including craniophyarngiomas and metastatic disease, can produce pituitary stalk compression and thereby elevate prolactin levels. Empty sella syndrome often causes hyperprolactinemia, possibly related to pituitary compression by the hydrostatic pressure of cerebrospinal fluid. There are isolated reports of ectopic prolactin production by bronchogenic carcinoma, gonadoblastoma, and hypernephroma,[20,21] and other pituitary tumors or hypothalamic tumors can also cause hyperprolactinemia.

"Functional" elevations of prolactin (Chiari–Frommel syndrome) and idiopathic hyperprolactinemia are also seen. With the advent of sensitive pituitary-imaging techniques, it has become apparent that many so-called functional hyperprolactinemics harbor small microadenomas. However, recent long-term studies have confirmed the existence of hyperprolactinemia in the absence of a pituitary tumor (or other cause).[22] Studies with long-term follow-up as well as autopsy series suggest that this is usually a nonprogressive disorder with pathophysiology similar to that seen in tumors.[23–25] Because of the variety of causes of hyperprolactinemia, idiopathic hyperprolactinemia becomes a diagnosis of exclusion.[26,27]

Hyperprolactinemia is sometimes seen with other endocrinopathies. Appropriately 11% to 40% of patients with polycystic ovarian disease (PCO) have associated hyperprolactinemia.[28–31] Some of the pathophysiological features of PCO are thought to contribute to the pathogenesis of hyperprolactinemia, specifically hyperestrogenemia, hyperandrogenemia, and a relative deficiency in central dopamine.[32] Shoupe and Lobo[28] reported that elevated serum unbound estradiol levels correlated with GnRH-stimulatable prolactin in a group of women with PCO. However, other investigators have found similar levels of both estrone and estradiol in PCO patients with or without hyperprolactinemia.[29,30] Dopamine, a potent inhibitor of prolactin, can also inhibit LH secretion, suggesting that a deficiency of dopamine could contribute to the elevated LH levels seen in PCO.[33] For example, administration of L-DOPA caused obliteration of the hyperprolactinemic response to GnRH in a group of PCO women.[28] Another report describes induction of ovulation with bromocriptine in hyperprolactinemic PCO patients.[34] These common pathogenetic features suggest common therapy for some subsets of PCO patients.[35]

Other endocrinopathies are less commonly associated with hyperprolactinemia. Thyroid disease can cause prolactin elevations both through increased levels of TRH (seen in hypothyroidism) and through the increased prolactin metabolic clearance rate seen in hyperthyroidism.[36-38] Cushing's syndrome or an ACTH-secreting tumor may stimulate prolactin release through elevations in endogenous opioids. Similarly, Addison's disease is sometimes associated with hyperprolactinemia. These endocrinopathies are rarely causes of hyperprolactinemia.

Other causes of hyperprolactinemia act by changing prolactin metabolism. These include chronic renal failure and hepatic disease. Patients with renal failure have a reduced metabolic clearance rate and an increased production rate of prolactin.[39] Whereas patients with hepatic disease also have abnormal metabolism of sex steroids (which can stimulate prolactin release), these disorders act primarily through prolongation of prolactin metabolism.[40]

Effects of Altered Prolactin Physiology on Fertility

Most patients with hyperprolactinemia are infertile because prolactin can cause hypogonadism in men and women. There is evidence that this occurs at the pituitary as well as the gonadal level.

Prolactin can interfere with normal GnRH pulsatility.[14] The exact mechanism is unknown, but it may include changes in hypothalamic dopamine and endogenous opiates. Despite the lack of normal GnRH pulses, pituitary response to GnRH is usually normal or even enhanced.[41] However, large tumors may directly cause pituitary insufficiency through compression. In addition to the central affects of prolactin, which disturb gonadotropin secretion, prolactin also has direct gonadal effects.

Prolactin can affect ovarian follicular maturation, as shown by studies of experimentally induced hyperprolactinemia as well as studies of the transient hyperprolactinemia seen with hyperstimulation.[42,43] This probably occurs by inhibition of granulosa cell steroidogenesis, an important factor in follicular development.[44] The impact of these gonadal effects is also important for luteal function.

The effects of prolactin on corpus luteum function are controversial. Some reports have found an association between mild hyperprolactinemia and luteal defects, as diagnosed by serum progesterone levels and/or endometrial biopsies.[45,46] Although this makes sense for theoretical reasons, other investigators have found that elevated serum prolactin is rare as a cause for luteal insufficiency.[47,48] In fact, some studies suggest that too low a prolactin level may be deleterious to corpus luteum function.[49,50] Thus, it seems that hyperprolactinemia may be an uncommon cause of luteal-phase insufficiency and that this should not be overvigorously treated.

Diagnosis of Hyperprolactinemia

Clinical Presentation

Classically, the hyperprolactinemic woman is a relatively hypoestrogenic patient with secondary amenorrhea and galactorrhea. Moreover, abnormal levels of prolactin with or without galactorrhea have been described in association with defective luteal phase, primary amenorrhea, hirsutism, polycystic ovarian disease, and endometriosis.[29,30,51-55] Furthermore, galactorrhea may be associated with normal prolactin levels.[27] For this reason, the prolactin level is fundamental in the evaluation of menstrual abnormality and infertility. This level is best obtained after the patient has fasted and in the morning, taking advantage of the daily nadir and avoiding the postprandial spikes.

The history and physical examination of the patient often suggest the etiology of hyperprolactinemia. Headaches or visual or neurological abnormalities lead one to suspect parasellar or pituitary masses. Vague systemic symptoms such as severe fatigue, constipation, and depression might suggest thyroid insufficiency. Any of a wide range of medications may provoke mild to moderately increased prolactin (Table 9-1). For most of the patients with idiopathic hyperprolactinemia, the symptoms usually include amenorrhea (or menstrual irregularity) with or without galactorrhea.[12,47,56]

The physical examination may provide additional clues. An undiagnosed pregnancy should always be considered. Other endocri-

TABLE 9-1. Pharmacological causes of hyperprolactinemia[a]

General class	Specific type
Anesthetics	All inhalation
Antimetics	Metoclopromide, sulpiride
Antihypertensives[b]	α-Methylodopa, reserpine
Histamine₂ receptor blockers	Cimetidine
Hormones[c]	Estrogens, progestins, oral contraceptives, testosterone
Opiates[c]	Methadone, morphine
Tranquilizers	Butyrophenones, dibenzoxazepines, meprobamate, phenothiazines, tricyclic antidepressants

[a] Many of these drugs act by blockage of receptors for prolactin inhibitors (e.g., tranquilizers, antiemetics, and blockers).

[b] The antihypertensives act by depletion of central catecholamine storage.

[c] The hormones and opiates act to stimulate prolactin release, directly or indirectly.

nopathies associated with hyperprolactinemia might also cause physical signs (e.g., Cushing's disease, Nelson's disease, or Graves' disease). Hirsutism or even virilization could be a sign of polycystic ovarian disease. To this end, it is useful to assess the patient's estrogenization, which will be evident in the vaginal mucosal texture and cervical mucus characteristics. Mucosal and labial atrophy with absent cervical mucus indicate hypoestrogenism, common in hyperprolactinemic patients.

The elicitation of galactorrhea requires careful milking of the mammary glands, with gentle pressure applied from the periphery to the areola. Microscopic examination of the secretions, which are usually clear or white, will demonstrate fat globules and confirm galactorrhea. Blood or colored or purulent secretions are seen with local processes and should be evaluated by mammogram and/or culture.[57] Breast disease per se is not a described cause of hyperprolactinemia; however, chronic irritation of thoracic nerves T2 through T6 by chest wall trauma and subsequent scarring is a well-known stimulus to prolactin.[58] In fact, any surgical procedure can result in temporary mild hyperprolactinemia and galactorrhea as well.[59] Because of the known physiological responses to suckling and sympathetic thoracic nerve stimulation, it is recommended that prolactin not be evaluated after breast examination.

Laboratory Evaluation

In general, two fasting morning prolactin levels above 20 ng/mL are sufficient to establish the diagnosis of hyperprolactinemia. The level itself is not particularly predictive of the existence of an adenoma, although it has often been stated that a prolactin level over 100 ng/mL is most likely to reflect tumor secretion. However, several series have found that as many as 40% to 50% of patients with surgically proven adenomas have modest elevations of serum prolactin levels (20 to 100 ng/mL).[18,26,41,60]

However, because hyperprolactinemia is seen in association with a variety of endocrinopathies, prolactin should always be measured in anovulatory patients. In addition, obtaining a β-hCG level to diagnose unsuspected pregnancy is prudent and frequently productive. A serum TSH level will allow diagnosis of primary hypothyroidism, which causes hyperprolactinemia in around 5% of patients.[36,37] Levels of LH and FSH are generally in the low normal range; however, because of preferential LH inhibition by prolactin, the FSH-to-LH ratio is 1 or more.[61] Inversion of this ratio as well as increased androgens are suggestive of PCO. However, patients with hyperprolactinemia tend to have increased adrenal androgens and decreased SHBG (even without hirsutism).[34,62]

Dynamic Testing

Before good imaging techniques were available, attempts were made to characterize pituitary responses and prolactin secretion patterns in an effort to predict which women had adenomas. Tests were devised based on the fact that a number of pharamacological challenges can elicit prolactin secretion in normal women, and dopamine, the most potent prolactin inhibitory factor, can lower prolactin levels (Table 9-2). In addition to

testing prolactin release, some of these tests examine other aspects of pituitary function.

In an effort to distinguish between functional and tumor-derived hyperprolactinemia, Chang and others administered a battery of anterior pituitary secretegogues to hyperprolactinemic amenorrheic women and controls. The tests included the administration of physiological prolactin-stimulating hormones—TRH and insulin—as well as GnRH to test for that aspect of pituitary responsiveness.[63,64] They found that patients with tumors had high baseline levels of prolactin that changed very little, whereas normoprolactinemic women had a brisk spike, on the order of a sixfold increase in prolactin levels. Gonadotropin response to GnRH produced somewhat greater response among the hyperprolactinemics. In particular, the FSH responses of hyperprolactinemics were greater than those of normoprolactinemics despite similar estradiol levels. In some of these women, hyperprolactinemia also blunted the response of GH to insulin-induced hypoglycemia. In general, other aspects of anterior pituitary function are normal in these patients. The blunted response of prolactin to TRH is the only known exception.

Some tests compare the response to pro-

TABLE 9-2. Dynamic tests for pituitary function[a]

Test hormone	Dose and route	Sample drawn	Results
1. TRH	500 μg, slow IV push	0, 20, 30, 45, 60, 90 min TSH, PRL	TSH normal at least doubled within 30 minutes Hypothyroidism: Baseline is elevated and response exaggerated Hyperthyroidism: Attenuated response, high T_3/T_4 PRL doubles within 30 min (normal) Hyperprolactinemia: High baseline with blunted response
2. Insulin	0.1 U/kg, IV push	0, 20, 30, 45, 60, 90 min GH, PRL, glucose, cortisol	Glucose must fall to less than 40 mg/dL GH should double by 60 min Cortisol should rise to more than 20 g/dL at 60 min PRL doubles within 30 min
3. Metoclopromide	10 mg IV bolus	0, 60, 120, 180 min PRL, LH, FSH	Normals: Prolactin triples at 60 to 120 min; no change in LH, FSH Hyperprolactinemics: Blunted response of prolactin.
4. Levodopa	500 mg po	0, 30, 60, 120, 180 min PRL	Normal: 50% decrease in PRL

[a] Each of these tests has be used to distinguish patients with pituitary tumors. Their use is now limited because of improved imaging techniques.

lactin inhibitors of normals and patients with tumors. For example, L-DOPA has been given to both groups; however, it caused a similar drop in prolactin in both normals and patients with tumors.[64] Metoclopramide, a dopamine receptor antagonist, has also been used to evaluate central dopaminergic tone. Some investigators have suggested that patients with prolactin-secreting adenomas secrete maximal amounts of prolactin and therefore cannot respond to such a stimulus. In normal women, prolactin increases to 100 ng/mL or more, whereas most patients with tumors show no increase. However, some patients with tumors may show a moderate response; thus, the discriminatory value of this test, like that of the other dynamic tests, is incomplete.[65,66]

At present, the use of these tests is generally limited to research protocols. They are not helpful clinically in patients with idiopathic hyperprolactinemia or microadenomas. Their use is reserved for patients with evidence of hypopituitarism or a history suspicious for it, e.g., extensive surgery, radiation therapy, or a macroadenoma.

There is some evidence that these dynamic tests may identify anovulatory women with occult hyperprolactinemia who will benefit from bromocriptine therapy. Suginami et al.[67] studied a group of euprolactinemic anovulatory women with metaclopramide stimulation tests, followed by treatment with bromocriptine. Clomiphene was added if no ovulation occurred after 2 months. Bromocriptine alone induced ovulation in 13 out of 34 patients; With clomiphene seven more patients ovulated. Those patients who responded to bromocriptine tended to have a greater maximal prolactin response to metoclopramide (twice normal). They also had a higher unstimulated nocturnal prolactin level than nonresponders. Other groups have found that some anovulatory patients who demonstrate an exaggerated prolactin response to TRH will ovulate when treated with bromocriptine.[68,69] Although there is much overlap between groups, these studies suggest that some anovulatory women may have occult hyperprolactinemia, seen only in response to pro-

vocative tests. Further data are needed before these observations can be clinically useful.

Pituitary Imaging

Once the diagnosis of hyperprolactinemia is made, the pituitary should be imaged to look for a tumor (Table 9-3). This includes not only prolactin-secreting adenomas but also craniopharyngiomas, meningiomas, or other brain tumors as well as granulomas or empty sella syndrome. Macroadenomas are often nonfunctioning and may cause mild to moderate hyperprolactinemia. It is therefore essential to establish the size and nature of any pituitary mass, since some tumors, including malignancies, cause prolactin secretion by local disruption of the tuberoinfundibular dopaminergic neurons.

In the past, polytomography of the sella turcica was used to look for evidence of a pituitary tumor (e.g., thinning or sloping of the sellar floor from compression by a tumor). However, this technique is insensitive and difficult to interpret (Fig. 9-2). For example, in one report the tomograms of 40 out of 50 euprolactinemic normal women of reproductive age were interpreted as being abnormal by the majority of four experienced radio-

TABLE 9-3. Outline of work-up for hyperprolactinemia

Evaluation of galactorrhea and menstrual dysfunction or amenorrhea

1. Fasting AM serum prolactin, rule out pregnancy
2. If prolactin elevated, repeat
3. Serum TSH, LH, FSH, T_3, and T_4

Evaluation of hyperprolactinemia
1. Thin-section MRI, high field strength, or coronal contrast-enhanced CT
2. If MRI shows extrasellar extension, thyroid tests are normal:
   a. Baseline formal field of vision testing by neuro-ophthalmologist
   b. TRH stimulation of prolactin and TSH
   c. Insulin tolerance test of GH[a] and cortisol response to ACTH

[a] GH, growth hormone.

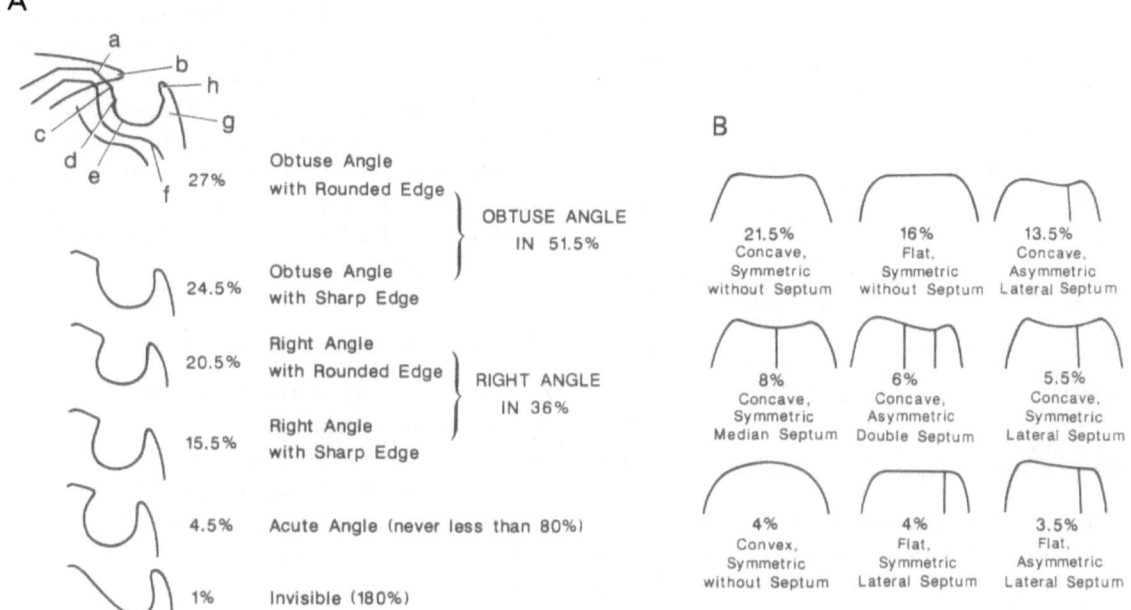

FIGURE 9-2. (A) The anterior sella turcica (a) and tuberculum sella (c), as seen on tomograms and the lateral view, demonstrating the many normal variants that are responsible for the low specificity of hypocycloidal tomograms. a, sella turcica; b, anterior clinoid process; c, tubercululm sella; d, middle clinoid process; e, sella floor; f, sphenoid sinus; g, dorsum sella; h, posteroid clinoid process. (B) Anterior projections of the tuberculum sella and anterior sella turcica, showing the percentages of each form present in the general population. Reprinted with permission from Bruneton et al.[70]

logists.[70] In addition, autopsy series have shown that tomograms are an extremely insensitive means of diagnosis.[71,72] Therefore, this technique is rarely used today, having been replaced by computerized tomography (CT) or magnetic resonance imaging (MRI).

Computerized Tomographic Scanning

During the last decade, CT scan resolution of the pituitary has been progressively improved. This is the result of the use of direct coronal views with intravenous contrast material to provide pituitary enhancement as well as thinner sections, constantly improving CT technology, and intrathecal metrizamide to provide CSF contrast around the gland and stalk.[72,73] Imaging performed shortly after intravenous injection of iodinated contrast material makes the adenoma, which is underperfused, appear as a defect in the enhanced pituitary. In microadeno-

mas, the diagnosis often depends on the mass effect, specifically gland enlargement (Fig. 9-3). Subtle change in the upper or lower contour of the gland from concave to convex, shifts in the pituitary stalk, or deviation of the stalk vessels with rapid imaging during contrast injection (the "tuft sign") can also be seen.[74–76] Although these radiologic features are much more reliable than polytomography for diagnosis of pituitary tumors, false positives (and negatives) are still seen.

The normal gland demonstrates slight heterogeneity of texture and variations in size and contour, making the interpretation of small lesions difficult and inaccurate, even by experienced radiologists.[77] Davis and others reported accurate diagnosis and location in 24 of 51 excised microadenomas, with false-negative studies in the others.[78] On the other hand, in a series of 34 patients with suspected microadenomas, 28 focal lesions and their locations were described based on CT find-

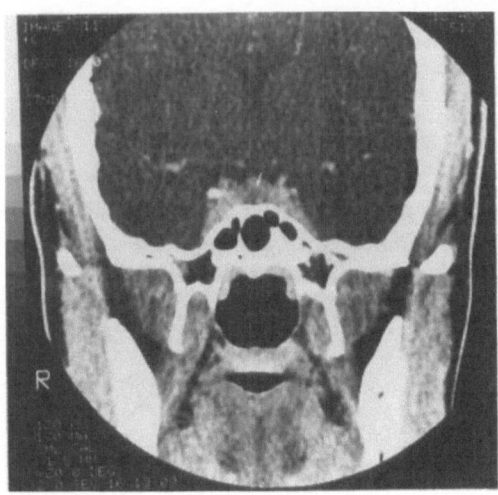

FIGURE 9-3. A 22-year-old woman with amenorrhea and galactorrhea: a radiolucent microadenoma on CT scan (arrow). The upper border on the gland is convex and bulging.

ings, and only 20 of these proved to be tumors. Twenty-nine tumors were excised, nine from sites considered radiologically normal. Three radiologists made 102 independent observations in these 34 patients, and the authors noted that they disagreed on the site of a lesion only once, when two radiologists considered that there was a lesion on one side while the third radiologist thought there was one on the opposite side. At surgery, a tumor was found, but at neither of the predicted sites.[79] They concluded that there was a 50:50 chance that a lesion of 5 mm or less seen on CT scan really existed but that diagnostic correlation between the radiographic and surgical findings was excellent in lesions of more than 6 mm. Unfortunately, half of the tumors found were 5 mm or less in size. Three out of five patients with radiologically normal glands proved to have tumors. Mass effects were unreliable in localizing the microadenomas in both studies.

Some of the false positives can be explained by nonadenomatous but real lesions. Chambers et al.[80] examined 50 normal patients and 100 cadavers with high-resolution CT. There were 22 lesions of 3 mm or less in the patients. In the cadavers, there was a 14% rate of mi-

croadenomas, 20% pars intermedia cysts, 4% metastatic tumors, and 3% infarcts, with no false positives, inferior bony irregularity, or infundibular displacement. Measurements of the sella and pituitary were similar to those of normal patients. They concluded that some of the small lesions seen in normal patients must have etiologies other than prolactin-secreting adenomas.

Magnetic Resonance Imaging

A good imaging method must first diagnose the tumor and then measure it accurately in order to detect changes following treatment or observation. Computerized tomographic scanning does not always meet these needs, although this method is invaluable for detecting intracranial calcification and skull abnormalities.[79,81]

Magnetic resonance imaging (MRI) has now become the imaging method of choice for intracranial pathology, and although its use and interpretation are still evolving, MRI will probably afford the most information for evaluation of patients with symptomatic hyperprolactinemia.[82-85] It has several advantages. First, it does not require ionizing radiation, especially important in long-term follow-up of medical treatment requiring repeated scans. Second, tissue definition is improved since imaging depends on four behavior characteristics of tissue protons, which are peculiar to the protons in each substance, rather than the mechanical absorption of x-rays dependent on tissue density. Third, as with CT scanning, when tissue sections become thinner (5 to 7 mm), the resolution of smaller lesions improves. In addition, higher-strength magnetic fields (1.5 Tesla or more) allow fairly routine imaging of the hypophyseal stalk, the optic chiasm and tracts, as well as identification of blood flow, without additional invasive procedures.[82] Fourth, MRI distinguishes among CSF, soft tissue, air, fat, and hemorrhage. It can accurately discriminate a CSF-filled empty sella from cystic degeneration of an intrasellar mass (Fig. 9-4). Fifth, imaging is possible in literally any plane, thus obviating the discomfort of hyperexten-

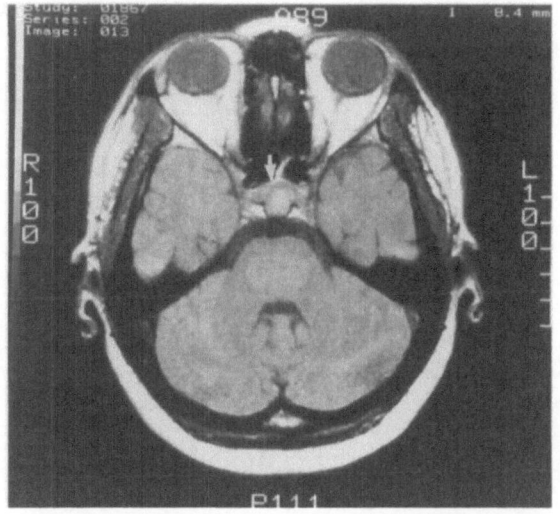
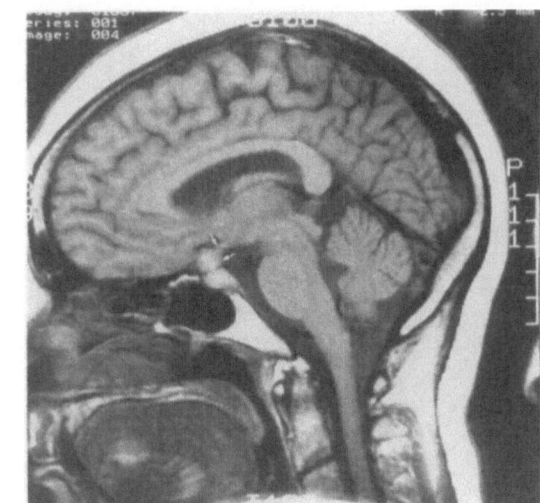

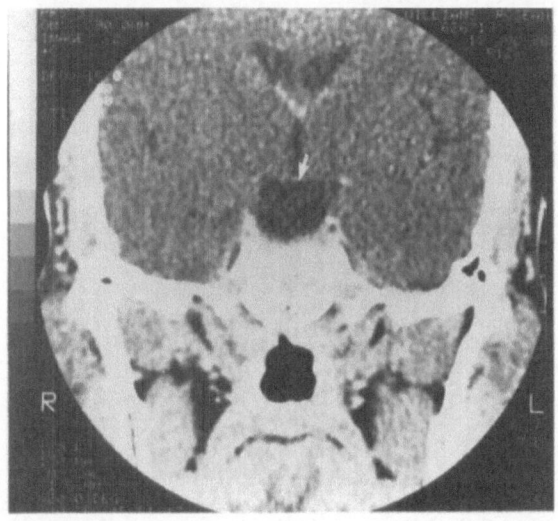

FIGURE 9-4. A 36-year-old woman with a prolactin level of 300 ng/mL. A craniopharyngioma (arrow) is identifiable as a hyperintense lesion on proton-weighted coronal (A) and T_1 sagittal views (B), appearing typically as a mucus-filled cystic structure involved with the optic chiasm (top arrow, B). (C) The CT version of the same lesion shows what appears to be a large cystic structure (arrow). A cystic adenoma cannot be distinguished from a noncalcified craiopharyngioma on high-resolution CT.

sion of the neck necessary for direct coronal views on CT (Fig. 9-5). Furthermore, intravenous administration of contrast material is not necessary for good pituitary visualization as it sometimes is with CT scanning. Lastly, dental fillings do not obscure the image with artifact, as they can on CT scans.

Studies with low-field-strength MRI have shown variable results in terms of accurate identification of pituitary tumors. Using relatively thick sections and low field strength, Glaser et al.[84] studied 22 patients with known pituitary tumors or empty sella, as well as 17 normal subjects. Measurements of the heights of normal glands were 6 to 9 mm, slightly greater than the original CT-determined reports (up to 0.7 mm) but in agreement with more recent measurments in young women.[86,87] The appearance of macroadenomas compared well with CT images, but microadenomas not seen on CT were suspected in 10 patients with elevated prolactin or ACTH.

By contrast, Davis et al.[78] found minimal correlation between CT and MRI. They also used a low-strength field of 0.5 T and 2- or 5-mm images but found poor agreement with CT scan in a small group of patients. Contrast-enhanced CT visualized three microadenomas, one at an incorrect site, one that was

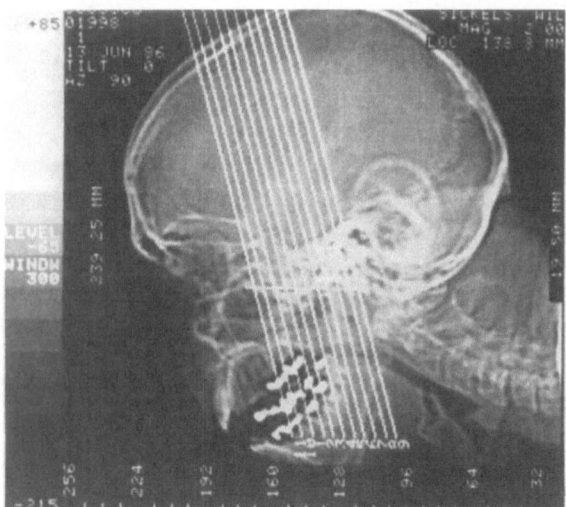

FIGURE 9-5. The scout film from a CT scan of the pituitary marking the coronal sections. This patient's neck is hyperextended, and the x-rays will pass through his dental fillings, unavoidably producing unacceptable artifacts.

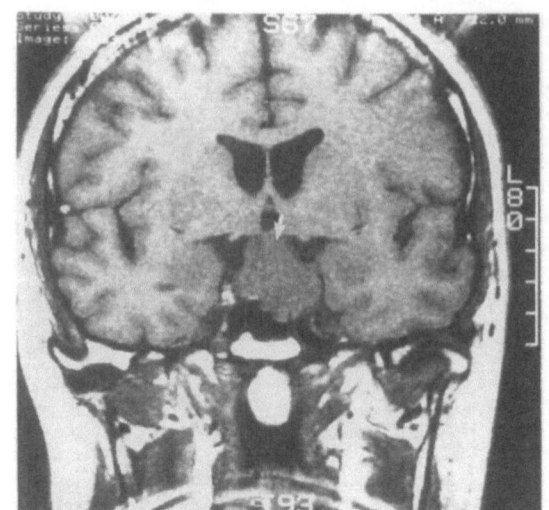

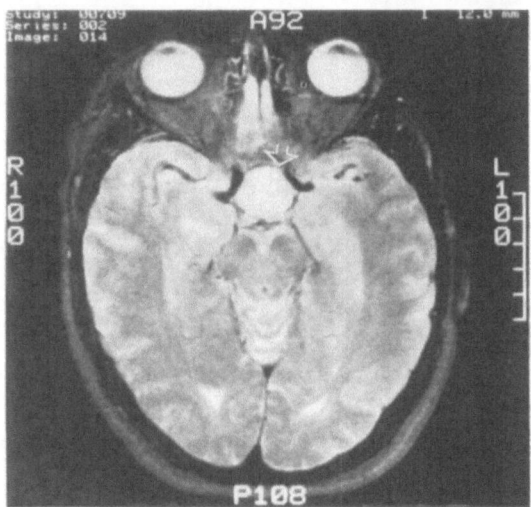

FIGURE 9-6. A large pituitary adenoma (arrows), hyperintense on the T_2 (A) image and hypointense on T_1 (B), extending well above the sella and down into the sphenoid sinus.

also seen on MRI, and one 8-mm microadenoma that was missed on MRI. On MRI, one microadenoma that was not noted on CT was found. Two patients with negative studies (CT and MRI) had no tumor at operation. The MRI demonstrated optic chiasm compression in six patients that could not be confirmed by CT. Davis concluded that CT was superior for microadenoma detection, and MRI for macroadenomas.

On the other hand, using a higher-field-strength unit (1.5 T) and 3-mm sections, Kucharczyk et al.[83] identified 10/11 known microadenomas and all 17 macroadenomas on T_1-weighted coronal images, again clearly demonstrating suprasellar extension and chiasm compression. All except one microadenoma appeared hypointense on T_1 weighting (600/25 msec), and seven demonstrated a convex superior surface. Three showed only an intraglandular hypointensity. The sellar floor could not be seen because of the signal void of bone, but actual herniation of the gland into the cavernous sinus was visible. Unfortunately, CT was not used in this study for comparison, and the population was al-

ready known to have abnormal pituitary function. However, they concluded that high-field MRI was useful as a sole method to diagnose and follow up suspected micro- and macroadenomas (Fig. 9-6).

Similarly, Bilaniuk et al.[85] found that CT and high-field (1.5-T) MRI compared well with each other in the imaging of four macroadenomas, one microadenoma, and one empty sella. They found that only MRI demonstrated asymptomatic optic chiasm compression as well as the intracavernous carotids and the anterior cerebral artery displacement by a large suprasellar mass. Their preference for MRI was based on a lack of radiation, exquisite supra- and parasellar detail of vital structures, and demonstration of an empty sella without intrathecal metrizamide. The low-field system (0.12 T) used by Davis[78] and Glaser[84] was inferior to both CT and the 1.5-T magnet. As MRI technology matures, its noninvasiveness and biological safety in repeated scans, multiplanar versatility, and remarkable tissue resolution will make it the first choice for evaluating the sella and its environs. High-resolution CT will always have its place as a complementary examination, particularly for evaluation of the skull and in patients with metallic clips, implants, and pacemakers.

Therapy of Hyperprolactinemia

Medical therapy of hyperprolactinemia is highly successful in anovulatory women. Not surprisingly, the ergot derivatives with dopamine agonist activity are the cornerstone of this therapy. In addition, other ovulation induction agents have been used (e.g., clomiphene, hMG, and GnRH). These are reviewed and compared to surgery.

Ergot Derivatives

Ergot drugs date back to the Middle Ages, when epidemics of ergotism occurred in groups who ate bread made from contaminated flour. The ergot alkaloids are obtained from a fungus (*Claviceps pupurea*) that grows on rye. Several other medications can be derived from this fungus, including tyramine, histamine, and acetylcholine, in addition to the three groups of ergot alkaloids.[88] Ergocryptine contains the condensation product of three amino acids in the amide nitrogen of its lysergic acid nucleus. Manipulation of ergocryptine has lead to the development of bromocriptine and several other drugs with selective dopaminergic activity.[89]

Bromocriptine is the most widely used drug of this class and has long been known to inhibit prolactin secretion. It acts by specific binding to dopamine receptors in the anterior pituitary as well as direct stimulation of neuronal dopamine receptors.[89,90] In addition, bromocriptine causes shrinkage of micro- and macroadenomas by reducing the number of secretory granules in the cell cytoplasm. Consequently, there is a decrease in cell size while the proportion of the tumor occupied by fibrous tissue is increased.[91,92] This tumor shrinkage may result in normal pituitary function as well as lowering of serum prolactin.[93] Interestingly, ovulaton may occur despite abnormal prolactin secretory patterns.[14] Apparently, these effects are mediated primarily by the dopaminergic actions of the ergot alkaloids.

Bromocriptine: Pharmacology

Bromocriptine is a semisynthetic ergot alkaloid that is usually administered orally, and about 28% is rapidly absorbed from the GI tract. Most (94%) of the absorbed drug undergoes first-pass hepatic metabolism and is subsequently excreted in the feces.[89] A single oral dose results in peak drug serum levels after 1 to 3 hours and suppresses prolactin levels for up to 14 hours (when the drug is no longer detectable in the serum).

Alternate routes of administration have also been tried in order to circumvent side effects and improve therapy. There is an intramuscular, long-acting suspension of bromocriptine polylactic acid microspheres. A preliminary trial showed an excellent therapeutic response in a small group of patients. Side effects were mild and transient, and prolactin remained suppressed for 4 to 6 weeks after a single injection.[94] Bromocriptine has also been administered vaginally in a preliminary study on a small group of normal women.[95] Absorption is apparently less rapid, since maximum prolactin inhibition was achieved at 11 hours. However, prolactin levels were suppressed to 63% of baseline levels, and this suppression lasted for 24 hours. Further data are needed before this can be reliably used for clinical purposes.

However, both vaginal and intramuscular administration may be useful alternatives in some patients intolerant to oral side effects.

The usual dose is 2.5 to 10 mg daily, in two or three divided doses. Most practitioners advise patients to start with 1.25 mg (half tablet) at night for 1 to 2 weeks and gradually increase the dose as needed. Some patients may be very sensitive to bromocriptine and respond adequately to even this low dose, particularly if they have only mild hyperprolactinemia.[96] Furthermore, one group reports excellent prolactin suppression with a single daily dose (instead of tid).[97] In general, adherence to as low a dose as possible may help improve compliance and minimize side effects.

The most common side effects are GI disturbances and postural hypotension. These are seen in about half of the patients with initiation of therapy. In about 20% of patients, headaches and dizziness occur as well. To minimize these problems, which, by the way, tend to lessen with time, the drug is usually given at night. In rare instances other side effects may include fatigue, depression, anxiety, and hallucinations.[89]

Treatment Outcome

Serum prolactin can be lowered by bromocriptine therapy in 80% to 90% of patients with hyperprolactinemia.[98] As a result, ovulatory menses return, usually within the first few weeks of treatment. Pregnancy rates are similarily impressive, 50% to 80%.[8,91–100]

If the etiology of the hyperprolactinemia is a pituitary tumor, shrinkage usually occurs, and complete disappearance is not uncommon. Prospective studies have noted a 60% to 75% tumor reduction rate. Changes in serum prolactin levels usually correlate with tumor size; however, there have been increases seen in tumor size despite a lowering of the serum prolactin.[98,101] Cessation of the drug may result in rapid reexpansion of the tumor.[102]

Other Ergot Derivatives

Since the synthesis of bromocriptine, several other drugs have been developed that have

TABLE 9-4. Efficacy of bromocriptine alternatives[a]

Drug	Dose	Return of gonadal function	Normalization of prolactin
Cabergoline	0.3–0.7 mg every 5–7 days	56%	61%
Lisuride	0.1–2.0 mg daily (divided doses)	46%	64%
Tergeride	0.2–3.0 mg daily (divided doses)	80%	47%
Metergoline	2–24 mg daily (divided doses)	53%	39%
Pergolide	50–500 μg (single daily dose)	69%	77%
Mesulergine	0.25–2.0 mg daily (divided doses)	57%	58%

[a] The range of dosages is shown as well as average reported efficacy (in terms of function and normalization of prolactin levels).

similar activity (Table 9-4). Some of these are ergoline derivatives (e.g., lacking the peptide side chain of bromocriptine), and others have been modified to provide a longer duration of therapeutic action.[88] Metergoline is an ergoline derivative with primarily antiserotonergic properties as well as some dopaminergic activities. It has been successfully used to treat hyperprolactinemia of various etiologies. Ovulation rates are quoted as 40% to 72%, and pregnancy rates are approximately 10% to 24%.[103–106] Although there are no direct trials comparing the efficacy of bromocriptine and metergoline, the latter appears less effective. Nonetheless, it sometimes works in patients who do not respond to bromocriptine.

The long-acting dopamine agonist pergolide is a synthetic ergoline that has been very effective for treatment of hyperprolactinemia. It can be given orally once a day in a 50- to 100-μg dose. Treatment has resulted in resumption of menses in 50% to 100% of women and shrinkage of adenomas in 33% to 75% of patients, depending on the size of the tumor. Most of the complications seen are similar to those of bromocriptine.[107-109] However, disturbing elevations of enzymes in liver function tests have been seen in a few patients who subsequently were found on biopsy to have eosinophilic hepatitis. Liver enzyme levels returned to normal on discontinuation of the drug.[107]

Lisuride is a semisynthetic ergot derivative that is interesting because it exhibits mixed dopamine agonist/antagonist activity in some systems.[88] It is effective in reduction of serum prolactin as well as tumor shrinkage.[103,110,111] Little information is available about pregnancy rates; however, one study cites a 38% pregnancy rate and a 61% ovulation rate. Side effects are similar to those of bromocriptine, although probably more common and more severe.[112] A new lisuride derivative, terguride, may circumvent this problem, since it was indistinguishable from placebo in a double-blind crossover study.[113] Preliminary data suggest that its effectiveness is similar to that of bromocriptine, although a formal trial to compare the two has not been published.[113-115]

Mesulergin is another aminoergoline that, like bromocriptine, works by binding to dopamine receptors. Early trials have shown that prolactin can be normalized in 50% to 65% of patients and that menses return in 50% to 90% women.[116,117] Mesulergin was administered once or twice daily in doses of 0.5 to 1.5 mg daily. The side effects were somewhat similar in nature and frequency to those of bromocriptine, although in one study almost half of the patients dropped out because of the severe nausea and vomiting.[109,116-118]

Cabergoline is the longest-acting dopamine agonist to date. In doses of 0.3 to 0.6 mg, it reliably suppresses prolactin for at least 5 days.[119,120] When it was given once weekly to a group of hyperprolactinemic women, 68% ovulated. Interestingly, prolactin was suppressed to normal levels in only about half of these women.[120] The usual dopamine agonist side effects were seen but were uncommon.

Its efficacy and ease of administration make cabergoline an appealing alternative.[119-122]

Other Medical Treatments

Before the introduction of the ergot derivatives, ovulation was induced in these patients with clomiphene citrate or human menopausal gonadotropins (hMG). There may still be a place for selective use of these agents as well as gonadotropin-releasing hormone (GnRH). In one retrospective study, the use of clomiphene alone resulted in a 57% pregnancy rate compared with 68% pregnancy rate with bromocriptine.[123] This is somewhat surprising, given that hyperprolactinemic women are usually hypoestrogenic, which would generally be associated with poor responsiveness to clomiphene. However, some of these patients could have had PCO. This study also shows that ovulation can be achieved in the face of hyperprolactinemia. This contention is further supported by studies of hMG therapy in hyperprolactinemic women. Although these studies are mostly retrospective, they show a 60% to 75% pregnancy rate in hyperprolactinemic women treated with hMG alone.[124,125] In one report bromocriptine was added in the luteal phase, but there is no evidence that this improved pregnancy rates. Most recently, isolated reports of pulsatile GnRH therapy have shown that this is also successful for induction of ovulation in hyperprolactinemic women.[126,127] Consequently, all of these traditional methods of ovulation induction have been successfully used in hyperprolactinemic women. For selected patients who do not ovulate when given an ergot derivative alone, one of these agents can be used.

Surgery

Transsphenoidal resection of prolactin-secreting adenomas was a very popular treatment at one time because of its rapid relief of symptoms, low rates of associated morbidity, and extremely rare mortality. Early reports described return of menses, normalization of prolactin, and pregnancy in 60% to 80% of women with microadenomas.[100,128,129] Macroadenomas were considered much more difficult to treat, and resection resulted in symptomatic relief in only about 10% to 30% of patients. Morbidity has included transient diabetes insipidus, hemorrhage, meningitis, CSF leakage, and panhypopituitarism, all of which are more common and more severe with the large tumors. Long-term follow-up studies have shown a recurrence rate of 40% to 50% in patients with microadenomas and as high as 80% with macroadenomas.[130,131] This remarkable failure rate has lead most experts to recommend medical therapy as the treatment of choice while reserving surgery for selected cases of macroadenomas.[129]

For example, a recently described "silent" pituitary macroadenoma that was associated with moderately elevated prolactin and growth hormone levels grew rapidly despite bromocriptine-induced normalization of hormone levels.[132] Surgery was necessary in this case to prevent loss of vision. Another proposed role for surgery is in patients who have had some shrinkage of a macroadenoma from bromocriptine and who plan a pregnancy. For these patients, surgical reduction of the tumor might prevent complications from pituitary expansion during pregnancy.[100]

Pregnancy

Although the normal endocrine changes of pregnancy induce hyperprolactinemia in all women, those patients who were hyperprolactinemic prior to pregnancy generally suffer from few complications. As in normal women, estrogens stimulate lactotroph growth. However, symptomatic enlargement of microadenomas is rare (about 1.6%) and for macroadenomas, uncommon (about 15% to 35%).[100,133–135] For the patients with microadenomas, these symptoms included headaches and/or visual disturbances, though not severe enough to warrant surgery. However, these complications tended to be more severe (as well as more common) in macroadenoma patients. Intrapartum bromocriptine or surgery is required more commonly for patients with macroadenomas regardless of whether

they have had antepartum therapy or not.[100,103] Prolactin levels are not valuable in these patients during pregnancy, as they do not always reflect tumor growth.[133,134] Instead, monitoring is usually clinical, with frequent visits to check for symptoms of tumor growth (e.g., headache) and formal visual field studies.

After pregnancy, prolactin levels usually return to prepregnancy levels, and the tumor to its prepregnancy size.[136,137] There is no contraindication to nursing. In addition, some patients will have spontaneous resumption of menses.[138–140] Some authors feel that a lack of the normal pregnancy increment in serum prolactin may correlate with spontaneous normal menstruation postpartum,[140,141] though this is based on small numbers of patients.

References

1. Suh HK, Frantz AG. Size heterogeneity of human prolactin in plasma and pituitary extracts. J Clin Endocrinol Metab. 1974;39:928–35.
2. Makoff E, Lee DW. Glycosylated prolactin is a major circulating variant in human serum. J Clin Endocrinol Metab. 1987;65:1102–06.
3. Niall HD. The chemistry of prolactin. In: Jaffe RB, ed. Prolactin. New York: Elsevier/North Holland, 1981:1–18.
4. Whittaker PG, Wilcox T, Lind T. Maintained fertility in a patient with hyperprolactinemia due to big-big prolactin. J Clin Endocrinol Metab. 1981;53:863–66.
5. Maurer RA. Estradiol regulates transcription of the prolactin gene. J Biol Chem. 1982;157:2133–36.
6. Ben-Jonathan N. Dopamine: a prolactin-inhibiting hormone. Endocr Rev. 1985;6:564–89.
7. Leong DA, Frawley LS, Neill JD. Neuroendocrine control of prolactin secretion. Ann Rev Physiol. 1983;45:109–27.
8. Martin MC, Weiner RI, Monroe SE, et al. Prolactin-secreting adenomas in women VII. Dopamine regulation of prolactin secretion. J Clin Endocrinol Metab. 1984;59:485–90.
9. del Pozo E, Brownell J. Prolactin: I. mechanism of control. Horm Res. 1979;10:143–72.
10. Lamberts SWJ, Verleun T, Hofland L et al.

Differences in the interaction between dopamine and estradiol on prolactin release by cultured normal and tumorous human pituitary cells. J Clin Endocrinol Metab. 1986;63:1342–47.

11. Nickolics K, Mason AJ, Szenyi E, et al. A prolactin-inhibiting factor within the precursor for human gonadotropin releasing hormone. Nature. 1985;316:511–17.

12. Frantz AG. Prolactin. N Engl J Med. 1978;198:201–07.

13. Weitzman E, Boyar RM, Kaper S, et al. The relationship of sleep and sleep stages to neuroendocrine secretion and biological rhythms in man. Recent Prog Horm Res. 1975;31:399–446.

14. Klibanski A, Beitins IZ, Merriam GR, et al. Gonadotropin and prolactin pulsations in hyperprolactinemic women before and during bromocriptine therapy. J Clin Endocrinol Metab. 1984;58:1141–46.

15. Cronin MJ, Cheung CY, Wilson CB, et al. [^{3}H]Spiperone binding to human anterior pituitaries and pituitary adenomas secreting prolactin, growth hormone and adrenocorticotropic hormone. J Clin Endocrinol Metab. 1980;50:387–91.

16. Quigley ME, Judd SJ, Gilliland GB, et al. Functional studies of dopamine control of prolactin secretion in normal women and women with hyperprolactinemic pituitary microadenomas. J Clin Endocrinol Metab. 1980;50:994–98.

17. Crosignani PG, Reschini E, Peracchi M, et al. Failure of dopamine infusion to suppress the plasma prolactin response to sulpuride in normal and hyperprolactinemic subjects. J Clin Endocrinol Metab. 1977;45:841–44.

18. Kleinberg DL, Noel GL, Frantz AG. Galactorrhea: a study of 235 cases, including 48 with pituitary tumors. N Engl J Med. 1977;296:589–600.

19. Conenblum B, Sirek AMT, Horvath E, et al. Human mixed somatotrophic and lactotrophic pituitary adenomas. J Clin Endocrinol Metab. 1976;42:857–63.

20. Hoffman WH, Gala RR, Kovacs K, et al. Ectopic prolactin secretion from a gonadoblastoma. Cancer. 1987;60:2690–95.

21. Rees IH, Bloomfield GA, Rees GM, et al. Mutiple hormones in a bronchial tumor. J Clin Endocrinol Metab. 1974;38:1090–93.

22. Corenblum B, Taylor PJ. Idiopathic hyperprolactinemia may include a distinct entity with a natural history different from that of prolactin adenomas. Fertil Steril. 1988;49:455–546.

23. Martin TL, Kim M, Markey WB. The natural history of idiopathic hyperprolactinemia. J Clin Endocrinol Metab. 1985;60:855–58.

24. Burrow GN, Wortzman G, Newcastle NB, et al. Microadenomas of the pituitary and abnormal sellar tomograms in an unselected autopsy series. N Engl J Med. 1981;304:156–58.

25. March CM, Kletzky OA, Davajan V, et al. Longitudinal evaluation of patients with untreated prolactin-secreting pituitary adenomas. Am J Obstet Gynecol. 1981;139:835–41.

26. Wiebe RH, Hammond CB, Borchert LG. Diagnosis of prolactin secreting microadenoma. Am J Obstet Gynecol. 1976;126:993–96.

27. Turksoy RN, Fairber M, Mitzhell GW. Diagnostic and therapeutic modalities in women with galactorrhea. Obstet Gynecol. 1980;56:323–28.

28. Shoupe D, Lobo RA. Prolactin response after gonadotropin-releasing hormone in the polycystic ovary syndrome. Fertil Steril. 1985;43:549–53.

29. Lunde O. Hyperprolactinemia in polycystic ovary syndrome. Ann Chir Gynaecol 1981;70:197–201.

30. Luciano AA, Chapler FK, Sherman BM. Hyperprolactinemia in polycystic ovary syndrome. Fertil Steril. 1984;41:719–25.

31. Futterweit W, Krieger DT. Pituitary tumors associated with hyperprolactinemia and PCO disease. Fertil Steril. 1979;31:608–13.

32. Alger M, Vasquez-Matute L, Mason M, et al. PCOD associated with hyperprolactinemia and defective metoclopramide response. Fertil Steril. 1980;34:70–71.

33. Quigley ME, Rakoff JS, Yen, SSC. Increased luteinizing hormone sensitivity to dopamine inhibition in polycystic ovary syndrome. J Clin Endocrinol Metab. 1981;52:231–34.

34. Blum I, Bruhis S, Kaufman H. Clinical evaluation of the effects of combined treatment with bromocriptine and spironolactone. Fertil Steril. 1981;35:629–33.

35. Buvat J, Buvat-Herbant M, Marcolin G, et al. Acute effects of bromocriptine on gonadotropin secretion in PCO. Fertil Steril. 1985;44:356–60.

36. Silverman AY, Schwartz SL, Steger RW. A quantitative difference between immunologically and biologically active prolactin in hy-

pothyroid patients. J Clin Endocrinol Metab. 1982;55:272–75.

37. Keye WR, Yuen BH, Knopf RF, et al. Amenorrhea, hyperprolactinemia and pituitary secondary to primary hypothyroidism. Obstet Gynecol. 1976;48:697–702.

38. Cooper DS, Ridgway EC, Kliman B, et al. Metabolic clearance and production rates of prolactin in man. J Clin Invest. 1979;64:1669–80.

39. Sievertsen GD, Lim VS, Nakawatase C, et al. Metabolic clearance and secretion rates of human prolactin in normal subjects and in patients with chronic renal failure. J Clin Endocrinol Metab. 1980;50:846–50.

40. Van Thiel DH, McClain CJ, Elson MK, et al. Evidence for autonomous secretion of prolactin in some alcoholic men with cirrhosis and gynecomastia. Metabolism. 1978;27:1778–84.

41. Monroe SE, Levine L, Keye WR, et al. Prolactin secreting pituitary adenomas in women V. Increased gonadotrope sensitivity in hyperprolactinemic women with pituitary adenomata. J Clin Endocrinol Metb. 1981;52:1171–78.

42. Kauppilla A, Leinonen P, Vihko P, et al. Metoclopromide-induced hyperprolactinemia impairs follicle maturation and corpus luteum function in women. J Clin Endocrinol Metab. 1982;54:955–60.

43. Reinthaller A, Bieglmayer C, Deutinger C, et al. Transient hyperprolactinemia during cycle stimulation: influence on the endocrine response and fertilization rate of human oocytes and effects of bromocriptine treatment. Fertil Steril. 1988;49:432–36.

44. Cutie ER, Andino NA. Prolactin inhibits the steroidogenesis in midfollicular phase human granulosa cells cultured in a chemically defined medium. Fertil Steril. 1988;49:632–37.

45. del Pozo E, Wyss H, Tolis G, et al. Prolactin and deficient luteal function. Obstet Gynecol. 1979;53:282–85.

46. Saunders DM, Hunter JC, Haase HR, et al. Treatment of luteal phase inadequacy with bromocriptine. Obstet Gynecol. 1979;53:287–89.

47. Pepperell RJ. Prolactin and reproduction. Fertil Steril. 1981;35:267–74.

48. Vanrell JA, Balasch J. Prolactin in the evaluation of luteal phase in infertility. Fertil Steril. 1983;39:30–33.

49. Kauppila A, Martikainen H, Puistola U, et al. Hypoprolactinemia and ovarian function. Fertil Steril. 1988;49:437–41.

50. Schulz KD, Gerger W, del Pozo E, et al. Pattern of sexual steroids, prolactin and gonadotropic hormones during prolactin inhibition in normally cycling women. Am J Obstet Gynecol. 1978;132:561–66.

51. Wallace A, Lees DAR, Roberts ADG et al. Danazol and prolactin status in patients with endometriosis. Acta Endocrinola. 1984;107:445–49.

52. Bahamondes L, Saboya W, Tramascia M, et al. Galactorrhea, infertility and short luteal phases in hyperprolactinemic women: early stage of amenorrhea–galactorrhea? Fertil Steril. 1979;32:476–77.

53. Sadeghi-Nejad A, Wolfdorf JI, Biller B, et al. Brief clinical and laboratory observations: hyperprolactinemia causing primary amenorrhea. J Pediatr. 1981;99:592–93.

54. Ferrari C, Telloli P, Rampini P, et al. Hyperprolactinemic primary amenorrhea. Gynecol Obstet Invest. 1980;11:317–26.

55. Keye WR, Chang RJ, Wilson CB, et al. Prolactin-secreting adenomas. III. Frequency and diagnosis in amenorrhea galactorrhea. JAMA. 1980;244:1329–32.

56. Bohnet HG, Dahlen HG, Wuttke W, et al. Hyperprolactinemic anovulatory syndrome. J Clin Endocrinol Metab. 1975;42:132–43.

57. Barnes AB. Diagnosis and treatment of abnormal breast conditions. N Engl J Med. 1966;275:1184–87.

58. MacFarlane IA, Rosen MD. Galactorrhea following surgical procedures to the chest wall: the role of prolactin. Postgrad Med J. 1980;56:23–25.

59. Noel GL, Sutt HK, Stone JG, et al. Human prolactin and growth hormone release during surgery and other conditions of stress. J Clin Endocrinol Metab. 1972;35:840–51.

60. Tolis G, Somma M, Van Casppenhout J, et al. Prolactin secretion in 65 patients with galactorrhea. Am J Obstet Gynecol. 1974;118:91–101.

61. Sarkar DK, Yen SSC. Hyperprolactinemia decreases the LHRH concentration in pituitary portal plasma, a possible role for β-endorphin as a mediator. Endocrinology. 1985;116:2080–84.

62. Higuchi K, Nawata H, Maki T, et al. Prolactin has a direct effect on adrenal androgen secretion. J Clin Endocrinol Metab. 1984;59:714–18.

63. Keye W, Chang J, Wilson C, et al. Prolactin-

secreting pituitary adenomas. JAMA. 1980;244:1329–32.

64. Chang RJ, Keye W, Monroe S, et al. Prolactin-secreting pituitary adenomas in women IV. Pituitary function in amenorrhea associated with normal or abnormal serum prolactin and sellar polytomography. J Clin Endocrinol Metab. 1980;51:830–35.

65. Quigley ME, Judd SJ, Gilliland GB, et al. Effects of a dopamine antagonist on the release of gonadotropin and prolactin in normal women and women with hyperprolactinemic anovulation. J Clin Endocrinol Metab. 1979;48:718–720.

66. Quigley ME, Sheehan KL, Casper RF, et al. Evidence for increased dopaminergic and opioid activity in patients with hypothalamic hypogonadotrophic amenorrhea. J Clin Endocrinol Metab. 1980;50:949–54.

67. Suginami H, Hamada K, Yano K, et al. Ovulation induction with bromocriptine in normoprolactinemic anovulatory women. J Clin Endocrinol Metab. 1986;62:899–902.

68. Corenblum B, Taylor PJ. A rationale for the use of bromocriptine in patients with amenorrhea and normoprolactinemia. Fertil Steril. 1980;34:239–42.

69. Peillon F, Vincens M, Cesselin F, et al. Exaggerated prolactin response of TRH in women with anovulatory cycles: possible role of endogenous estrogens and effect of bromocriptine. Fertil Steril. 1982;37:530–33.

70. Bruneton JN, Drovillard JP, Sabatier JC, et al. Normal variants of the sella turcica. Radiology. 1979;131:99–104.

71. Muhr G, Bergstrom K, Grimelias L, et al. A parallel study of roentgen anatomy of the sella turcica and the histopathology of the pituitary gland in 205 autopsy specimens. Neuroradiology. 1981;21:55–65.

72. Kendall B. Current approaches to hypothalamic pituitary radiology. Clin Endocrinol Metab. 1983;12:353–66.

73. Ghigo E, Ciccarellie, Bianchi SD, et al. Comparison between pituitary computed tomographic findings and tests of hypothalamo-pituitary function in 72 patients with hyperprolactinemia. Acta Endocrinol. 1986;112:20–27.

74. Hankins CA, Zamini AA, Rumbaugh CL. Prolactinomas, clinical presentation radiologic assessment and therapeutic options. Invest Radiol. 1985;20:345–54.

75. Wolpert SM, Molitch ME, Goldman JA, et al. Size, shape and appearance of the normal female pituitary gland. Am J Neuro Rad. 1984;5:263–67.

76. Schwartz JD, Russel KB, Basile BA, et al. High resolution computed tomographic appearance of the intrasellar contents in women of child-bearing age. Radiology. 1983;147:115–17.

77. Ropollo H, Atchaw R, Meyer J, et al. Normal pituitary gland: 1. Macroscopic anatomy—CT correlation. Am J Neurorad. 1983;4:927–35.

78. Davis PC, Hoffman JC, Spencer T, et al. MR imaging of pituitary adenoma: CT, clinical and surgical correlation. Am J Radiol. 1987;148:797–802.

79. Teasdale E, Teasdale G, Mohsen F, et al. High resolution computed tomography in pituitary microadenoma: is seeing believing? Clin Radiol. 1986;37:227–32.

80. Chambers RE, Turski PA, LaMasters D, et al. Regions of low density in the contrast-enhanced pituitary gland: normal and pathologic process. Radiology. 1982;144:109–13.

81. Taylor CR, Jaffe CC. Methodological problems in clinical radiology research: pituitary microadenoma detection as a pradignm. Radiology. 1983;147:279–83.

82. Kaufman B. Magnetic resonance imaging of the pituitary gland. Radiol Clin North Am. 1984;22:795–803.

83. Kucharczyk W, Davis DO, Kelly WM, et al. Pituitary adenomas: high resolution MR imaging at 1.5T. Radiology. 1986;161:761–65.

84. Glaser B, Sheinfield M, Benmair J, et al. Magnetic resonance imaging of the pituitary gland. Clin Radiol, 1986;37:9–14.

85. Bilaniuk LT, Zimmerman RA, Wehrli FW, et al. Magnetic resonance imaging of pituitary lesions using 1.0 to 1.5 T field strength. Radiology. 1984;153:415–18.

86. Syvertson A, Haughton VM, Williams AL, et al. The computed tomographic appearance of the normal pituitary gland and pituitary microadenomas. Radiology. 1979;133:385–91.

87. Swartz J, Russell K, Basile B. Resolution computed tomographic appearance of the intrasellar contents in women of child bearing age. Radiology. 1983;147:115–17.

88. Muller EE, Panarai AE, Cocchi D, et al. Endocrine profile of ergot alkaloids. Life Sci. 1977;21:1545–58.

89. Vance ML, Evans WS, Thorner MO. Bromocriptine . Ann Intern Med. 1984;100:78–91.

90. Corrodi H, Fuxe K, Hokfelt T, et al. Effect of ergot drugs on central catecholamine

neurons: evidence for a stimulation of central dopamine neurons. J Pharm Pharmacol. 1973;25:409–12.

91. Esiri MM, Bevan JS, Burke CW, et al. Effect of bromocriptine treatment on the fibrous tissue content of prolactin-secreting and nonfunctioning macroadenomas of the pituitary gland. J Clin Endocrinol Metab. 1986;63:383–88.

92. Bassetti M, Spada A, Pezzo G, et al. Bromocriptine treatment reduces the cell size in human macroprolactinomas: a morphometric study. J Clin Endocrinol Metab. 1984;58:268–73.

93. Warfield A, Finkel DM, Schatz NJ, et al. Bromocriptine treatment of prolactin-secreting pituitary adenomas may restore pituitary function. Ann Intern Med. 1984;101:783–85.

94. Montini M, Pagani G, Gianola D, et al. Long-lasting suppression of prolactin secretion and rapid shrinkage of prolactinomas after a long-acting, injectable form of bromocriptine. J Clin Endocrinol Metab. 1986;63:266–68.

95. Vermish M, Fossum GT, Kletzky DA. Vaginal bromocriptine: pharmacology and effect on serum prolactin in normal women. Am J Obstet Gynecol. 1988;72:693–98.

96. Soto-Albors C, Randolph J, Ying YK, et al. Medical management of hyperprolactinemia: a lower dose of bromocriptine may be effective. Fertil Steril. 1987;48:213–17.

97. Ciccarelli E, Mazza E, Ghigo E, et al. Long term treatment with oral single administration of bromocriptine in patients with hyperprolactinemia. J Endocrinol Invest. 1987;10:51–53.

98. Molitch ME, Elton RL, Blackwell RE, et al. Bromocriptine as primary therapy for prolactin-secreting macroadenomas: results of a prospective multicenter study. J Clin Endocrinol Metab. 1985;60:698–705.

99. Badano AR, Miechi HB, Mirkin A, et al. Bromocriptine in the treatment of hyperprolactinemic amenorrhea. Fertil Steril. 1979;31:124–29.

100. Molitch ME. Pregnancy and the hyperprolactinemic woman. N Engl J Med. 1985;312:1364–70.

101. Daughaday WH. The anterior pituitary. In: Wilson JD, Foster DW, eds. Williams textbook of endocrinology, Philadelphia: W. B. Saunders. 1985:568–613.

102. Thorner MO, Perryman RL, Rogol AD, et al. Rapid changes in prolactinoma volume after withrdrawal of and re-institution of bromocriptine. J Clin Endocrinol Metab. 1981;53:480–83.

103. Crosignani PG, Ferrari C, Liuzzi A, et al. Treatment of hyperprolactinemic states with different drugs: a study of bromocriptine, metergoline and lisuride. Fertil Steril. 1982;37:61–67.

104. Casson IF, Walker BA, Hipkin LJ, et al. Intolerance of bromocriptine: is metergoline a satisfactory alternative? Br Med J. 1985;290:1783–84.

105. Crosignani PG, Peracchi M, Lombroso GC, et al. Antiserotonin treatment of hyperprolactinemic amenorrhea: long-term follow-up with metergoline, methysergide and cyprokeptadine. Am J Obstet Gynecol. 1978;132:307–12.

106. Bohnet HG, Kato K, Wolf AS. Treatment of hyperprolactinemic amenorrhea with metergoline. Obstet Gynecol. 1986;67:249–52.

107. Kleinberg DL, Boyd AE, Wardlaw S, et al. Pergolide for the treatment of pituitary tumors secreting prolactin or growth hormone. N Engl J Med. 1983;309:704–09.

108. Blackwell RE, Bradley EL, Kline LB, et al. Comparison of dopamine agonists in the treatment of hyperprolactinemic syndromes: a multicenter study. Fertil Steril. 1983;39:744–48.

109. Grossman A, Bouloux PMG, Loneragan R, et al. Comparison of the clinical activity of mesulergine and pergolide in the treatment of hyperprolactinemia. Clin Endocrinol. 1985;22:611–16.

110. Stracke H, Heinlein W, Horowski R, et al. Dopamine agonists in the treatment of hyperprolactinemia, comparison between bromocriptine and lisuride. Arzneim Forsch/Drug Res. 1986;36:1834–36.

111. Liuzzi A, Dallabonzana D, Oppizzi G, et al. Low doses of dopamine agonists in the long term treatment of macroprolactinomas. N Engl J Med. 1985;313:656–59.

112. Bouloux PMG, Besser GM, Moult PJA, et al. Clinical evaluation of lysuride in the management of hyperprolactinemia. Br Med J. 1987;294:1323–24.

113. Ciccarelli E, Touzel R, Besser M, et al. Terguride—a new dopamine agonist drug: a comparison of its neuroendocrine and side effect profile with bromocriptine. Fertil Steril. 1988;49:589–94.

114. Graf KJ, Kohler D, Horowski R, et al. Rapid regression of macroprolactinomas by the new

dopamine agonist terguride. Acta Endocrinol. 1986;111:460–66.

115. Dallabonzana D, Liuzzi A, Oppizzi G, et al. Effect of the new ergot derivative on plasma prolactin and GH in patients with pathological hyperprolactinemia or acromegaly. J Endocrinol Invest. 1985;8:147–51.

116. Hesla JS, Rodman EF, Molitch ME, et al. The effect of the ergoline derivative, CU 32-085, on prolactin secretion in hyperprolactinemic women. Fertil Steril. 1987;48:555–59.

117. Dewailly D, Thomas P, Buvat J, et al. Treatment of human hyperprolactinemia with a new dopamine agonist: CU32085 (mesulergin). Acta Endocrinol. 1985;110:433–39.

118. Poulsen HK, Rasmussen P, Petersen MR, et al. Puerperal lactation inhibition with a novel 8 alpha aminoergoline (CU32/085). Gynecol Obstet Invest. 1984;17:139–44.

119. Ferrari C, Barbieri C, Caldar E, et al. Long-lasting prolactin-lowering effect of carbergoline, a new dopamine agonist, in hyperprolactinemic patients. J Clin Endocrinol Metab. 1986;63:941–45.

120. Mattei AM, Ferrari C, Baroldi P, et al. Prolactin-lowering effect of acute and once weekly repetitive oral administration of cabergoline at two dose levels in hyperprolactinemic patients. J Clin Endocrinol Metab. 1988;66:193–98.

121. Pontiroli AE, Cammelli L, Baroldi P, et al. Inhibition of basal and metoclopramide-induced prolactin release by cabergoline, an extremely long-acting dopaminergic drug. J Clin Endocrinol Metab. 1987;65:1057–59.

122. Melis AB, Gambacciani M, Paoletti AM, et al. Dose-related prolactin inhibitory effect of the new long-acting dopamine receptor agonist carbergoline in normal cycling, puerpera, and hyperprolactinemic women. J Clin Endocrinol Metab. 1987;65:541–45.

123. Radwanska E, McGarrigle HHG, Little V, et al. Induction of ovulation in women with hyperprolactinemic amenorrhea using clomiphene and human chorionic gonadotropin or bromocriptine. Fertil Steril. 1979;32:187–92.

124. Farine D, Dor J, Lupovici N, et al. Conception rate after gonadotropin therapy in hyperprolactinemia and normoprolactinemia. Obstet Gynecol. 1985;65:658–60.

125. Archer DF, Josimovich JB. Ovarian responses to exogenous gonadotropins in women with elevated serum prolactin. Obstet Gynecol. 1976;48:155–57.

126. Jansen RPS, Handelsman DJ, Boylan LM, et al. Pulsatile intravenous gonadotropin-releasing hormone for ovulation-induction in infertile women. I. safety and effectiveness with outpatient therapy. Fertil Steril. 1987;48:33–38.

127. Gindoff PR, Loucapoulos A, Jewelewicz R. Treatment of hyperprolactinemic amenorrhea with pulsatile gonadotropin releasing hormone. Fertil Steril. 1986;46:1156–58.

128. Chang RJ, Keye WR, Young JR, et al. Detection, evaluation and treatment of pituitary microadenomas in patients with galactorrhea and amenorrhea. Am J Obstet Gynecol. 1977;128:356–63.

129. Kletzky OA, Kawajan V. Hyperprolactinemia. In: Mishell DR, Davajan V, eds. Infertility, contraception and reproductive endocrinology. New Jersey: Medical Economics, 1986:275–99.

130. Schlechte JA, Sherman BM, Chapler FK, et al. Long term follow-up of women with surgically treated prolactin secreting pituitary tumors. J Clin Endocrinol Metab. 1986;62:1296–1301.

131. Serri O, Rasio E, Beaugard H, et al. Recurrence of hyperprolactinemia after selective transsphenoidal adenomectomy in women with prolactinoma. N Engl J Med. 1983;309:280–83.

132. Horvath E, Kovacs K, Smyth AS, et al. A novel type of pituitary adenoma: morphological features and clinical correlation. J Clin Endocrinol Metab. 1988;66:1111–18.

133. Gemzell C, Wang CF. Outcome of pregnancy in women with pituitary adenoma. Fertil Steril. 1979;31:363–72.

134. Divers WA, Yen SSC. Prolactin producing microadenomas in pregnancy. Obstet Gynecol. 1983;62:425–29.

135. Daya S, Shewchuk AB, Bryeland N. The effect of multiparity on intra-sellar prolactinomas. Am J Obstet Gynecol. 1984;148:512–15.

136. Rasmussen C, Bergh T, Nillius S, et al. Return of menstruation and normalization of prolactin in hyperprolactinemic women with bromocriptine-induced pregnancy. Fertil Steril. 1985;44:31–34.

137. Samaah N, Leavens ME, Sacca R, et al. The effects of pregnancy on patients with hyperprolactinemia. Am J Obstet Gynecol. 1984;148:466–73.

138. Crosignani PG, Ferrari C, Scarduelli C, et

al. Spontaneous and induced pregnancies in hyperprolactinemic women. Obstet Gynecol. 1981;58:708–13.

139. Crosignani PG, Matteir AM, Cavioni V. Is pregnancy the best permanent cure for hyperprolactinemia? Paper presented at the conjoint annual meeting of the American Fertility Society and the Canadian Fertility and Andrology Society, 1986.

140. Rjosk HK, Fahlbusch R, von Werder K. Influence of pregnancies on prolactinomas. Acta Endrocinol. 1982;100:337–46.

141. Andersen AN, Starup J, Tabor A, et al. The possible prognostic value of serum prolactin increment during pregnancy in hyperprolactinemic patients. Acta Endocrinol. 1983;102:1–5.

10
Surgical Management of Polycystic Ovarian Disease

JAMES F. DANIELL

Polycystic ovarian disease (PCO) was first described in 1935 by Stein and Leventhal.[1] Their first ovarian wedge resection was performed successfully in 1929. A follow-up article by Stein et al.[2] reported long-term results in 75 cases treated with his surgical procedure. Although hormonal therapies were suggested and used throughout the 1940s and 1950s, it was not until clomiphene citrate became commercially available that medical treatment of PCO became satisfactory. With the popularity of clomiphene citrate and later human menopausal gonadotropins (hMG), the need for surgical treatment of PCO has become less frequent. With the reports in the 1970s of significant number of patients undergoing laparotomy and ovarian wedge resection who developed postoperative adhesions, the classic operation of wedge resection fell into disfavor. Over the last decade laparoscopic techniques for performing various ovarian traumatizing procedures have been reported with varying degrees of successful subsequent ovulation and pregnancy. Because of these two facts (the success of ovulation induction therapy for PCO and the knowledge of post-wedge-resection adhesion formation), techniques for surgical treatment of PCO have fallen into disrepute, and the surgical skills are not often learned by physicians in training today. This chapter reviews the history of surgical treatment of PCO and discusses the techniques and results obtained by investigators over the last 60 years.

History of Surgical Treatment of PCO

In 1935 Stein and Leventhal[1] first reported their experience treating PCO, describing the condition that is well known to gynecologists today. Because of the high morbidity associated with laparotomy during the first part of this century and the absence of effective drug therapy for PCO, most patients went without treatment. Stein himself was able to accumulate a series totaling only 75 cases over a 30-year period.[2] With long-term follow-up of this initial group of patients, he was able to report a 65% conception rate. His method consisted of sharp resection of the ovarian cortex, removal of a wedge from each ovary, puncture of the cysts from within, and careful approximation the edges with fine catgut. He felt this was superior to other more traumatic surgical techniques that had been described and practiced for treatment of polycystic ovaries. Of his 75 patients, 47 were married and attempted pregnancy with no other significant fertility factors; 26 of these patients (65%) conceived one or more times, with a total of 46 pregnancies. There were 35 live births (one set of twins), seven miscarriages, one stillbirth, and four who were pregnant at the time of his last report.

It is interesting that Stein noted that the long-term effect on hirsutism in his patients was minimal but that the majority of patients did maintain regular menses for his long follow-up. Stein made no mention of looking again at the ovaries in any of his patients; therefore, we have no information concerning postoperative adhesion formation Goldzieher and Green[3] gleaned 1,097 cases from 187 references published in the world literature prior to 1962. Published conception rates ranged from 95% down to only 13%, with normalization of menstrual cycles from 93% to 6%. Improvement in hirsutism was generally poor, with positive results obtained in fewer than 10% of patients.

A more recent review from Johns Hopkins Hospital describes a 10-year follow-up of 90 consecutive ovarian wedge resections for PCO.[4] The Hopkins group reported 91% ovulation, but only 68% had persistent regular menses. The conception rate was 60%. The number of these patients who were clomiphene citrate failures is not clear, but the study did contribute the observation that there was a 23% rate of concurrent tubal peritoneal adhesive disease discovered at the time of the wedge resection. When these adhesions were present, the subsequent pregnancy rate was cut in half. Unfortunately, in the Hopkins study, there was no evaluation of postoperative adhesions based on repeat evaluation at laparotomy or laparoscopy.

It was not until the 1970s that reports began to appear suggesting a high incidence of postoperative adhesion formation and its role in postoperative infertility. The possibility of premature menopause secondary to ovarian fibrosis and atrophy also became recognized. In 1975, two reports from Israel brought worldwide attention to the problem of adhesion formation after wedge resection for PCO. The first, by Toaff et al.,[5] reported seven cases of wedge resection who underwent follow-up laparoscopy. All seven patients had extensive periovarian and peritubal adhesions. Four of these patients were treated surgically, and three of four later conceived. The investigators concluded that ovarian wedge resection should be done only in patients who were resistant to clomiphene citrate and/or hMG therapy and that meticulous surgical techniques should always be utilized. They suggested laparoscopic follow-up in cases in which pregnancy did not occur fairly soon.

In the same year, Weinstein and Polishuk[6] reported follow-up of 72 patients who had undergone wedge resection. All had the classic Stein–Leventhal syndrome. Fifty-seven patients who were followed for 8 years were reported to have a 67% pregnancy rate. Of 19 patients who did not conceive and who underwent a subsequent laparoscopy, eight were found to have significant ovarian adhesions. This resulted in a 14% incidence of pelvic adhesions, which impaired fertility after induction of ovulation in these patients. Interestingly, the authors also reported that the use of intraperitoneal hydrocortisone or rheomacrodex had no beneficial effect on the prevention of adhesion formation. In the same article, they reported 198 women found to have mechanical infertility caused by adhesions. Of these patients, 28 gave a history of prior bilateral ovarian wedge resection because of Stein–Leventhal syndrome. These two bits of information led the authors to conclude that meticulous hemostasis and atraumatic handling of pelvic organs during surgery are very important for preventing postoperative adhesions and that intraperitoneal steroids or dextran was of no benefit.

Portuondo et al.[7] in 1984 reported their experience at the University of Bilbao, Spain. In this interesting article, the effects of laparotomy wedge resection were compared with those of laparoscopic ovarian biopsy by the same surgeons. Twelve patients who underwent classic laparotomy wedge resection had a 92% postoperative adhesion rate, whereas 24 patients who underwent laparoscopic ovarian biopsy had a 0% adhesion rate at laparoscopic reevaluation. In this article, several photographs illustrated the typical postsurgical adhesions now recognized to occur after ovarian wedge resection in some cases. These authors concluded that laparoscopic multiple ovarian biopsies produced no adhesions, whereas ovarian wedge resection by laparotomy had a high rate of postoperative periovarian adhesion formation. They recommended laparoscopic treatment as the treatment of choice in patients in whom hormonal stimulation therapy achieved no response.

Palmer and Brux,[8] from France, were the

first to report experience with laparoscopic treatment of polycystic ovaries. Results included a 60% ovulation rate and a 20% pregnancy rate after simple ovarian biopsy with unipolar cautery as indicated for control of bleeding. The first report in the North American literature was from Neuwirth in 1972.[9] He described a patient with the classic PCO phenotype who was resistant to clomiphene citrate stimulation. He used the technique described by Palmer and included a series of photographs in his case report. The patient ovulated spontaneously postoperatively and conceived on the third cycle. Unfortunately, the pregnancy terminated in a spontaneous abortion at 10 weeks, and no follow-up was reported. Neuwirth suggested that this technique might be useful as an alternative to laparotomy and wedge resection in patients in whom there is no response to clomiphene or gonadotropin therapy.

Campo et al.,[10] in 1983, reported on 12 patients who underwent laparoscopy with ovarian biopsy and use of unipolar cautery at times. They reported postoperative ovulation in 45% of the patients, with 42% becoming pregnant. They analyzed the hormonal changes after the biopsy and noted that results were similar to those reported after laparotomy wedge resection. They felt the technique had much to offer because of the lesser surgical risk compared with laparotomy and the possibility of repeating the procedure and of performing subsequent laparotomy if ovulation could not be induced with ovarian biopsy.

A larger series was reported in 1984[11] by Gjonnaess from Norway. He reported on 62 women who underwent laparoscopic ovarian cautery without biopsy. Postoperative ovulation occurred within 3 months in 92% of the patients, with 86% establishing regular cycles. The pregnancy rate was 69% postoperatively without clomiphene citrate and 80% when postoperative clomiphene citrate was given to the patients who did not ovulate spontaneously after laparoscopic ovarian cautery.

Early second-look laparoscopy after ovarian wedge resection has been suggested by several authors, including Pittaway et al.,[12] who reported benefits of performing second-look laparoscopy within the first 6 weeks after ovarian surgical procedures such as wedge resection or excision of endometrioma. This and other articles[13-15] suggested that judicious use of second-look laparoscopy after laparotomy for ovarian wedge resection is probably a good idea in patients who have associated adhesions or other pathological conditions requiring extensive dissection of the pelvis.

Recently, the advent of surgical lasers has led to the suggestion by some authors that use of the laser at laparotomy for wedge resection may be of benefit in reducing bleeding and postoperative adhesions. McLaughlin[16] reported his results and suggested that the use of laser led to greater hemostasis and formation of fewer postoperative adhesions. Unfortunately, there has been no prospective evaluation of use of the laser compared with cautery for wedge resection of ovaries. The most recent studies of other types of infertility surgery suggest that there are no benefits of surgical laser over cautery in carefully done reconstructive surgery via laparotomy.[17,18]

Laparoscopic use of laser energy, however, does appear to be effective in treating polycystic ovaries. The advantage we have seen is that it avoids the laparoscopic use of cautery and can effectively vaporize ovarian tissue under direct vision. Over the last several years, we have used CO_2, argon, and KTP lasers for laparoscopic vaporization of polycystic ovarian tissue.[19]

Wedge Resection or Laparoscopic Ovarian Treatment: Mechanism of Ovulation

The classic study of hormonal changes after wedge resection by Judd et al.[20] in 1976 has been confirmed by other authors, including Katz et al.[21] and Mahesh et al.[22] for laparotomy wedge resection. Additional studies[23,24] have reported hormonal changes after laparoscopic trauma to the ovary for treating PCO.

Since the changes seen after laparotomy are the same as those seen after laparoscopy, they are both discussed as one common method for correction of the ovulation defect. There is profound temporary reduction of ovarian steroid secretion and persistent postoperative reduction of testosterone secretion. Transient decreases in estradiol are observed as well as declines in 17α-alphahydroxyprogesterone, dehydroepiandrosterone (DHA), and androstenedione (A). There appears to be no immediate change in FSH or LH. However, approximately 10 to 18 days after surgery, there is an LH surge preceded by an estradiol surge and followed by onset of progesterone rise. The mean time to ovulation appears to be 22 days after surgical trauma to the ovary. Falling intraovarian androgen levels combined with reduction in intrafollicular substances may relieve the block to ovulation and thus allow the initiation of folliculogenesis and spontaneous ovulation. With improved understanding of other peptides present in the follicular fluid (such as inhibin[25]), it seems reasonable to conclude that by decreasing the overall volume of follicular fluid in the ovary and traumatizing the stroma, an acute reduction in active ovarian steroidogenesis may ensue. Inhibin has been demonstrated to be increased in follicular fluid in patients with polycystic ovarian disease,[26] the reduction of which by local trauma may play an important role in removing the block to ovulation.

Technique of Surgical Treatment of Polycystic Ovaries

Laparotomy Technique

Numerous techniques for ovarian trauma have been described. We feel that in rare instances when a laparotomy and wedge resection are necessary in the patient with PCO, the most important surgical rule is to limit tissue trauma. These patients are often obese, which usually requires a fairly large incision, packing of the bowel, and use of retractors. The ovaries are usually fairly mobile and can be brought up to the abdominal wall without much difficulty unless there is associated disease. We try to limit trauma to the ovary by picking it up gently and limiting tissue handling. We use heparinized Ringer's solution for irrigation throughout the procedure (5,000 units of heparin in 1 L of Ringer's solution). A fine-needle electrode is used to excise a wedge of the ovary, being careful to avoid the hilus. Internal sutures are then placed. Our preference is for absorbent suture, either PDS, Dexon, or Vicryl. We use the smallest suture that will successfully pull the ovarian tissue together without tearing through. This may vary from case to case depending on the consistency of the ovary but is usually either 4-0 or 3-0 in size.

After the ovarian stroma has been approximated, the surface of the ovary should be closed. Our preference is to use an imbricated stitch that buries the ovarian edge with the knot tied inside the incision. We do not use any intraabdominal adjuvants other than the heparinized Ringer's. We do use perioperative antibiotics and high-dose antiprostaglandins postoperatively. Discussion with the patient about consideration of early second-look laparoscopy should be held, particularly when the patient has adhesions inthe pelvis. If a second-look laparoscopy is to be done, it should be done within the first 6 weeks postoperatively so that any adhesions formed will be thin and avascular and can be easily lysed. Patients are told to expect spontaneous ovulation between 3 and 5 weeks postoperatively. We instruct patients to begin coitus on a regular basis at that time so they will not miss any ovulations. We tell patients that the effects of a wedge resection are probably transient, and, because of this, they should make every effort to conceive each month and not put off conception in the immediate postoperative period.

Laparoscopic Treatment of Polycystic Ovaries

Because of our interest over the last few years in evaluating various surgical lasers, we began in 1984 to use the CO_2 laser for laparoscopic treatment of polycystic ovaries.[27] We felt that we should be able to accomplish the same results as had been reported by Gjonnaess[11] and others for laparoscopic cautery. Our technique for laparoscopic treatment with the CO_2 laser has included the following: The patients are all operated on in Trendelenburg's position with a drained bladder. A three-puncture technique is used. The laser is either brought in through the operating channel laparoscope or through a special 7-mm second puncture probe. A third probe is used to grasp the ovary to roll it about and lift it up. A high-flow insufflator is preferable, since copious amounts of smoke will be generated when the CO_2 laser is used to vaporize polycystic ovaries. The new Wolf variable-flow electronic insufflator is outstanding for suctioning off this high volume of smoke (Wolf Instrument Company, Chicago, IL). To irrigate and suction the smoke, we use a Pumpvac system (Lastech, Joelton, TN). This disposable device allows copious irrigation and smoke suction by the scrub nurse while the surgeon is performing the procedure. This combination of a high-flow insufflator and immediate suction from the point of origin of the smoke allows us to use high power densities with the CO_2 laser to accomplish the vaporization of polycystic ovaries effectively and rapidly.

Each ovary is treated by drilling anywhere from 20 to 40 holes on each ovary. Each hole is symmetrically placed, either over a follicle or over the thickened stroma (Fig. 10-1). We are careful to avoid the hilus and try not to penetrate any deeper than 4 to 5 mm in each hole. Each ovary is treated in a similar fashion, and rarely small bleeding sites require coagulation with either unipolar or bipolar cautery. We recommend monitoring of basal body temperature, beginning at 2 weeks postoperatively, and active coitus so that pregnancy can be accomplished as expeditiously as possible.

Recently, we have begun to use the KTP laser for this procedure and have been pleased with the ease and speed with which we can accomplish vaporization of polycystic ovaries. The KTP laser can be passed through a flexible fiber, which simplifies the delivery of

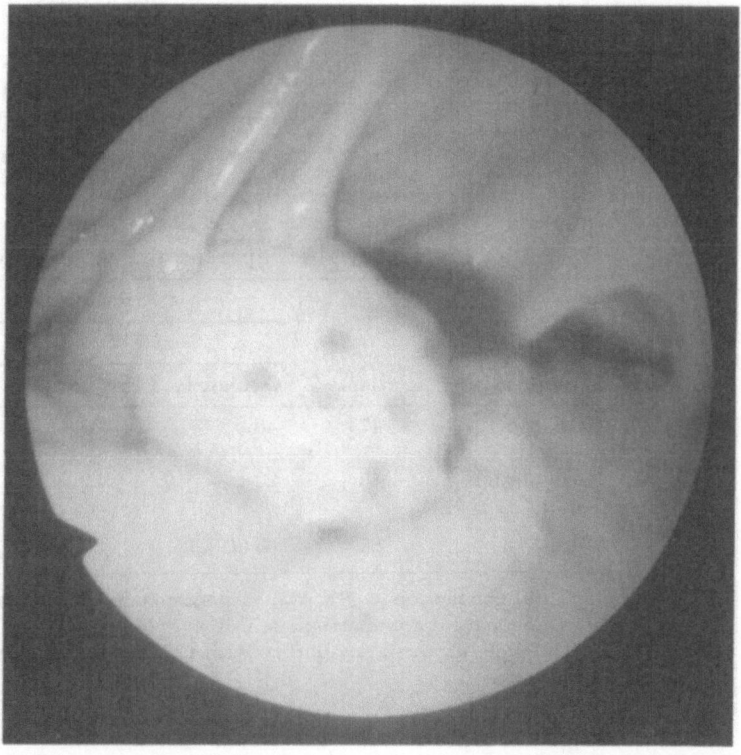

FIGURE 10-1. A typical white smooth polycystic ovary that has been partially treated with CO_2 laser vaporization is seen in this photograph. Further vaporization will continue to produce a uniform dimpled appearance.

the laser energy into the pelvis. In addition, this laser penetrates to a depth of 2 mm, which allows more rapid ovarian stromal damage with less smoke accumulation and less propensity to bleeding. Lomano[28] reported use of the Nd:YAG laser for laparoscopic surgery, but we have no experience with this laser during laparoscopy. The Nd:YAG laser can be used either with sapphire tips, which allow direct contact with the tissue, or with the naked fiber under laparoscopic control. The laparoscopic use of the Nd:YAG laser has not yet been approved by the FDA. The CO_2, KTP, and also the argon laser, which has tissue effects similar to those of the KTP, are all approved clinically for laparoscopic treatment of polycystic ovaries. Tables 10-1 and 10-2 give our results over the last 4 years in our initial group of patients treated with laser energy for PCO. In this series we have had no complications and have had only one

patient who has needed gonadotropin therapy postoperatively to induce ovulation.

We have not performed any organized second-look laparoscopy after laparoscopic laser treatment of polycystic ovaries. However, we have occasionally performed repeat laparoscopy or have observed the ovaries at laparotomy or cesarean section. We have yet to see any ovarian adhesions and have in all cases found the ovaries to have small dimpled craters with few carbon particles present. We have seen more carbon particles in patients treated with the CO_2 laser than with the KTP laser.

Present Recommendations for Surgical Treatment of PCO

With today's availability of clomiphene, gonadotropin therapy, and gonadotropin-releasing hormones, the need for surgical treatment of PCO has become less common. There are, however, patients who are resistant to clomiphene citrate and who are afraid of, cannot afford, or do not elect to undergo ovulation induction therapy with gonadotropins, pure FSH, or gonadotropin-releasing factors. For this group, initial treatment of controlled ovarian damage with laparoscopic techniques should be attempted before proceeding to a laparotomy. The obvious advantages of laparoscopic treatment are that there

TABLE 10-1. Ovulation after laparoscopic vaporization in PCO[a]

Ovulatory status	Preop status	Postop status
Spontaneous	0	60 (71%)
CC nonresponder[b]	38	1
CC responsive	47	24
Total	85	85

[a] Polycystic ovarian disease.
[b] CC, clomiphene citrate.

TABLE 10-2. Pregnancy after laparoscopic vaporization for PCO[a]

		Postoperative results			
		No CC		CC given	
Presurgery	Patients	Ovulated	Pregnant	Ovulated	Pregnant
Ovulation on CC	47	40	20	7	2
No ovulation on CC	38	20	15	17[b]	10
Total	85	60 (71%)	35	24	12

[a] Total conception = 48 (56%) − spontaneous, clomiphene citrate, (CC), or human menopausal gonadotropins (hMG).
[b] One patient was anovulatory with CC and required hMG for ovulation and conception.

is less pain and discomfort for the patient, more rapid return to regular activity, less postoperative morbidity, less likelihood for postoperative adhesion formation, and it can be performed safely as an outpatient procedure. In our opinion, the only candidates for open laparotomy and wedge resection are rare PCO patients who have another reason for laparotomy and who also are planning pregnancy. The data suggest that laparoscopic treatment with either biopsy, ovarian cautery, or laser energy can give satisfactory results in the majority of patients without the necessity of laparotomy.

Conclusions

Surgical treatment of PCO, although not common, still has a role in the management of some patients who desire pregnancy. It behooves all gynecologists to become familiar with and understand the principles of meticulous pelvic surgery before undertaking laparotomy and wedge resection of the ovaries. Certainly in this day of cost containment in medicine and interest in operative laparoscopy, it seems reasonable for gynecologists who have the skills of operative laparoscopy to consider the various forms of laparoscopic treatment now available for PCO. Whether laser vaporization will be more effective than cautery remains to be investigated in a prospective controlled study design. Both techniques appear to give good results when selectively applied to patients with PCO who meet the proper criteria for laparoscopic treatment and who are attempting conception.

References

1. Stein IF, Leventhal ML. Amenorrhea associated with bilateral polycystic ovaries. Am J Obstet Gynecol. 1935;29:181–91.
2. Stein IF, Cohen MR, Elson R. Results of bilateral ovarian wedge resection in 47 cases of sterility. Am J Obstet Gynecol. 1949;58:267–74.
3. Goldzieher JW, Green JA. The polycystic ovary: I. clinical and histological features. J Clin Endocrinol Metab. 1962;22:325–38.
4. Adashi EY, Rock JA, Guzick D, et al. Fertility following bilateral ovarian wedge resection: A critical analysis of 90 consecutive cases of the polycystic ovary syndrome. Fertil Steril. 1981;36:320–24.
5. Toaff R, Toaff ME, Peyser MR. Infertility following wedge resection of the ovaries. Am J Obstet Gynecol. 1975;124:92–96.
6. Weinstein D, Polishuk WC. The role of wedge resection of the ovary as a cause of mechanical sterility. Surg Gynecol Obstet. 1975;141:417–18.
7. Portuondo JA, Melchor JC, Neyro JL, et al. Periovarian adhesions following ovarian wedge resection or laparoscopic biopsy. Endoscopy. 1984;16:143–45.
8. Palmer R, Brux J. Resultats histologiques, biochimiques et therapeutiques obtenus chez les femmes dont les ovaires avalent ete diagnostiques Stein–Leventhal a la coeliscopie. Bull Fed Gynec Obstet Fr. 1967;19:405–08.
9. Neuwirth RS. A method of bilateral ovarian biopsy at laparoscopy in infertility and chronic anovulation. Fertil Steril. 1972;23:361–65.
10. Campo S, Garcea N, Caruso A, et al. Effect of celioscopic ovarian resection in patients with polycystic ovaries. Gynecol Obstet Invest. 1983;15:213–22.
11. Gjonnaess H. Polycystic ovarian syndrome treated by ovarian electrocautery through the laparoscope. Fertil Steril. 1984;41:20–25.
12. Pittaway DE, Daniell JF, Maxson WS. Ovarian surgery in an infertility patient as an indication for a short-interval second-look laparoscopy: a preliminary study. Fertil Steril. 1985;44:611–14.
13. Daniell JF, Pittaway DE. Short-interval second-look laparoscopy after infertility surgery. J Reprod Med. 1983;28:281–83.
14. Raj SG, Hulka JF. Second-look laparoscopy in infertility: therapeutic and prognostic value. Fertil Steril. 1982;38:325–28.
15. Surrey MW, Friedman S. Second-look laparoscopy following reconstructive surgery for infertility. J Reprod Med. 1982;27:658–61.
16. McLaughlin DS. Evaluation of adhesion reformation by early second-look laparoscopy following microlaser ovarian wedge resection. Fertil Steril. 1984;42:531–35.
17. Diamond MP, Daniell JF, Martin DC, et al. Tubal patency and pelvic adhesions at early second-look laparoscopy following intra-

abdominal use of the carbon dioxide laser: initial report of the intra-abdominal laser study group. Fertil Steril. 1984;42:717–22.

18. Diamond MP, Daniell JF, Feste J, et al. Pelvic adhesions at early second-look laparoscopy following carbon dioxide laser surgery procedures. Infertility. 1984;7:39–42.

19. Daniell JF, Miller W, Tosh R, et al. Laparoscopic use of the KTP/532 laser in nonendometriotic pelvic surgery. Colpo Gyn Laser Surg. 1986;2:107–11.

20. Judd HL, Rigg LA, Anderson DC, et al. The effects of ovarian wedge resection on circulating gonadotropin and ovarian steroid levels in patients with polycystic ovary syndrome. J Clin Endocrinol Metab. 1976;43:347–55.

21. Katz M, Carr PJ, Cohen BM, et al. Hormonal effects of wedge resection of polycystic ovaries. Obstet Gynecol. 1978;51:437–44.

22. Mahesh VB, Toledo SPA, Mattar E. Hormone levels following wedge resection in polycystic ovary syndrome. Obstet Gynecol. 1978;51:64s–69s.

23. Aakvaag A, Gjonnaess H. Hormonal response to electrocautery of the ovary in patients with polycystic ovarian disease. Br J Obstet Gynecol. 1985;92:1258–64.

24. Gjonnaess H, Norman N. Endocrine effects of ovarian electrocautery in patients with polycystic ovarian disease. Br J Obstet Gynecol. 1987;94:779–83.

25. DiZerega GS, Goebelsmann U, Nakamura RM. Identification of protein(s) secreted by the preovulatory ovary which suppresses the follicle response to gonadotropins. J Clin Endocrinol Metab. 1982;54:1091–92.

26. Tanabe K, Sagliano P, Channing CP, et al. Levels of inhibin-F activity and steroids in human follicular fluid from normal women and women with polycystic ovarian disease. J Clin Endocrinol Metab. 1983;57:24–31.

27. Daniell JF. Polycystic ovaries treated by laparoscopic laser vaporization. Fertil Steril. 1989;51:232–36.

28. Lomano JM. Photocoagulation of early pelvic endometriosis with the Nd:YAG laser through the laparoscope. J Reprod Med. 1985;30:77–81.

11
Pharmacologically Enhanced Follicular Recruitment for In Vitro Fertilization

MARTIN M. QUIGLEY

The ultimate goal of any program treating infertility by means of in vitro fertilization (IVF) and embryo transfer is to maximize the number of patients who become pregnant in any treatment cycle. To achieve a pregnancy, there must be successful accomplishment of several individual steps including oocyte collection, fertilization, embryo replacement, and subsequent implantation, none of which has a 100% success rate. In order to maximize the chances of pregnancy, all successful IVF treatment programs currently utilize some combination of ovulation-inducing agents to control the spontaneous menstrual cycle, making fertilizable eggs available at the time of scheduled oocyte recovery, and, most important, modifying the normal spontaneous menstrual cycle so that several preovulatory oocytes are potentially recoverable. It is the purpose of this chapter to review the current use of ovulation-inducing agents in IVF and to describe the reported success rates with the commonly used regimens.

Historical Background

The oocytes used for the first successful fertilization in vitro of preovulatory human oocytes were collected by laparoscopy after treatment of the patients with human menopausal gonadotropins (hMG) and human chorionic gonadotropin (hCG) to induce follicular growth and maturation.[1] However, after 5 years' experience with variations of this regimen, and in the absence of any continuing pregnancies, these original investigators abandoned the use of ovulation-inducing agents. They believed that such agents resulted in the disruption of the luteal phase of the cycle and accordingly began attempting oocyte recovery during spontaneous menstrual cycles.[2] This change resulted in the first successful human pregnancy initiated by fertilization in vitro followed by embryo replacement.[3]

With these same procedures, this success was duplicated by other investigators.[4] However, in view of the relatively low pregnancy rate, caused not only by the presence of usually a single preovulatory follicle in a spontaneous cycle but also by the difficulty of monitoring a spontaneous cycle and performing the oocyte retrieval 24 hours a day, several groups of investigators again adopted the use of ovulation-inducing agents,[5,6] in this case clomiphene citrate alone. These workers soon demonstrated not only that it was possible to produce pregnancies in cycles in which the patients received ovulation-inducing agents but that actually the percentage of patients successfully undergoing oocyte recovery and ultimately embryo replacement and pregnancy was substantially higher.[6]

Even though the results obtained with clomiphene citrate alone were superior to those of the natural or unstimulated cycle, several authors soon reported even more efficient follicular recruitment either with hMG alone[7,8] or with the addition of either concurrent[9-11] or sequential[12] hMG to the clomiphene citrate.

Therapeutic Regimens

Clomiphene–hMG Combination Regimens

Although there are almost as many individualized regimens for the combination of clomiphene and hMG as there are IVF programs, the combination regimens can be generally classified as concurrent, sequential, or both.

A typical concurrent regimen is the administration of 50 to 150 mg of clomiphene citrate per day on cycle days 5 to 9, with two ampules per day of hMG [containing 75 international units (IU) each of luteinizing hormone (LH) and follicle-stimulating hormone (FSH)] given on cycle days 6, 8, and 10.[9,10]

An example of a sequential regimen is clomiphene, 150 mg per day for 5 days, followed by hMG, two ampules per day for 3 to 5 days, depending on follicular response.[13]

A regimen combining these two approaches is to use clomiphene, 50 to 150 mg a day on cycle days 4 to 8, with one ampule of hMG given daily cycle days 4 to 8 and one to three ampules of hMG given from day 9 through the day before hCG depending on the follicular response.[14]

Regimens with hMG Alone

The group at the Eastern Virginia Medical School at Norfolk pioneered the use of hMG (Pergonal, Serono Laboratories, Randolph, MA) alone for enhanced follicular recruitment. Initially, two ampules of hMG were administered starting on the first, third, or fifth day of the cycle, depending on cycle length. After 3 days of treatment the dose was lowered to one ampule of hMG per day. With the appearance of the "clinical shift" (estrogenic effects on the cervical mucus and exfoliated vaginal epithelial cells), hMG was discontinued, and 10,000 IU of hCG was admin-

istered 2 to 3 days later (depending on when the largest follicle reached 18 mm in diameter as measured by ultrasound).[15]

Subsequently, their hMG protocol was individualized according to the estrogen level at the time of the clinical estrogen shift. Two ampules of hMG were administered starting on the third or fifth day depending on cycle length. Further management was based on serum estradiol levels and the occurrence of the "clinical shift." For low responders (E_2 less than 300 pg/mL on the day of clinical shift), hMG was continued for three additional days after the shift. In normal responders (E_2 between 300 and 600 pg/mL), hMG was discontinued if the shift had occurred, or the dosage was lowered to one ampule per day until the shift occurred. In high estrogen responders, hMG was discontinued once the E_2 level exceeded 600 pg/mL even if the clinical shift had not occurred. The ovulatory dose of hCG was administered 50 hours after the last hMG injection.[8]

Regimens Using hMG–FSH Combinations

In the Norfolk group's early experience, the pregnancy rate in the normal and high responders was higher than that in the low-responder group. An attempt was made to increase follicular response in the previous low-responder group by the addition of supplemental FSH on cycle days 3 and 4. Encouraging results were reported using this "FSH-sweetened" protocol in patients who had previously exhibited poor response.[16] Other than the supplemental FSH on cycle days 3 and 4, this protocol was similar to the hMG-alone protocol.

Regimens Using FSH Alone and in Combination with Clomiphene

In view of the better results obtained in some patients treated with hMG and FSH combinations, various regimens utilizing FSH alone[17,18] and in combination with clomiphene[19,20] were devised. In general, these protocols were similar to those using hMG but substituting FSH for the hMG.

Published Results

Several studies have been performed comparing clomiphene citrate, clomiphene citrate combined with hMG, and hMG alone. Vargyas et al.[13] compared four protocols to which patients were randomly assigned. Group 1 consisted of 31 patients receiving clomiphene, 150 mg per day for 5 days. Group 2 consisted of 33 patients receiving clomiphene, 150 mg per day for 5 days, followed by hMG, two ampules per day for 3 to 5 days depending on follicular growth. Group 3 consisted of 16 patients who received clomiphene, 150 mg per day for 5 days, plus hMG, two ampules per day on cycle days 3, 5, and 7. In addition, the patients in group 3 also received two ampules of hMG daily following cessation of the clomiphene. Group 4 consisted of 25 patients who received two ampules per day of hMG for 6 to 8 days. In group 1 significantly fewer follicles per patient (a mean of 2.9) developed than in groups 2, 3, and 4 (4.4, 4.4, and 4.2, respectively). Likewise, significantly fewer oocytes were obtained in group 1 (a mean of 1.9) than in groups 2, 3, or 4 (2.8, 3.0, and 2.5, respectively). No pregnancies occurred in the group receiving clomiphene alone, while sim-

ilar pregnancy rates were achieved with the clomiphene–hMG combinations and the hMG- alone regimen.

Johnston et al.[6] reported similar results. In his report, group A received clomiphene citrate, 100 to 150 mg per day on cycle days 5 to 9. Group B received the same dose of clomiphene citrate followed by four ampules of hMG daily until adequate follicular development had occurred. Group C took clomiphene citrate, 50 to 100 mg per day on days 5 to 9, followed by an individualized dose of hMG depending on follicular size and response to clomiphene. The average numbers of follicles per patient were 3, 6.4, and 5.6, and the average numbers of oocytes recovered per laparoscopy were 1.7, 5.0, and 4.7 for groups A, B, and C, respectively.

In a prospective, randomized comparison of two groups of patients treated concurrently, Quigley and co-workers[21] found that hMG alone produced significantly higher follicular-phase E_2 levels (Fig. 11-1) compared to clomiphene alone. However, their hMG stimulation protocol produced an abnormal luteal phase as manifested by foreshortened progesterone production (Fig. 11-2), unphysiologically elevated E_2 levels (Fig. 11-3), and a shortened luteal phase (Table 11-1).

Quigley[22] compared four groups treated at the University of Texas at Houston during 1983. Forty-five patients received 50 mg of

FIGURE 11-1. Daily follicular-phase serum E_2 measurements [mean ± standard error of the mean (SEM)] for the two patient groups. Data have been normalized to the day of hCG administration (day 0). The values were significantly different on cycle days −2, −1, and 0 (*$P < 0.05$; **$P < 0.001$).

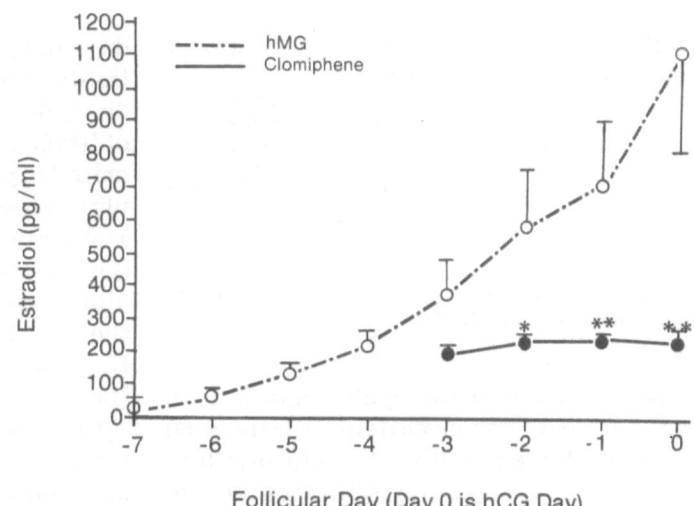

Follicular Day (Day 0 is hCG Day)

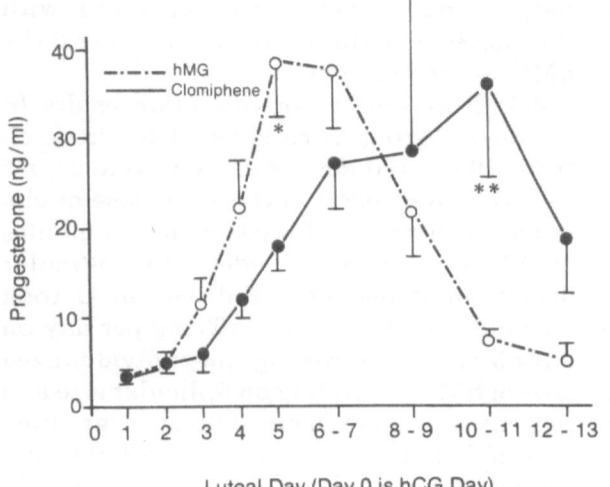

FIGURE 11-2. Daily luteal-phase serum progesterone levels in the two patient groups (mean ± SEM). The data have been normalized to the day of hCG administration (day 0). The values were significantly different on luteal days +5 and +10/+11 (*$P < 0.05$; **$P < 0.01$).

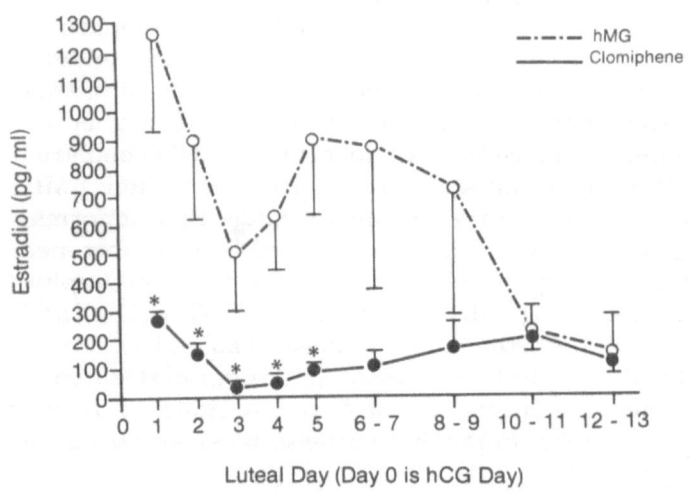

FIGURE 11-3. Daily luteal-phase serum E_2 levels in the two patient groups (mean ± SEM). The data have been normalized to the day of hCG administration (day 0). The values were significantly different on luteal days +1 through +5 (*$P < 0.05$).

TABLE 11-1. Cycle lengths for the treatment groups (means ± standard deviations)[a]

Treatment group	Total cycle length	Length of luteal phase
hMG ($n = 19$)	21.2 ± 1.5 days	11.6 ± 1.5 days
Clomiphene ($n = 18$)	26.8 ± 2.3 days	14.3 ± 2.3 days
Significance	$P < 0.001$	$P < 0.001$

[a] Modified from Quigley et al.[21] Reproduced with permission of the publisher, The American Fertility Society.

clomiphene per day on cycle days 5 to 9 (group A). Forty-seven patients received 50 mg of clomiphene per day for cycle days 5 to 9 plus two ampules per day of hMG on cycle days 6, 8, and 10 (group B). Thirty-three patients received 50 mg of clomiphene per day on cycle days 5 to 9 plus one ampule per day of hMG on cycle days 5 to 9 and one to three ampules per day of hMG, depending on follicular growth and development, from day 10 through the day of hCG administration (group C). Twenty patients received hMG alone, four ampules per day, from day 3 to the day before hCG administration (group D). The results obtained in these groups are shown in Table 11-2 and Fig. 11-4.

Plachot and co-workers[23] attempted to correlate the follicular response with the clomiphene dosage and the total dosage of hMG

TABLE 11-2. Comparison of four follicular recruitment regimens used during 1983 at the University of Texas, Houston[a]

	Follicles aspirated per laparoscopy	Oocytes recovered per patient	Embryos transferred per patient	Number of clinical pregnancies
Clomiphene alone	4.3 ± 1.3[b] $(n = 39)$	1.7 ± 0.9 $(n = 38)$	1.8 ± 0.7 $(n = 23)$	3
Clomiphene plus fixed hMG	4.5 ± 1.1 $(n = 43)$	4.4 ± 2.0 $(n = 42)$	2.1 ± 1.1 $(n = 23)$	3[c]
Clomiphene plus variable hMG	5.5 ± 1.5 $(n = 33)$	4.9 ± 2.0 $(n = 30)$	2.3 ± 1.1 $(n = 23)$	6[d]
hMG alone	5.2 ± 1.4 $(n = 19)$	4.7 ± 2.2 $(n = 18)$	3.5 ± 1.5 $(n = 14)$	0

[a] From Quigley,[22] reproduced with permission of the publisher, Lippincott/Harper & Row.
[b] Mean ± standard deviation.
[c] One twin pregnancy.
[d] One triplet pregnancy.

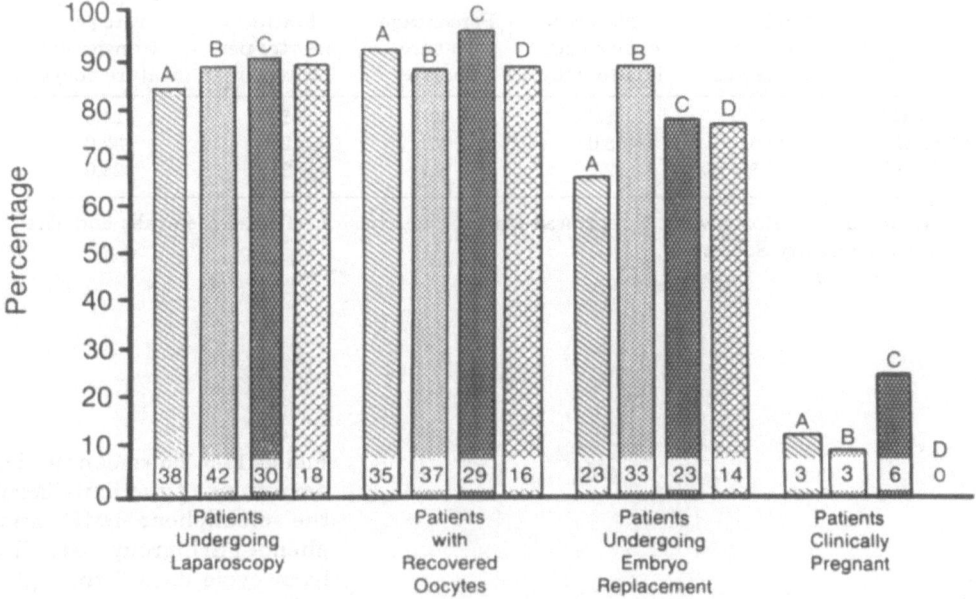

FIGURE 11-4. Summary of the clinical outcomes of the treatment cycle for the four groups. Illustrated are the percentage of patients beginning a treatment cycle who underwent laparoscopy, the percentage of patients undergoing laparoscopy who had at least one oocyte recovered, the percentage of patients with at least one oocyte recovered who underwent embryo replacement, and the percentage of patients who underwent embryo replacement who achieved clinical pregnancies. The number of patients in each group is shown at the bottom of each bar. See text for description of the different patient groups. From Quigley,[27] reproduced with permission of the publisher, The New York Academy of Sciences.

in several combination regimens. Their data are summarized in Table 11-3. These data indicate that there was no statistically significant effect of the increase in clomiphene dose. However, in the patients who received

TABLE 11-3. Mean number of preovulatory follicles in various clomiphene and hMG combinations[a]

Clomiphene dose per day	Total amps hMG	Number of patients	Number of follicles
100 mg	6	33	3.0 ± 1.3[b]
100 mg	9–12	51	3.7 ± 1.4[b]
150 mg	6	14	3.4 ± 1.8
150 mg	9–12	12	4.3 ± 1.5

[a] Modified from Plachot et al.,[23] reproduced with permission of the publisher, The American Fertility Society, Birmingham, Alabama.
[b] $P < 0.02$.

100 mg clomiphene per day, those who received greater amounts of hMG had significantly greater follicular development.

Bayly and co-workers[24] compared patients receiving clomiphene, 50 mg per day for 5 days with hMG beginning on the fifth day of clomiphene, to patients receiving 100 mg per day of clomiphene per day for 5 days with the same hNG regimen. In the group receiving 50 mg clomiphene, there was a 34% incidence of spontaneous LH surges that was reduced to 20% with the higher dose of clomiphene. Follicular development, oocyte recovery, and pregnancy rates were not different between the groups.

Rosenwaks[25] has reported the results from the Norfolk Program in respect to the agents used for enhanced follicular recruitment (Table 11-4). Although the groups are not strictly comparable, and the studies were not con-

TABLE 11-4. Mature occytes and outcome by method of stimulation[a]

	Number of oocyte recoveries	Mature oocytes per laparoscopy	Percentage Mature oocytes	Mature oocytes per transfer	Pregnancy rate per transfer of mature oocyte
hMG	453	1.6	41	1.4	24.3
FSH/hMG	228	3.0	47	2.6	32.0
FSH	55	2.7	51	2.4	25.0

[a] Modified from Rosenwaks,[25] reprinted with the permission of Dr. Rosenwaks and The American Fertility Society.

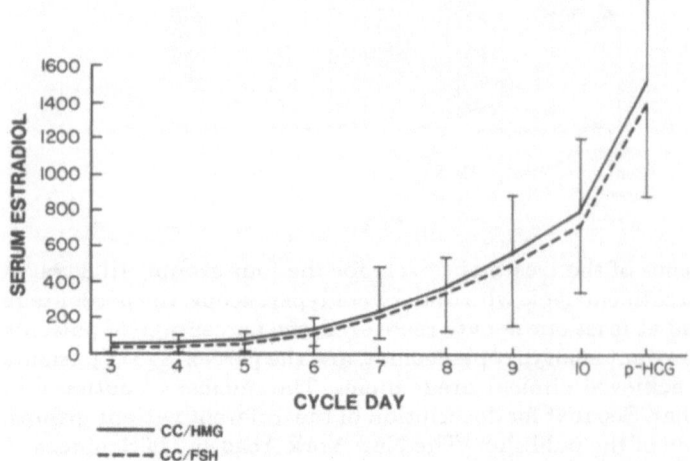

FIGURE 11-5. The means and standard deviations of the daily serum E_2 in the clomiphene–hMG and clomiphene–FSH groups are illustrated from cycle days 3 through 10. The daily samples from cycle days 3 and 4 were drawn before any follicular recruitment agents were given. Also illustrated are the mean and standard deviation of the E_2 level on the day after hCG administration. None of the differences between the groups are statistically significant.

ducted concurrently, the combination of FSH with hMG appeared to give marginally better results than either hMG or FSH alone. The differences in pregnancy rates, however, were not statistically significant.

Scoccia and co-workers[26] reported the outcome of a randomized trial of hMG alone versus FSH alone. There were minor differences between treatments, including cycle day for starting therapy, last gonadotropin dose to hCG interval, and luteal-phase support (progesterone). There were no statistically significant differences between groups with respect to number of oocytes recovered, embryos transferred, or pregnancy rate.

Quigley and co-workers[20] reported the results of a randomized, prospective, double-blind comparison of clomiphene (100 mg/day, cycle days 4 through 8) and either FSH or hMG (1 ampule/day, cycle days 4 through 8, then continued in an individualized fashion until the day before hCG administration). There were no statistically significant differences between groups in the percentages of dropped cycles, follicular response as measured by serum E_2 (Fig. 11-5) or ultrasound imaging, cycle day for hCG administration, number of oocytes recovered, or the rate of clinical pregnancy establishment.

Timing of hCG Administration

Most patients undergoing enhanced follicular recruitment are monitored with a combination of daily measurements of serum E_2 and daily ultrasound imaging of ovarian follicular diameters. The hCG is usually administered on the basis of one or both of these criteria. For example, Vargyas and co-workers[13] primarily relied on E_2 levels to determine time of hCG administration. If E_2 concentration doubled from day to day, hCG was withheld. When E_2 concentration did not double from the previous day and correlated with approximately 300 to 600 pg per follicle 18 mm or greater, hCG was administered. Quigley[27] primarily administered hCG on the evening of the day that the largest follicle reached or exceeded 20 mm in mean diameter by ultrasound measurements.

TABLE 11-5. Patient outcome by E_2 rise day[a]

Day of E_2 rise	Outcome	Number of patients
5	Transfer/not pregnant	1
	Clinical pregnancy (twins)	1
	Total	2
6	Laparoscopies (LH surge)	1
	Oocytes fertilized	6
	Transfer/not pregnant	28
	Clinical pregnancy (one twin; four singleton)	5
	Total	40
7	Oocytes recovered	1
	Oocytes fertilized	3
	Transfer/not pregnant	2
	Total	6
	Total	48

[a] From Quigley et al.,[29] reproduced with permission of the publisher, The American Fertility Society, Birmingham, Alabama.

Investigators from the University of Melbourne[28] presented a novel schema for timing hCG administration. They observed that their best pregnancy rate was achieved when hCG had been administered on the sixth day of sustained E_2 rise. Quigley and co-workers[29] subsequently confirmed those observations (Table 11-5). In that study, patients had baseline blood samples for E_2 drawn on cycle days 3 and 4. They then received 100 mg per day of clomiphene from cycle days 4 to 8, concurrently with one ampule per day of hMG. From cycle day 9 through the day before hCG administration, one to three ampules per day of hMG were administered depending on follicular response. The first day of E_2 rise was defined as the day on which the E_2 level exceeded 150% of the base line (the mean of cycle day 3 and 4). On the evening of the sixth day of sustained E_2 rise, hCG was usually administered.

Premature LH Surges

Clomiphene, particularly when added to hMG at a dosage of 100 mg per day, seems to result in a diminution in the incidence of premature spontaneous LH surges.[24] Contrary to the experience of Kerin et al.[10] (that when clomiphene alone was used, the best pregnancy rate occurred when the oocyte recovery was timed after a spontaneous LH surge), Fishel and co-workers[30] reported that in clomiphene–hMG combinations the best pregnancy rate is obtained when hCG is given after appropriate follicular development has been achieved. In stimulation with hMG alone, premature LH surges rarely occur.[15] Further improvements in follicular response may be attainable with pretreatment by gonadotropin hormone-releasing hormone (GnRH) agonists, which prevent premature exposure of the follicle to elevated levels of endogenous LH.

Poor Responders

Largely because of poor follicular response, between 10% and 20% of all patients beginning a follicular recruitment cycle do not reach oocyte recovery. In the subhuman primate, it has been shown that hMG therapy in the early follicular phase, before the completion of the selection process, increased the number of follicles recruited.[31] In an attempt to apply this observation to humans, Blankstein and co-workers[32] administered increased hMG (two versus one ampule per day, cycle days 4 through 8) in combination with clomiphene, 100 mg/day, to 18 patients who previously had responded poorly to the one ampule per day regimen. Contrary to the experience in the first cycle, where none out of 18 patients had attempted oocyte retrieval, 10 of the 18 patients had oocytes recovered, and two out of the six patients who had embryos placed in their uterus conceived and delivered at term. Comparison of the daily serum E_2 levels between the two treatments demonstrated that the augmented gonadotropins resulted in significantly higher E_2 levels on cycle days 8 and 9 (Fig. 11-6).

An alternative attempt to improve follicular recruitment by administering hMG from the first day of the menstrual cycle did not result in the intended effect. Dlugi and co-workers[33] compared two different groups of patients and found that the initiation of hMG therapy on cycle day 1 was associated with diminished sensitivity to FSH, which they speculated might be related to an inadequate number of receptor sites at the beginning of therapy.

Gonadotropin-Releasing Hormone Agonists

Gonadotropin-releasing hormone agonists are compounds that act similarly to native GnRH in that they initiate the release of LH and FSH from the pituitary. Paradoxically,

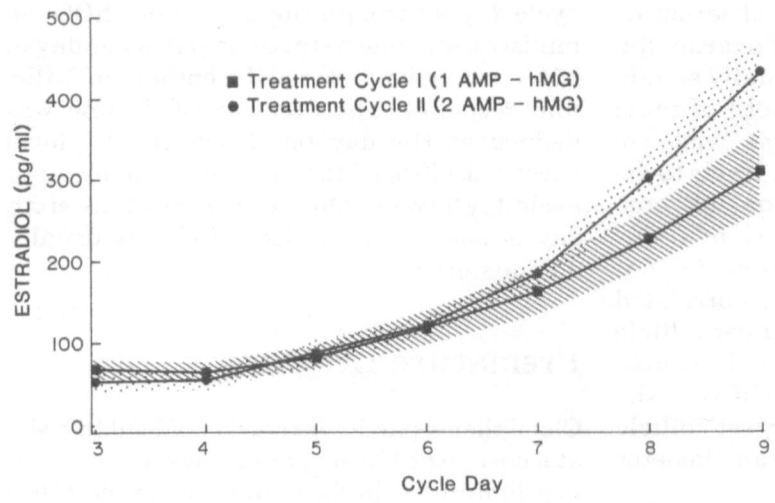

FIGURE 11-6. Mean ($\pm$ SEM) E_2 levels in response to hMG, one ampule per day (treatment cycle I) or two ampules per day (treatment cycle II). Note that the increases in E_2 on cycle days 8 and 9 are significantly higher in treatment cycle II.

because of their extremely long duration of action (when compared to native GnRH), following the initial release of gonadotropins, the GnRH agonists produce a down-regulation of the pituitary. Continued administration of these compounds leads to the production of a "medical hypophysectomy."

Recently, several groups have been investigating the pretreatment of previous "poor responder" patients with GnRH agonists, followed by follicular recruitment with gonadotropins alone once a "medical hypophysectomy" has been produced. Buserelin, a compound with about a 4-hour duration of action that can be administered either parenterally or by nasal spray, has been used in Europe. Use of GnRH agonist pretreatment increased the number of oocytes collected, fertilization rate, length of the luteal phase, and pregnancy rate in one report.[34] In the United States the only GnRH agonist presently available is leuprolide acetate (Lupron, TAP Pharmaceuticals, North Chicago, IL) (Fig. 11-7), which is currently approved only for the treatment of prostatic cancer. The available formulation requires once-daily subcutaneous administration, but a 30-day depot preparation has recently been released. Preliminary experience with pretreatment of "poor responders" with leuprolide acetate followed by hMG alone for follicular recruitment has yielded mixed results. Some patients have responded with very normal follicular response,[35,36] but other patients have re-

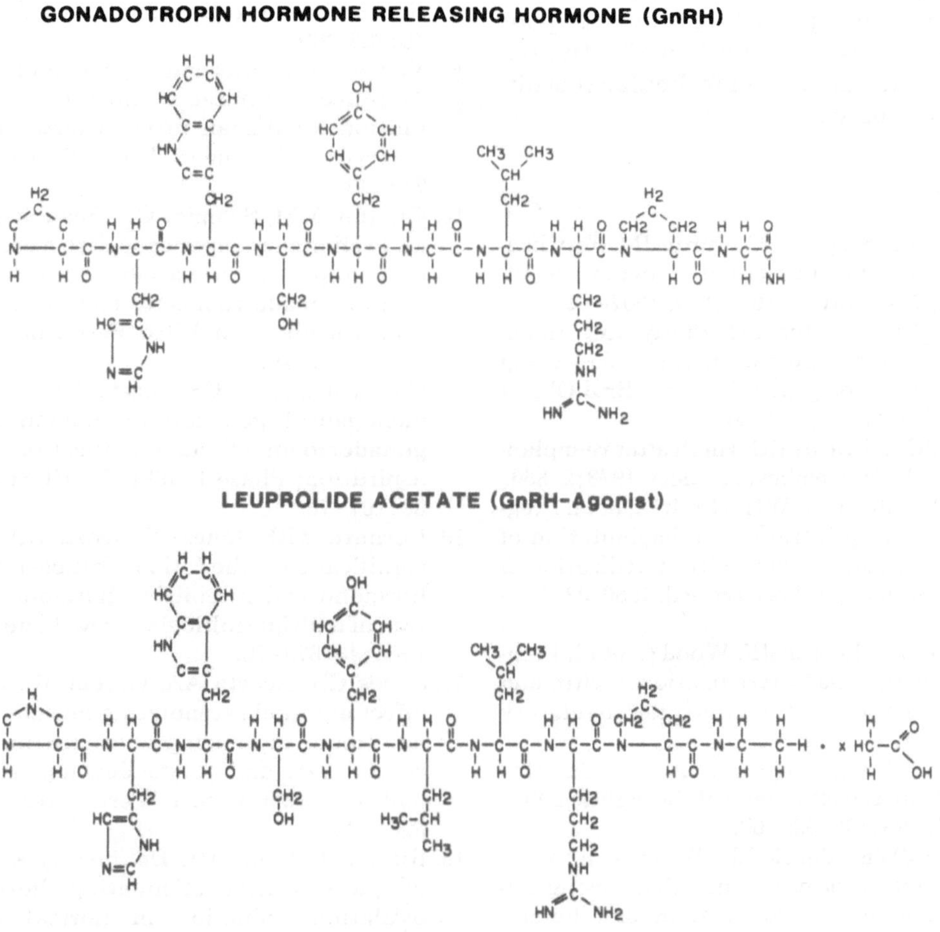

GONADOTROPIN HORMONE RELEASING HORMONE (GnRH)

LEUPROLIDE ACETATE (GnRH-Agonist)

FIGURE 11-7. Illustration of the structural formulas of native GnRH (above) and the commercially available GnRH agonist leuprolide acetate (below).

quired extraordinarily high levels of exogenous gonadotropins.[37]

Summary

Just as the use of clomiphene alone for follicular recruitment was shown to have substantial advantages over oocyte collection in spontaneous cycles, the combination of clomiphene and hMG or FSH, hMG, or FSH alone, and hMG–FSH combinations have resulted in increased efficacy of follicular recruitment when compared to clomiphene alone, as evidenced by an increased number of recovered oocytes and improved pregnancy rate. Prestimulation pituitary suppression with GnRH agonists, followed by hMG stimulation, has allowed successful follicular recruitment in a portion of previous "poor responders." However, the "ideal" stimulation regimen for enhanced follicular recruitment is still elusive.

References

1. Edwards RG, Steptoe PC, Purdy JM. Fertilization and cleavage in vitro of preovulatory human oocytes. Nature. 1970;227:1307–09.
2. Edwards RG, Steptoe PC, Purdy JM. Establishing full-term human pregnancies using cleaving embryos grown in vitro. Br J Obstet Gynaecol. 1980;87;737–56.
3. Steptoe PC, Edwards RG. Birth after reimplantation of a human embryo. Lancet. 1978;2:366.
4. Lopata A, Johnston IWH, Hoult IJ, et al. Pregnancy following intrauterine implantation of an embryo obtained by in vitro fertilization of a preovulatory egg. Fertil Steril. 1980;33:117–20.
5. Trounson AO, Leeton JF, Wood C, et al. Pregnancies in humans by fertilization in vitro and embryo transfer in the controlled ovulatory cycle. Science. 1981;212:681–82.
6. Johnston I, Lopata A, Speirs A, et al. In vitro fertilization: the challenge of the eighties. Fertil Steril. 1981;36:699–06.
7. Wortham JWE, Veeck LL, Witmyer J, et al. Vital initiation of pregnancy (VIP) using human menopausal gonadotropin and human chorionic gonadotropin ovulation induction: Phase I, 1981, Fertil Steril. 1983;39:785–92.
8. Jones HW, Jones GS, Andrews MC, et al. The program for in vitro fertilization at Norfolk. Fertil Steril. 1982;38:14–21.
9. Quigley MM, Schmidt CL, Beauchamp PJ, et al. Enhanced follicular recruitment in an in vitro fertilization program: clomiphene alone versus a clomiphene/human menopausal gonadotropin combination. Fertil Steril. 1984;42:25–33.
10. Kerin JF, Warnes GM, Quinn PJ, et al. Incidence of multiple pregnancy following human fertilization in vitro fertilization and embryo transfer. Lancet. 1983;2:537–40.
11. Mandelbaum J, Plachot M, Cohen J, et al. The use of Clomid and hMG in human in vitro fertilization: consequences for egg quality and luteal phase adequacy. In: Beier HM, Lindner HR, eds. Fertilization of the human egg in vitro. Berlin: Springer-Verlag, 1983:123–30.
12. Lopata A. Concepts in human in vitro fertilization and embryo transfer. Fertil Steril. 1983;40:289–301.
13. Vargyas JM, Morente C, Shangold G, et al. The effect of different methods of ovarian stimulation for human in vitro fertilization and embryo replacement. Fertil Steril. 1984;42:745–49.
14. Quigley MM, Schmidt CL, Beauchamp PJ, et al. Preliminary experience with a combination of clomiphene and variable dosages of menopausal gonadotropins for enhanced follicular recruitment. J In Vitro Fert Emb Transfer. 1985;2:11–16.
15. Garcia JE, Jones GS, Acosta AA, et al. Human menopausal gonadotropin/human chorionic gonadotropin follicular maturation for oocyte aspiration: Phase I, 1981. Fertil Steril. 1983;39:167–73.
16. Bernardus RE, Jones GS, Acosta AA, et al. The significance of the ratio in follicle stimulating hormone and luteinizing hormone in induction of multiple follicular growth. Fertil Steril. 1985;43:373–78.
17. Jones GS, Acosta AA, Garcia JE, et al. The effect of follicle stimulating hormone without additional luteinizing hormone on follicular recruitment and oocyte development in normal ovulatory women. Fertil Steril. 1985;43:696–702.
18. Russel JB, Polan ML, DeCherney AH. The use of pure follicle stimulating hormone for ovulation induction in normal ovulatory women in an in vitro fertilization program. Fertil Steril. 1986;45:829–33.

19. Martikainen H, Ronnberg L, Puitola U, et al. Comparison of the effects of follicle-stimulating hormone and human menopausal gonadotropin on peripheral serum and follicular fluid hormones during ovarian stimulation. Fertil Steril. 1986;46:317–20.

20. Quigley MM, Collins RL, Blankstein J. Pure follicle stimulating hormone (FSH) does not enhance follicular recruitment in clomiphene citrate/gonadotropin combinations. Fertil Steril. 1988;50:562–66.

21. Quigley MM, Schmidt CL, Beauchamp PJ, et al. Menopausal gonadotropins compared with clomiphene citrate for enhanced follicular recruitment in an in vitro fertilization program. Fertil Steril. 1984;41:42S.

22. Quigley MM. The use of ovulation inducing agents in in vitro fertilization. Clin Obstet Gynecol. 1984;27:983–92.

23. Plachot M, Mandelbaum J, Cohen J, et al. Sequential use of clomiphene citrate, human menopausal gonadotropins and human chorionic gonadotropins in human in vitro fertilization. I. follicular growth and oocyte suitability. Fertil Steril. 1985;43:255–62.

24. Bayly CM, McBain JC, Clarke GA, et al. Ovarian stimulation regimens in an in vitro fertilization program: a comparative analysis. Ann NY Acad Sci. 1985;442:123–27.

25. Rosenwaks Z. Multiple follicle development utilizing hMG–FSH–HCG combinations. Postgraduate Syllabus Material, American Fertility Society Annual Meeting, September 1986.

26. Scoccia B, Blumenthal P, Wagner C, et al. Comparison of urinary human follicle-stimulating hormone and human menopausal gonadotropins for ovarian stimulation in an in vitro fertilization program. Fertil Steril. 1987;48:446–49.

27. Quigley MM. Selection of agents for enhanced follicular recruitment in an vitro fertilization and embryo replacement treatment program. Ann NY Acad Sci. 1985;442:96–111.

28. Levran D, Lopata A, Nayudu PL, et al. Analysis of the outcome of in vitro fertilization in relation to the timing of human chorionic gonadotropin administration by the duration of estradiol rise in stimulated cycles. Fertil Steril. 1985;44:335–41.

29. Quigley MM, Sokoloski JE, Richards SI. Timing human chorionic gonadotropin administration by days of estradiol rise. Fertil Steril. 1985;44:791–95.

30. Fishel SB, Edwards RG, Purdy JM, et al. Implantation, abortion, and birth after in vitro fertilization using the natural menstrual cycle or follicular stimulation with clomiphene citrate and human menopausal gonadotropin. J In Vitro Fert Emb Transfer. 1985;2:123–31.

31. diZerega GS, Hodgen GD. Folliculogenesis in the primate ovarian cycle. Endocr Rev. 1981;2:27–49.

32. Blankstein J, Collins RL, Easley KA, et al. Increased human menopausal gonadotropin during the follicular phase: Effect on follicular recruitment and treatment outcome. Presented at The Endocrine Society, Annual Meeting, New Orleans, LA, June 9, 1988.

33. Dlugi AM, Laufer N, DeCherney AH, et al. The day of initiation of human menopausal stimulation affects follicular growth in in vitro fertilization cycles. J In Vitro Fert Emb Transfer. 1985;2:33–40.

34. Neveu S, Hedon B, Bringer J, et al. Ovarian stimulation by a combination of gonadotropin-releasing hormone agonist and gonadotropins for in vitro fertilization. Fertil Steril. 1987;47:639–43.

35. de Ziegler D, Cedars MI, Randle D, et al. Suppression of the ovary using a gonadotropin releasing-hormone agonist prior to stimulation for oocyte retrieval. Fertil Steril. 1987;48:807–10.

36. Awadalla SG, Friedman CI, Chin NW, et al. Follicular stimulation for in vitro fertilization using pituitary suppression and human menopausal gonadotropins. Fertil Steril. 1987;48:811–15.

37. Barnes RB, Scommegna A, Schreiber JR. Decreased ovarian response to human menopausal gonadotropin caused by subcutaneously administered gonadotropin-releasing hormone agonist. Fertil Steril. 1987;47:512–15.

Index

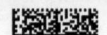